An
Alternative
Medicine
Definitive Guide to

HEADACHES

Headaches Can Be Eliminated. This Book Tells
How, Using Natural Alternative Therapies.

ROBERT D. MILNE, M.D.

AND BLAKE MORE

WITH BURTON GOLDBERG

ALTERNATIVEMEDICINE.COM BOOKS
TIBURON, CALIFORNIA

AlternativeMedicine.com, Inc.
1640 Tiburon Blvd., Suite 2
Tiburon, CA 94920
www.alternativemedicine.com

Cover design by Amparo Del Rio Design
Book Design and Production: Amparo Del Rio Design

Manufactured in the United States of America.

9 8 7 6 5 4 3

Library of Congress Cataloging-in-Publication Data

Milne, Robert D.,
        An alternative medicine definitive guide to headaches / Robert
D. Milne and Blake More with Burton Goldberg.
        p. cm.
        Includes bibliographical references and index.
        ISBN: 1-887299-03-3 (hardcover)
        1. Headache—Alternative treatment. I. More, Blake
II.Goldberg, Burton,   III. Title.
RB128.M54   1997   96-46914
616.8,49106—dc21   CIP

Dedication

To the millions of people who

suffered from headaches because

they thought there was nothing

they could do about them. And to

those who will suffer no more.

Icons Used in This Book

An Alternative Medicine Definitive Guide to Headaches is an interactive book. The icons below appear throughout. They alert you to an important piece of information or tell you where you can find out more. Use them to get the most out of this book.

 Turn to another place in this book for more information on the same subject.

 Please give this point your special attention.

 An especially important point to remember.

 This sign tells you there may be some risks, uncertainties, side effects, or special contraindications regarding a procedure or substance.

 Telephone numbers and addresses of organizations, publications, or professionals whom you can contact immediately.

 Self-care options you can put into practice yourself to improve your health.

 This icon tells you where to look for additional information in Future Medicine Publishing's 1,100-page encyclopedia, *Alternative Medicine: The Definitive Guide.* To order, call 800-333-HEAL.

 Alternative Medicine Yellow Pages lists alternative practitioners throughout the U.S. by type of therapy and location. To order, call 800-333-HEAL.

 Consult this icon for a quick definition of scientific terms, alternative medicine procedures and techniques, or other terms that appear in the text.

 This icon tells you where to look for additional information in Future Medicine Publishing's bimonthly magazine, *Alternative Medicine Digest.* To subscribe or order back issues, call 800-333-HEAL.

Acknowledgments

BURTON GOLDBERG, Dr. Robert D. Milne, and Blake More would like to express thanks and special recognition to mentor John Renner (1890-1989) for his special clinical skills and his vision to make alternative medicine mainstream. We sincerely appreciate the following individuals and organizations, without whose help this book would not have been possible:

Don Ash, R.P.T.

Anne Barber, O.D.

Joseph Carter, L.Ac., C.M.T.

Dennis Crawford, D.C.

Eleanor Criswell
Hanna, Ed.D.

Ellen W. Cutler, D.C.

Stefan Hagopian, D.O.

Paul Herscu, N.D.

Jay Holder,
D.C., Ph.D.

Michael Gelb, D.D.S., M.S.

Dwight Jennings, D.D.S.

Patricia Kaminski

David Krofcheck,
O.M.D., D.Ac., C.A.

William LaVelle, M.D., L.Ac.

Lita Lee, Ph.D.

Nancy Lonsdorf, M.D.

Kathleen Merikangas, Ph.D.

Herbert Miller, D.O.

Devi Nambudripad, D.C.,
L.Ac., R.N., Ph.D.

Christiane Northrup, M.D.

William Philpott, M.D.

Janiece Piper. M.S.W.,
C.A.M.T.

James R. Privitera, M.D.

Harold E. Ravins,
D.D.S., C.Ac.

Judyth Reichenberg-Ulman,
N.D.

Sherry Rogers, M.D.

Amy Rothenberg, N.D.

Joseph Schames, D.M.D.

Vivek Shanbhag, M.D.

Benjamin Shield, Ph.D.

Jan Henry Sultan, L.M.T.

Kelly Sutton, M.D.

John Upledger, D.O.

Julian Whitaker, M.D.

Rick Williams, N.M.T., B.S.

Contents

PART II

Each individual headache chapter covers:
- Causes and Triggers
- Diagnosing and Treating Underlying Causes
- Alternative Treatments
    Metabolic/Bioenergetic/Biochemical-based Therapies
    Structurally Oriented Therapies
    Psycho/Emotional Therapies
- Self-Care Options
- Recommended Reading

Contents

DISCLAIMER

This book is intended as an educational tool to acquaint the reader with alternative methods of preventing and treating headaches. Future Medicine Publishing hopes the book will enable you to improve your well-being and to better understand, assess, and choose the appropriate course of treatment. Because the methods described in this book are for the most part alternative methods, by definition, many of them have not been investigated and/or approved by any government or regulatory agency. National, state, and local laws vary regarding the use and application of many of the treatments that are discussed. Accordingly, this book should not be substituted for the advice and treatment of a physician or other licensed health care professional. Pregnant women in particular are especially urged to consult with their physician before using any therapy. Throughout the book, icons appear in many instances where caution is especially necessary.

Your health is important. Use this book wisely. Discuss the alternative treatment options that are described with your doctor. Ultimately, you, the reader, must take full responsibility for your health and how you use this book.

Future Medicine Publishing and the authors have no financial interest in any of the health care products discussed in this book.

Foreword

LET ME REVEAL TWO SECRETS about headaches. A headache is not an aspirin deficiency. A headache is not something you must learn to live with. If you suffer from headaches, the book you hold in your hands could change your life. It is entirely possible that with the invaluable practical information contained in this book, you may well put headaches behind you as something you once suffered from, but no more.

No matter what kind of headache you have, alternative medicine has a solution to bring you relief. When you find the root cause of your condition, then you can remove the cause and allow healing to take place. Robert Milne, M.D., and Blake More expertly guide you through the root causes and multiple treatment options for 11 major types of headaches, from sinus to migraine, cluster to tension.

We have made every effort possible to make this book practical and user-friendly for you. For a quick reference to headache types, symptoms, treatment options, and where to find this information in the book, please refer to the Master Symptom Chart in the Introduction. If you suffer from tension headaches, you may turn directly to Chapter 6; if migraines are your millstone, you may turn directly to Chapter 7; and if you're not sure what type of headache you have, study the symptoms list in the Master Symptom Chart until you find the clinical term that best matches your condition.

So say goodbye to headaches for the rest of your life. No matter what kind of headache you used to have, thanks to the proven and effective alternative medicine health information in this book, your head may never pain you again.

God Bless,

BURTON GOLDBERG

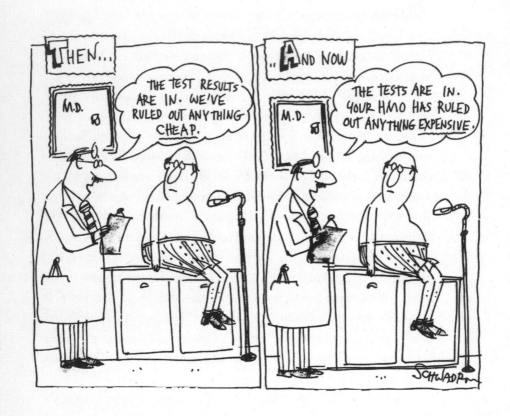

Preface

FIFTEEN YEARS AGO, as a recently graduated, board-certified physician, I was personally confronted with an extremely difficult medical problem: how to help my newborn daughter Brooke, who was suffering from severe, medically unresponsive colic. For the first 6 months of her life, Brooke cried virtually 20 hours a day—a problem many of you no doubt have experienced to some degree. After consulting, without success, many able and well-meaning pediatricians and professors, I became desperate. I asked myself a difficult question: What right do I have to treat other patients if I can't help my own daughter?

In my frustration, I happened across a book entitled *The Science of Homeopathy* in the medical bookstore. This book advocates a nontoxic system of medicine using highly diluted plant and mineral extracts, with no side effects, stimulating the body to heal itself by enacting the principle "Like cures like." Although it sounded interesting, I was not convinced that the medicines could really work. After all, I had just completed one of the finest residency programs in the United States, the University of Texas-Southwestern program for family practice in Fort Worth. If the homeopathic form of medicine was so good, I remember asking myself, why hadn't I heard about it during my residency?

As fate had it, my daughter's condition continued to worsen, and with it, her suffering. Seeing that my choices were being rapidly exhausted, I decided to learn more about homeopathy. Once I convinced myself that homeopathy would at least not hurt Brooke, I gave it a try. I ordered some homeopathic medications but as soon as they arrived, I became anxious as to whether they would help. My wife and I began giving Brooke 2 tablets of the homeopathic remedy every hour. On the fourth hour, soon after receiving a dose of the remedy, Brooke stopped crying and began to smile. From this point on, she was never to suffer from colic again. My wife and I cried with relief. To us, it was a miracle.

From this personal experience, I wanted to find out if this medicine could help other patients who were suffering. Although my colleagues felt I was a bit crazy to want to explore these medications, I felt that I must. I gave up a teaching position to learn this alternative medicine. My journey to discover more about alternative medicine took me to many faraway places, until I met my 92-year-old mentor, John H. Renner, M.D., who had studied homeopathy in Chicago. Under his tough, brass-tacks tutelage, I was able to learn how to combine conventional and alternative medicine—and better help patients in need. Dr. Renner's clinical skills of listening and physical examination were exceptional. He taught me that the patient was more important than the remedy. Moreover, he had the vision that alternative and conventional medicine could work together—a vision that is just now starting to be realized. I am fortunate to have worked with this amazing man of medicine.

Now 15 years have passed, my daughter remains healthy, my wife no longer suffers from arthritic pains, and I no longer suffer from asthma. By studying and following a different path, I was able to gain the valuable knowledge that helped me and my family and is now helping hundreds of my patients every week. Thankfully, now that alternative medicine is proving its effectiveness and being used worldwide with more openness and success, the secret is out: The methods and medicines of alternative medicine work. Now it is your turn to learn these secrets.

When Burton Goldberg and his group at Future Medicine Publishing asked me to help write a book for them, I realized that this would be a great opportunity to share some of the wisdom I gained along my journey to help my family, myself, and my patients. For readers who suffer from headaches or have family members or friends who are suffering from headaches, this book will offer more than a pat on the back and a prescription. My talented coauthor, Blake More, and I have compiled a compendium of valuable information to give you real answers to your health problems. We are interested in teaching you about underlying causes, not just symptoms. We believe that if you read and follow these guidelines, you will learn, first, how you can heal yourself; second, how to take action; and third, how to empower yourself to be more in charge of your health for the rest of your life.

We invite you to make that important choice for wellness. And we hope this book will become your companion as you do so because, once you have finished reading it, you should truly be headache free.

Robert D. Milne, M.D.

Message to the Reader

THIS BOOK IS INTENDED as an educational tool to acquaint you with alternative ways to treat your headaches. The information provided herein will enable you to find whole-body wellness by supplying the means to better understand, assess, and choose the most effective solution to your head pain.

Because the methods in this book are by definition alternative methods, many may not have been investigated and/or approved by government or regulatory agencies. Regardless of government action or inaction, we have included treatment modalities that we believe have a successful track record and a verifiable approach. Other treatments may also be useful, but we have chosen to focus on the methods that we have found most valuable for headache sufferers.

We also urge you to use common sense. This book is not a substitute for the advice or treatment of a licensed medical practitioner. Use this book instead as an intermediary to guide you toward the most appropriate care for your needs. All readers, but especially pregnant women and those seeking help for children, are advised to consult a licensed medical practitioner or physician before undertaking any therapy.

Your health is important. You are fully responsible for it. So use this book wisely. Consult it as you discuss your treatment options with your doctor, refer to it when you need to, and remember that only you can heal yourself.

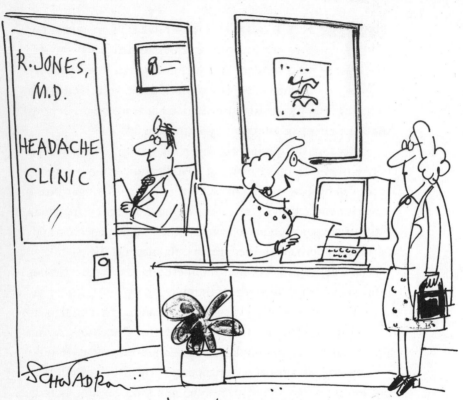

"ACTUALLY, DR. JONES' SPECIALTY IS HEADACHES CAUSED BY OTHER DOCTORS' PRESCRIPTIONS."

Introduction

EVER SINCE SHE TURNED 12 and started menstruating, Elizabeth, now in her early thirties, had been taking medication for her migraines. Over the years, doctors had also given her drugs for stomach ulcers, hyperthyroidism, fertility problems, difficult pregnancies, miscarriages, endometriosis, kidney stones, colitis, gallstones, fibromyalgia, chronic fatigue syndrome, insomnia, emotional breakdown, and depression. Since drugs didn't always work, Elizabeth's doctors had performed surgery on her gallbladder and surgically removed her thyroid and her uterus. When she first came to the Milne Medical Center, Elizabeth was on seven different medications. She told us she had "not come to be cured or healed, just to be helped enough to live out my life with less pain and fewer drugs."

Physical examination of Elizabeth suggested that she was suffering from multiple organ dysfunction which included severe intestinal congestion and inflammation brought on by toxic overload. In addition to her severe head pain, a line across the middle of her upper lip revealed ovarian weakness, her eyes were bloodshot, her nose was congested, her neck, shoulders, and lower back were stiff and painful to the touch, her abdomen and liver were swollen and tender, her hips were limited in motion, and the energy pathways along her legs corresponding to her gallbladder, liver, and spleen as described by acupuncture were blocked and painful. Thus, it was no surprise when allergy testing revealed that she was allergic to the medications that were supposed to be helping her—so allergic that she nearly vomited just by touching them.

Due to the complicated and painful nature of Elizabeth's headaches, we first devised a plan to relieve her pain while we took her off her medications. This included intravenous colchicine, a natural anti-inflammatory agent derived from the plant, *Colchicum autumnale*. This gave her 50% improvement, so we began a detoxification program of enemas and herbal laxatives, which relieved her intestinal swelling. We then further reduced her pain through a series of trigger point injections with lidocaine and vitamin B12. We also tested her for allergies and found that she was highly sensitive to a large number of foods, so she was placed on a restricted, whole foods diet. All of this was supplemented with acupuncture and herbal medications. Elizabeth steadfastly adhered to our program and, within 6 weeks, she was off medications and her condition had improved 70 to 80%, at which time the symptomatic crisis was over and we were able to spend more time on her underlying conditions.

> *Headache roameth over the desert, blowing like the wind. Flashing like lightning, it is loosed above and below.*
>
> —Anonymous, Babylonia 3000-2000 B.C.

Almost everyone suffers from a headache at one time or another: headache ranks as the number-one health complaint in America, surpassing in occurrence even the common cold. It is estimated that approximately 90% of men and 95% of women suffer from headaches at some point in any given year.[1] Headaches affect both the young and the old, the somber and frivolous, fat and lean—making them among the most confounding conditions in the field of medicine. And they are costly: A 1994 U.S. Centers for Disease Control report measuring the economic impact of headaches states that each year headaches generate 80 million visits to the doctor and cost employers 157 million workdays, resulting in an estimated annual cost from absenteeism and medical bills of $50 billion.

Headaches are a huge problem that is rarely understood. One of the reasons for the lack of understanding, as you will see in the following chapters, is that there are as many types of headaches as there are contributing factors. Moreover, the frequency, severity, and duration of headaches varies dramatically. Some sufferers gain relief by stimulating a pressure point and going to bed early, while others endure pain so debilitating and recurrent that the minute one headache subsides, an even more incapacitating headache follows. Another challenge to our understanding is that, if not caused by a brain tumor or another recognizable medical cause, head pain is often assigned to the realm of the imaginary, psychological, or, worse yet, untreatable. Given the present approach of conventional medicine, many headache sufferers are left to fend for themselves as their headaches continue to impair the quality of their lives. This may explain why only 5 to

7% of the estimated 50 million Americans who suffer from chronic headaches bother to seek medical help.[2]

One might suppose that if headache sufferers bandaged their heads and wore red H's around their necks, they might be taken seriously by doctors, family members, coworkers, and friends. Barring that, and until perceptions change, it is essential to remember that headaches are not a character flaw. No matter what "experts" tell you, a headache is a legitimate biological disorder that deserves to be treated as such.

Forgoing medical attention for the disorder is rarely a wise approach, particularly because headaches often signal a potentially serious health condition. This is why we suggest alternative therapies that acknowledge the seriousness of head pain and seek to discover and treat the root conditions that are causing it. Contrary to common assumption, alternative therapies are actually better at treating headaches than conventional ones. Alternative therapies work to heal underlying causes as well as symptoms, providing both short- and long-term relief without the risks and side effects associated with conventional treatments. Furthermore, alternative therapies give you the opportunity to be an *active* participant in your healing process, helping you to see that *you* ultimately have control over your well-being.

> *The headache ranks as the number-one health complaint in America, surpassing in occurrence even the common cold. It is estimated that approximately 90% of men and 95% of women suffer from headaches at some point in any given year.*

What Is Alternative Medicine?

Alternative medicine is an umbrella term used to describe a wide range of health-care approaches, including acupuncture, homeopathy, herbal medicine, chiropractic, and others, that differ from the more commonly known, conventional medical treatments. Where conventional medicine primarily approaches problems from the outside in—often in a way that is drug-based and symptom-driven—alternative medical therapies work from the inside out, in a sensitive, balanced approach to whole-body health.

Conventional medicine says a prescription can cure your headache. When the pain recurs a few months later, the conventional response is a dosage adjustment or a different prescription. Alternative practitioners know

Basic Tenets of Alternative Medicine

Although alternative medicine includes a wide range of treatment options of varying approaches, all the therapies are based on a common philosophy that includes the following elements. Alternative medicine:

- focuses on empowering you to accept responsibility for the task of recovery and health maintenance in the future
- emphasizes the importance of nutrition as an essential requirement for good health
- considers a balanced lifestyle (proper exercise, sleep, relaxation, and emotional tranquility) a prerequisite for optimum health
- attempts to ensure the efficiency of your body's organs and organ systems (through detoxification, nutritional supplements, and related whole body approaches)
- recognizes that your musculoskeletal system provides a vital link between nerve transmission and energy pathways and is in direct relationship with internal and emotional states
- treats you rather than your symptoms.

better: they understand that a symptom stopped with drugs isn't an ailment cured. They want to heal headaches, not stop them for the time being. Antacids may seem to cure your indigestion until you eat again, but changing your diet may mean never needing another antacid again. In the world of alternative medicine, true health lasts.

Faced with the current decline in public health resources, many Americans are recognizing the need for medical alternatives for their health concerns. A landmark study published in 1993 by the *New England Journal of Medicine* showed that over one-third of all Americans were choosing alternative medicine over conventional methods.[3] It is increasingly apparent that what was once a "fringe" interest is becoming an integral part of the nation's health-care program. In recent years, even major health insurance companies have begun to cover alternative modalities such as chiropractic, acupuncture, and yoga classes based on stress-reduction.

The underlying concepts of alternative medicine aren't new. They are a return to the principles that shaped our understanding of health and disease thousands of years ago. Hippocrates, the father of Western medicine, linked health to a state of harmony or balance, and disease to one of disharmony or imbalance. He also looked at the underlying factors contributing to health and disease; he realized that each individual had unique needs and concerns and he tailored treatments accordingly. The genius of Hippocrates is not found in the drugs he used or even in his diagnostic skills but in his determination to help individuals reach a sustainable state of good health. He knew that certain elements were necessary to health, essentials such as good hygiene, peace of mind, proper diet, a sound work and home environment, and exercise. In addition, he recognized the harmony in Nature and taught that, to be healthy, humanity must be aligned with nature.

Western medical science, however, seems to have lost track of Hippocrates' ideas through the centuries. As a result, conventional medicine has become increasingly one-sided, particularly in the way it reduces the body to a series of isolated parts and ignores the imbalances which cause illness in the first place. A good analogy is to compare the body to a house with gaps in the foundation that are letting pests inside. Hippocrates would have located the "holes," repaired the foundation, and taught you how to prevent them from coming back. Today, many conventional doctors prescribe drugs which, in our opinion, act more like poisons.

A landmark study published in 1993 by the New England Journal of Medicine showed that over one-third of all Americans were choosing alternative medicine over conventional methods. What was once a "fringe" interest is becoming an integral part of the nation's health care program.

Fortunately for all of us, the concepts of Hippocrates are still alive in alternative medicine. To an alternative practitioner, health is far more than the absence of symptoms. When healthy, all systems of the body are integrated and working in equilibrium with each other, which means we can effectively handle the hazards presented by life—without headaches and, more importantly, without drugs.

Alternative Medicine Works

Whether you consult Hippocratic texts or alternative practitioners, you will be awakened to the fact that you are born with an innate, powerful, life-affirming wisdom that can accomplish anything you let it. Your body is designed to repair, regenerate, and renew itself every day without your conscious consent. Your blood cells replenish themselves every 28 days, you grow a completely new liver every 6 months, and each cell in your body is brand-new every 7 years. When you cut yourself, you heal, and when you get a cold, your immune system sends it away.

This self-regulation process is called homeostasis, and it is a natural by-product of good health. When your body is called on to deal with a crisis, it often causes symptoms—a headache, for example. Under normal conditions, your body will try to heal itself without help, and your headache is its way of indicating what type of healing process is transpiring. Alternative medicine fully supports this process, recognizing and respecting your symptom as a clue to the homeostatic process occurring in your body. It then seeks to support this process first by finding out and eliminating the cause of the crisis, and then by ensuring that your body has everything it needs to heal itself.

Your Headache *Can* Be Healed

Although conventional physicians doubt that chronic headaches, particularly migraines, can be healed, you need not agree with them. The medical term "migraine" only refers to your most obvious symptom, one that often bears little relation to the problem that is causing it. Alternative health-care providers recognize this distinction and seek to treat the *root* cause, addressing your entire being, taking into account your mental, emotional, and physical makeup, as well as your structural, biochemical, and energy elements.

To be truly healthy, you must release whatever it is that is making you sick—even if that means giving up prescription drugs or the job that drives you mad—and accept the innate wellness that lives in your body. Every day, you have the opportunity to live in the remarkable simplicity of natural healing. Granted, this isn't easy given the way contemporary life is arranged, but, with determination and incentive (like a throbbing head), it can be done. The medical establishment often dubs natural healing "spontaneous remission," making it out to be some remarkable act unidentifiable by conventional medicine. Yet "spontaneous remission" is what is expected in alternative medicine. We see such miracles daily; the difference is that we see you as the miracle and let you take credit for your healing.

This book provides a greater understanding of the inner workings of your body, and how its dysfunctions express themselves as headaches, to empower you to take the first step in ridding yourself of head pain, forever. The book challenges conventional medicine with an alternative system based on scientific evidence, the most innovative medical thinking, and real-life case studies. We explain which therapies work best for your particular headache based upon the root causes rather than solely on categorical types. We include self-help techniques that you can use to supplement your therapies, as well as a list of organizations you can call to find the alternative health care you need.

For many of you, some of the information contained in this book may be new, foreign, or even controversial. If this is the case, we ask you to read with an open mind and to suspend judgment until after you have had the opportunity to experience personally and directly the treatment methods described. By taking this middle path, in contrast to either blind faith or outright dismissal, you will be on the road to health and well-being.

Chances are you have turned to alternative medicine because you followed every avenue conventional medicine had to offer, only to end up "incurable," facing the rest of your life dependent upon drugs and their side effects. Rest assured that you have finally reached the end of your search. By taking the first step of reading this book, you have set the course to find the answers you seek. Now you are ready to heal.

Medicine Doesn't Have to Be Either/Or

By the time you finish this book, you will have observed that alternative medicine is not interested in treating diseases *per se* but in preventing them. We do not prop up health; we build it. We are not concerned about only your headaches, for if that were the case, we would hand you a prescription and prepare to see you again in a few months, when your headache found a way around the drug and expressed itself anew. However, conventional medicine should not as a whole be dismissed. Many genuine, caring, conventional physicians employ techniques with the perspective of a balanced, holistic approach. Furthermore, some life-threatening conditions are best served by conventional medicine, at least until the initial crisis is over.

In our opinion, the most effective treatment approach is one that is driven by the needs of patients. This requires that conventional physicians and alternative practitioners alike be aware of all treatment options, whether conventional or alternative, and be ready to treat each patient as a unique individual. In the words of Thomas Edison, "The doctor of the future will give no medicine, but will interest his patients in the care of the human frame, in diet, and the cause and prevention of disease."

The Master Symptom Chart

The Master Symptom Chart is designed to allow ample room for different approaches and interpretations of headaches. Our intent is to give you a comprehensive yet easy-to-read overview and then to send you to the place in the book that will most help you. In this way, you need not flip from the table of contents to the index and back again looking for a solution to your headache. Instead, use the Master Symptom Chart as a map to the place of painless living: The Symptoms and Headache Type columns are your starting points, the Pain Location and Underlying Causes columns are your journey's landmarks, and the Primary Treatments and Self-Care Treatments columns are the jumping-off point to your final destination.

A detailed Master Symptom Chart appears at the beginning of each chapter (Chapters 5-15) on a specific headache type. A summary Master Symptom Chart (At a Glance) for all headaches appears at the end of this introduction. Self-Care Treatments does not appear as a heading in the summary chart, but is featured in the individual chapter charts.

HEADACHE SYMPTOMS

Accurately describing your headache symptoms is essential to finding the solution that eventually heals them. Symptoms are clues to the underlying cause, and you must be as specific and as thorough as possible when you describe them; otherwise you may miss something. Take extra time to determine exactly what you are experiencing: such as whether your head pain is piercing, aching, throbbing, crushing, boring, burning, pressing, squeezing, or dull; whether it is accompanied by vomiting, visual disturbances, or dizziness; and/or whether you get constipation, ear ringing, or numb and tingly legs. This will get you headache free a lot sooner than if you jump to the first healing modality that interests you.

HEADACHE TYPE

Although we use the terminology of headache classification, our approach focuses mainly on symptoms. Symptoms vary widely among sufferers— even among those who are considered within the same headache type. Therefore, the most effective way to understand and treat your headache is to view yourself as an individual with a headache rather than fitting your head pain into a preexisting category. Although we believe classifications are often more confusing than they are helpful and are probably one of our least concerns, we are structuring the book around headache types because we believe this will make finding a solution easier for you.

We gathered headache symptoms into the most widely accepted classifications: tension, migraine, cluster, trauma, exertion, allergy/food/chemical sensitivity, rebound, TMJ/dental, sinus, eyestrain, environmental, organic, and other. Be aware that among these general classifications there is a great deal of overlap as to which symptoms indicate which headache type.

PAIN LOCATION

Although the location of pain is obviously part of the symptom, the location of your head pain deserves a category of its own. This is because pinpointing exactly where your head pain is expressing itself brings you one step closer to discovering its origin.

As a general rule, the seat of your head pain corresponds to the location where you are feeling it, even though much of your pain is actually being transmitted or referred from arteries, veins, sinuses, and the upper spine. In addition, if your pain is intense, it may be felt both in the direct nerve supply of the affected area and in areas only indirectly related. Transferred or referred pain can exist at one point and be felt someplace else entirely, but, for classification purposes, pain is classified into one or more of the following areas:

- back of head (occipital) pain
- frontal pain
- side of head (temporal) pain
- top of head (vertex) pain
- eyeball pain
- upper jaw pain
- lower jaw pain
- total head pain.

UNDERLYING CAUSES

To permanently rid yourself of head pain, you must first determine what your headache symptoms mean and where they come from. As we say many times, headaches are a *symptom* of an imbalance or interference somewhere in one or more of the mechanical, organic, or bioelectric mechanisms of the body. In order to uncover this interference, you must learn to recognize the relationship between your headache and any other physiological symptoms you are experiencing. Once this connection is made, your headache

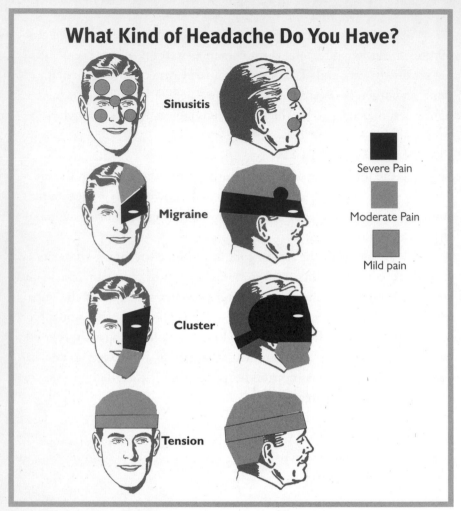

Figure 0.1—Pain locations.

can be treated from a position of understanding.

Rather than overwhelming you with an exhaustive list of possible causes, we have instead created 4 general categories. These categories cover the underlying bases for most headache-causing illnesses, and we refer to them elsewhere in the book before discussing more specific problems. The categories are as follows:

1. Metabolic/biochemical imbalances (digestive disorders, hormonal imbalance, circulatory problems);
2. Structural imbalances (which could be adjuncts of digestive or pelvic disorders);

3. Psycho/emotional imbalance;

4. Combination of one or more of the above.

PRIMARY TREATMENTS

Primary treatments are alternative healing modalities that are administered by qualified practitioners. The treatments listed for each headache type are carefully selected according to research and experience, and all are documented as effective treatments. Since the treatments are not equally useful in each case, be sure to refer for more information to the chapter listed for the best treatment modality for your particular set of symptoms.

SELF-CARE TREATMENTS

Self-care treatments are alternative healing techniques that you can administer on your own. Each of these techniques was specifically chosen because patients have reported relief while using them. Since self-care techniques are often less potent, they are generally used in conjunction with primary treatments—if you have only mild headaches, you might want to try these first, for some headache sufferers are able to rely solely on them.

If you decide to supplement your treatment with self-care, not only will you stand a better chance of recovering sooner, but you will witness your ability to heal at your own hand. And since these techniques pave the road for a balanced lifestyle, they should eventually be enough to keep you healthy and headache free.

Headache Trigger Chart

Your headache may be triggered, or started, by factors that fall into 8 broad categories: dietary sensitivity, environmental irritants, hormonal imbalances, digestive disturbances, problems in the immune system, lifestyle factors, structural imbalances, and mental stress.

The Headache Trigger Chart is a supplement to the Master Symptom Chart, specifically column 4, Underlying Causes/Triggers, as well as a brief overview of the information presented in Chapter 3. It was created to help you identify the range of conditions and problems most commonly cited as the underlying causes of headaches.

The chart is divided into 2 columns. The first column, Triggers, lists the general categories of underlying causes. The second column, Common

Headache Trigger Chart

TRIGGER	COMMON EXAMPLES
DIETARY SENSITIVITIES	**FOODS:** all dairy products, eggs, sugar, chocolate, alcohol, pickled or cured meat and fish, shellfish, game (hare, pheasant, venison, etc.), fatty and fried foods, pickles of any kind, chutneys, some seasonings (bay leaves, cinnamon, chilies, sassafras), some vegetables (onions, broad beans, capsicums, spinach, tomatoes, eggplant, avocados), some fruits (bananas, seed fruits such as peaches, plums, citrus fruits, pineapples, raspberries), nuts **CHEMICALS:** contaminated water, tyramine, MSG, sodium nitrate, aspartame, caffeine, tartrazine, dyes and food colorings, pesticides **MEDICATIONS:** birth control pills, diet pills, diuretics, painkillers, antihistamines, estrogen supplements, and heart, blood pressure, and asthma medications
ENVIRONMENTAL SENSITIVITIES	bright light, noise, high altitude, weather changes, exposure to poorly ventilated enclosures causing prolonged exposure to pollutants, cigarette smoke, carbon monoxide, heavy metals, and other pollutants (such as formaldehyde, phenol, gasoline, plastics, perfumes), pollen, mold, house dust, mercury dental amalgams
HORMONAL IMBALANCES	low progesterone levels (PMS, irritability, fluid retention, menopause), excess estrogen levels (breast tenderness, fluid retention), hypothyroid (cold extremities), hypoglycemia (low blood sugar which causes fainting, irritability, dizziness, sugar cravings), Hashimoto's Autoimmune Thyroiditis (HAIT)
DIGESTIVE DISTURBANCES	constipation, leaky gut syndrome, candidiasis, hypoglycemia, nutritional deficiencies
AUTOIMMUNE DISTURBANCES	chronic fatigue syndrome, candidiasis, blood clotting

LIFESTYLE FACTORS	sleep disturbances or disruptions in regular patterns (napping, too little or too much sleep), inadequate nutrition, changed meal patterns (hunger, missed or skipped meals, crash diets), overconsumption of sugar and junk food, smoking, fatigue, overworking, uncorrected faulty vision, astigmatism, excessive frowning or squinting, long periods of reading or close work (especially in dim light), constant use of computer, TV, or VCR
STRUCTURAL DISTURBANCES	musculoskeletal misalignments, head trauma, muscle trauma, coccyx bone trauma, overexertion, jaw clenching, grimaced face, teeth grinding, poor posture, dental problems, TMJ
PSYCHOLOGICAL STRESS	stress, anxiety, depression, repressed emotions, anger, boredom

Examples, suggests the actual health condition, substance, or lifestyle factors that may lead to each of the triggers. For example, Dietary Food and Chemical Sensitivity is the first listing in column 1; its related column discusses the specific foods and chemicals that are most often linked to headaches.

Master Symptom Chart—At a Glance

SYMPTOMS	HEADACHE TYPE	PAIN LOCATION
Intermittent, generalized pain that gradually becomes more frequent and severe; worse with head movement, stooping over, coughing, and/or straining; more pronounced in the morning (Note: brain tumors are not always accompanied by headaches.)	ORGANIC HEADACHES **Brain Tumor Headache**	near or around tumor site, usually one-sided
Intense, generalized headache of sudden on-set, often with considerable eye pain	**Meningitis Headache**	total head pain
Early symptoms similar to migraine or cluster headache **Symptoms of Small Rupture:** persistent neck pain and stiffness followed by mental confusion and pain in back and legs **Symptoms of Burst Vessel:** (leading to stroke) sudden unbearable headache, double vision, neck rigidity, and loss of consciousness	**Aneurysm Headache**	varies according to occurrence of clot or ruptured vessel
Intense stabbing pain that lasts from seconds to minutes; mainly in middle to old age	**Trigeminal Neuralgia Headache**	facial area, especially mouth and jaw
Jabbing pain like icepick stabs in back of the head; generally accompanied by neck and shoul-der tenderness; mainly in middle to old age	**Occipital Neuralgia Headache**	back of head and neck
Piercing, burning, or jabbing pain, especially when chewing or opening mouth	**Temporal Arteritis Headache**	temples, around ears, and on side of the jaw
Throbbing pain, reddened eyes; seeing halos or rings around lights	**Glaucoma Headache**	around or behind eye or in forehead
Localized or generalized pain after severe head injury; can mimic migraine or cluster headache symptoms	**Subdural Hematoma Headache**	at site of injury or total head pain
Dull, throbbing pain interspersed with brief but intense jabs of pain	**Hemicrania Continua Headache**	on one side of the head
Mild to severe throbbing pain, most severe in morning	**Hypertension (high blood pressure) Headache**	generalized total head pain or encircling "hat-band" pain

UNDERLYING CAUSES AND TRIGGERS	PRIMARY TREATMENTS	WHERE IN THE BOOK PAGE #
Causes: unknown	see medical doctor; can be supplemented by: ■ acupuncture ■ homeopathy ■ herbal medicine ■ neural therapy ■ nutritional therapy ■ traditional Chinese medicine	**Chapter 5** Page 157
Causes: inflammation of brain membranes brought on by bacterial or viral infection	see medical doctor	**Chapter 5** Page 157
Causes: rupturing or bursting of blood vessel **Triggers:** high blood pressure, heart disease, physical exertion	see medical doctor	**Chapter 5** Page 157
Causes: unknown nerve disorder	see medical doctor	**Chapter 5** Page 157
Causes: unknown nerve disorder	see medical doctor	**Chapter 5** Page 157
Causes: inflammation of the temporal arteries (located behind temple) due to an immune system reaction	see medical doctor	**Chapter 5** Page 157
Causes: inherited eye disease, digestive/liver dysfunction	see medical doctor; can be supplemented by: ■ acupuncture ■ homeopathy ■ neural therapy ■ nutritional therapy ■ traditional Chinese medicine	**Chapter 5** Page 157
Causes: injury to head	see medical doctor	**Chapter 5** Page 157
Causes: unknown	see medical doctor	**Chapter 5** Page 157
Causes: very high blood pressure (systolic over 200, diastolic over 100)	see medical doctor; can be supplemented by: ■ acupuncture ■ homeopathy ■ neural therapy ■ nutritional therapy ■ traditional Chinese medicine	**Chapter 5** Page 157

Master Symptom Chart—At a Glance

SYMPTOMS	HEADACHE TYPE	PAIN LOCATION
	ORGANIC (cont.)	
Throbbing or pounding pain with migraine-like symptoms and muscle spasms in neck	**Spinal Tap Headache**	head, neck, and/or shoulder area
Gradual onset, mild, steady or dull, aching, sometimes described as viselike squeezing or heavy pressure around head; usually does not throb	TENSION HEADACHES **Muscle Contraction Headache**	most often located on both sides of head or as band-like sensation around head or back of neck spreading to whole head
Throbbing headache, often synchronized with pulse, steady, but brief jolts of pain, aggravated by activity	MIGRAINE HEADACHES **Common Migraine**	generally one-sided, centered above or behind one eye
Like common migraine, with about a half hour before onset, a warning aura consisting of visual disturbances, sensory motor disturbances, and/or mental function disturbances	**Classic Migraine**	same as common
Migraine aura without headache, usually occurs in middle age or childhood	**Migraine Equivalent**	one side of the head
Paralysis and altered sensation on one side, often accompanied by double vision; most common in children and adolescents	**Hemiplegic and Ophthalmoplegic Migraine**	one side of the head
Severe throbbing, sometimes accompanied by lack of coordination, visual problems, hearing loss, vomiting; develops mainly in children and adolescents, especially in young women beginning menstruation	**Basilar Migraine**	same as common
Migraine with blindness or blurring in one eye	**Retinal Migraine**	same as common but with eye pain
Migraine with prolonged aura lasting up to 7 days or symptoms lasting longer than 1 week or continuously; auras continue past pain phase	**Complicated Migraine**	same as common

UNDERLYING CAUSES AND TRIGGERS	PRIMARY TREATMENTS	WHERE IN THE BOOK PAGE #
Causes: Lumbar Puncture Diagnostic Test	see medical doctor	**Chapter 5** Page 157
Causes: metabolic imbalances, structural disturbances, emotional/psychological factors **Triggers:** dietary and/or environmental sensitivity, hormonal imbalance, autoimmune disturbances, lifestyle factors, structural disturbances, psychological stress	■ acupuncture ■ detoxification ■ environmental medicine ■ homeopathy ■ naturopathy ■ neural therapy ■ nutritional therapy ■ psychotherapy ■ traditional Chinese medicine	**Chapter 6** Page 173
Causes: metabolic imbalances, structural disturbances, emotional/psychological factors **Triggers:** dietary and/or environmental sensitivity, hormonal imbalance, autoimmune disturbances, lifestyle factors, structural disturbances, psychological stress	■ acupuncture ■ detoxification ■ environmental medicine ■ homeopathy ■ naturopathy ■ neural therapy ■ nutritional therapy ■ traditional Chinese medicine	**Chapter 7** Page 197
		Chapter 7 Page 197
		Chapter 7 Page 197
		Chapter 7 Page 197
		Chapter 7 Page 197
		Chapter 7 Page 197
		Chapter 7 Page 197

Master Symptom Chart—At a Glance

SYMPTOMS	HEADACHE TYPE	PAIN LOCATION
Rapid onset, burning, boring, sharp or throbbing; can be knifelike; excruciating and among the worst pain known, affects men more frequently	CLUSTER HEADACHES	on one side of the head, felt most intensely behind or around one eye
Similar to above; chronic; mostly strikes in women	**Chronic Paroxysmal Hemicrania Headache (also called Atypical Cluster or Cluster Variant Headache)**	pain can occur in places other than behind eye and can shift locations
Dull, aching, stabbing, and sharp or excruciating pain at site of injury	TRAUMA HEADACHES	where the head injury occurred or can mimic location of tension or migraine headache
Persistent headache that worsens with time; sleepiness, confusion, disturbances of vision, nausea or vomiting; weakness or numbness in one part of body	**Subdural Hematoma Headache**	↓
Dull, aching, or throbbing, generalized pain, felt either continuously or in brief jolts; worsened by activity	ALLERGY/ SENSITIVITY HEADACHES **(Food/Chemical/ Environmental)**	anywhere on or all over head, although sometimes located in forehead, back of head and/or neck; above or behind one eye
Gradual onset, gnawing, dull, aching pain	SINUS HEADACHES	forehead or face; depending on which sinus group affected

UNDERLYING CAUSES AND TRIGGERS	PRIMARY TREATMENTS	WHERE IN THE BOOK PAGE #
Causes: metabolic imbalances, structural disturbances, emotional/psychological factors **Triggers:** dietary and/or environmental sensitivity, hormonal imbalance, autoimmune disturbances, lifestyle factors, structural disturbances, psychological stress	■ acupuncture ■ detoxification ■ environmental medicine ■ homeopathy ■ naturopathy ■ neural therapy ■ nutritional therapy ■ oxygen therapy ■ traditional Chinese medicine	**Chapter 8** Page 231
		Chapter 8 Page 231
Causes: blow to head or fall; can be worsened by metabolic imbalances, structural disturbances, emotional/psychological factors	■ acupuncture ■ bodywork ■ chiropractic ■ craniosacral therapy ■ homeopathy ■ neural therapy ■ osteopathy ■ traditional Chinese medicine	**Chapter 9** Page 257
	see medical doctor	**Chapter 9** Page 257
Causes: metabolic imbalances, structural disturbances, emotional/psychological factors **Triggers:** dietary and/or environmental sensitivity, hormonal imbalance, autoimmune disturbances, lifestyle factors, structural disturbances, psychological stress	■ acupuncture ■ detoxification ■ environmental medicine ■ homeopathy ■ naturopathy ■ nutritional therapy	**Chapter 10** Page 277
Causes: inflammation and/or infection of sinus worsened by metabolic imbalances, structural disturbances, emotional/psychological factors **Triggers:** dietary and/or environmental sensitivity, structural disturbances, psychological stress	(see medical doctor to rule out infection) ■ acupuncture ■ chiropractic ■ detoxification ■ environmental medicine ■ enzyme therapy ■ naturopathy ■ nutritional therapy ■ osteopathy	**Chapter 11** Page 303

Master Symptom Chart—At a Glance

SYMPTOMS	HEADACHE TYPE	PAIN LOCATION
Similar to tension headache, with dull, steady pain usually felt as pressure on top, often accompanied by clicking sound in jaw	TMJ/DENTAL HEADACHES	most often on both sides of head or as a band-like sensation around head; tenderness around jaw, within mouth, and where jaw meets skull (temporomandibular joints)
Can resemble tension headache, with mild steady pain usually felt as pressure on top of head or around head	EYESTRAIN HEADACHES	forehead and face; sometimes with pain at back of head and/or neck
Throbbing, generalized headache; steady jolts of pain; can be similar to migraine	REBOUND HEADACHES	one or both sides of the head, often felt as total head pain; can begin at back of neck and spread to entire head or side of head
Sharp, throbbing headache with either generalized or localized pain	EXERTION HEADACHES	anywhere on or all over head

Causes: dysfunction of one or both temporomandibular joints due to faulty bite; tooth infections, other dental problems;
Triggers: dietary and/or environmental sensitivity, hormonal imbalance, lifestyle, structural imbalances, psychological stress

- acupuncture
- biological dentistry
- bodywork
- chiropractic
- craniosacral therapy
- detoxification
- environmental medicine
- homeopathy
- neural therapy
- osteopathy

Chapter 12
Page 321

Causes: overuse of eyes; worsened by metabolic imbalances, structural disturbances, emotional/psychological factors
Triggers: lifestyle factors, dietary and/or environmental sensitivity, hormonal imbalance, autoimmune disturbances, structural disturbances, psychological stress

- acupuncture
- behavioral optometry
- bodywork
- environmental medicine
- homeopathy
- nutritional therapy
- osteopathy

Chapter 13
Page 347

Causes: overuse of narcotics, caffeine, or other stimulants; worsened by metabolic imbalances, structural disturbances, emotional/psychological factors
Triggers: dietary and/or environmental sensitivity, hormonal imbalance, autoimmune disturbances, lifestyle factors, structural disturbances, psychological stress

- acupuncture
- bodywork
- detoxification
- environmental medicine
- homeopathy
- neural therapy
- nutritional therapy

Chapter 14
Page 365

Causes: lactic acid accumulation, worsened by metabolic imbalances, structural disturbances, emotional/psychological factors
Triggers: structural disturbances, running, aerobics, sexual intercourse, sneezing, coughing, moving bowels, psychological stress

- acupuncture
- detoxification
- environmental medicine
- homeopathy
- naturopathy
- neural therapy
- nutritional therapy
- traditional Chinese medicine

Chapter 15
Page 387

Part One

Chapter 1

Head Pain—What's It All About?

Lord, how my head aches! What a head have I! It beats as if it would fall in twenty pieces.

Shakespeare, *Romeo and Juliet*

Although it may be little consolation, your headaches link you to a number of noteworthy individuals. Besides Shakespeare, you can count yourself in the company of Virginia Woolf, Frederic Chopin, Karl Marx, Ulysses S. Grant, Peter Tchaikovsky, Cervantes, Leo Tolstoy, and John Calvin. They all knew what it felt like to curl up and will the world to silence. They all knew the agony of head pain.

What Is Pain ?

Although the physiology of pain is still being debated, most doctors agree upon a few aspects of pain. Foremost among these theories is that pain, despite the anguish it causes, is an essential ally. We know that pain starts when the nervous system responds to tissue irritation or damage caused by an extrinsic stimulus, such as a ball in the face, a burned finger, or a disease. Nerve fibers convey this message to the spinal cord and then the brain. Upon learning that tissue damage has occurred, the brain orders the body to protect itself. In the case of a burned finger, it says: pull your hand away from the hot oven.

Many of the headache treatments on which most people rely only take away the pain rather than removing what caused it. This symptom-driven approach may work for a while, but it usually does not last.

Pain keeps your body alive and intact. If it were not for its signal, you would not know to protect yourself from whatever is hurting you. Unfortunately, many of the treatments on which most people rely only take away the pain rather than removing what caused it. This symptom-driven approach may work for a while, but it usually does not last.

For more information on Dr. Devi Nambudripad's approach to treating allergy headaches, see Chapter 17, An A-Z of Alternative Medicine, and Chapter 10, Allergy/Sensitivity Headaches.

This was the approach to Mala Moosad's headaches before Devi Nambudripad, D.C., L.Ac., R.N., Ph.D., discovered Mala's food allergy 5 years ago. Mala, a 41-year-old nurse who suffered from chronic migraine headaches for 20 years before she met Dr. Nambudripad, explains:

"Day in and day out, my head never stopped hurting. I was grouchy all the time. I saw many doctors and took even more medications. All gave me temporary relief, but my headaches always came back. Then I saw Dr. Nambudripad, who was the first to look for what caused them in the first place. It took her four treatments, and my headaches have been gone ever since."

Chronic pain like Mala's is generally much harder to pin down than acute pain. Pain may be saying you have a chemical or structural imbalance or that you need to change your diet. It may be trying to get you to let go of anger and relax more. It may be telling you all of these things. But before we consider your headache's message, it is necessary first to understand some of the current theories of head pain.

Types of Head Pain

Although head pain is felt differently by everybody, it can be categorized according to the following characteristics:

TYPE OF PAIN	POSSIBLE INDICATIONS
sharp, shooting pain	nerve problems
pulsating, throbbing, one-sided pain	abnormal swelling and constricting of blood vessels
dull, heavy, diffuse pain	digestive disturbances, infections, and fevers
pressing, blinding, squeezing pain	toxic overload, chronic fatigue, emotional difficulties
sore, hot, burning pain	rheumatic ailments and anemia-related deficiencies (low blood iron)
sharp, boring pain	epilepsy and other problems that overstimulate the nervous system

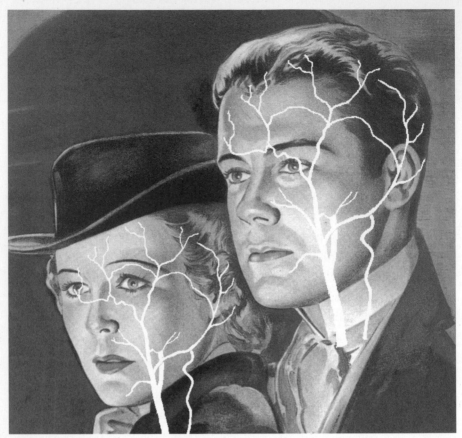

Figure 1.1—The carotid artery supplies blood to the brain.

A Look at Head Pain

Because there are no pain-sensitive nerves inside the brain, the brain itself does not feel pain. Rather, your pain is generally expressing itself on or around the skull and meninges (membranes covering the brain and spinal cord). Skull pain is grouped into two categories: extracranial pain, or pain felt outside the skull (which includes meningeal pain), and the rare intracranial pain, or pain produced inside the skull, which affects only about 1% of all headache sufferers. Thus, although it sometimes feels like your brain is exploding, your pain is most likely rooted someplace else.

Jes Oleson, M.D., a neurologist at the University of Copenhagen in Denmark, suggests that headaches result from nerve stimulation in three different sites on and around the head:

1. In constricting or dilating arteries and blood vessels surrounding the brain that become painful due to changes in blood flow patterns;
2. in the muscles in and around the head, such as those leading to the blood vessels and muscles around the neck, scalp, and face, that become painful when they contract too tightly;
3. in the nerve cells around the brain itself, including those associated with the eyes, jaw, sinuses, ears, teeth, and spinal cord, that become painful as a result of changes in blood chemistry.[3]

Other researchers attribute the sensation of head pain to alterations in fluid pressure within the skull; chemical imbalances resulting from blood sugar fluctuations, hormonal changes, or allergic reactions; spinal problems, pinched nerves or other structural difficulties that affect the way the nervous system functions; and movement restrictions in the cranial bones that make up the skull, including the temporomandibular joint in the jaw.

However, since all sensory input is ultimately interpreted by the brain's cerebral cortex, your brain is in many ways the real source of your head pain. Taking the long way around, head pain, or any other pain for that matter, is electrochemically relayed along neural pathways one nerve cell at a time until its message reaches the dorsal horn of the spinal cord, where it must wait alongside other sensory messages at a neurological "gate" before entering the brain.

The messages pressing to get past the gate then travel to the midbrain, where the brain's painkilling chemicals try to block them by deactivating a hormone called substance P, one of the chemical messengers (known as neurotransmitters) that carry pain impulses in the brain. If these natural opiates fail, pain moves on, through the hypothalamus and the pituitary glands and finally to the place responsible for the perception of pain, the cerebral cortex.

Conflicting Theories of Head Pain

Although no one really knows for certain exactly how headaches start, many doctors, researchers, and health practitioners uphold theories that attempt

QUICK DEFINITION

Substance P is a compound, called a polypeptide, made naturally in the body of several amino acids bonded together. It stimulates the expansion and contraction of the smooth muscles in the intestines and elsewhere. Substance P is also involved in the secretion of saliva and the functioning of the peripheral and central nervous system.

to offer an answer. Consider this partial sampling of currently held theories:

1. A neurosurgeon and dental school professional tell the public in a national weekly magazine that headaches are caused by a muscle connecting the top of the spinal column and the base of the skull.
2. A university specialist says headaches begin when an electric wave ripples across the nerve cells on the surface of the cortex.
3. A scientist believes that DNA, and thus your parents and their parents, holds the key to headaches.
4. A major research organization points to nerve impulses traveling the wrong way along the brain's major nerve, the trigeminal.

The list of causes seems endless. Serotonin, hormones, menstruation, blood vessels, the spinal cord, the neck, cranial alignment, digestion, smoking cigarettes, fatigue, allergies, stress, weather, alcohol, food reactions, alignment problems—all have been found responsible for the onset of headaches.

This is not to find fault with the research conventional doctors are conducting or the information they are releasing; chances are a day will come when every theory proves plausible. The problem is that what you hear tells you very little about your headache, and about how to treat it, particularly since causation theories tend to emphasize structural mechanisms one day and metabolic ones the next.

So what is a sufferer to do? The best advice is to relax, educate yourself, and look for doctors and practitioners who take the whole body into consideration. For example, a naturopath may find that your head pain is caused by faulty genes, a food allergy, and a misaligned spinal cord, whereas a physician may tell you your body does not produce enough serotonin because your mother's mother didn't either.

This is not to say that alternative doctors don't get attached to causation theories and particular treatments. Blaming a headache on allergies as has Dr.

> *Headaches are often caused by factors unrelated to the head itself. In such cases, remote pain, such as pain caused by pelvic or digestive irritations, is then transferred to corresponding areas in the head where it is experienced as a headache.*

Nambudripad; on dental problems as has Michael Gelb, D.D.S, M.S.; on energy blocks as has David Krofcheck, O.M.D., D.Ac., C.A.; or on a combination of physical and emotional stressors as has John Upledger, D.O., draws more attention toward a cure than a pharmacist's prescription.

Transferred or Referred Pain

Since only 12 pairs of cranial nerves (see Figure 1.3) carry information to and from your brain and 30 pairs of spinal nerves (see Figure 1.2) carry information to and from your spinal cord, messages from many parts of the body are being carried by the same nerves. This overlap means that stimulation can take place in one part of the body and be felt in another, suggesting that headaches are often caused by factors unrelated to the head itself. In such cases, remote pain, such as pain caused by pelvic or digestive irritations, is then transferred to corresponding areas in the head where it is experienced as a headache.

Ischemic Pain

Another major category of pain, ischemic (is-*key*-mick) pain, describes the type of pain felt when blood flow is cut off somewhere in the body. If you wrapped a cloth tightly around your wrist and stopped the blood flow to your hand, your hand would fall

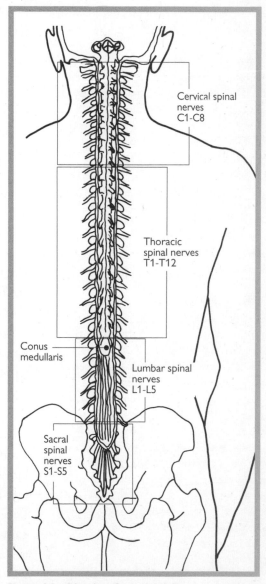

Cervical spinal nerves C1-C8

Thoracic spinal nerves T1-T12

Conus medullaris

Lumbar spinal nerves L1-L5

Sacral spinal nerves S1-S5

Figure 1.2—30 pairs of spinal nerves.

Hormones—Messengers of Pain and Relief

Without the chemical messengers called hormones traveling through your bloodstream, chances are you would never feel any pain. Hormones, in response to negative triggers or systemic imbalances, set off a chain of biochemical events that result in a wide variety of pain. Damaged cells secrete hormones, such as histamine, serotonin, and bradykinin, to induce pain responses along electrical networks of specialized nerve cells called neurons. Other hormones, known as prostaglandins, make nerve endings more sensitive to pain-inducing hormones, thus helping nerves fire off their initial pain signals.

Once activated, pain signals jump from nerve cell to nerve cell and talk to the brain via hormones called neurotransmitters, such as serotonin and norepinephrine. Luckily, as pain nears the brain, special pain-blocking cells called interneurons release other hormones—such as the brain's painkilling chemicals, the short-lived enkephalins, and the longer-lasting endorphins—which try to deactivate the neurotransmitters (particularly substance P) that are carrying the pain signals. These natural opiates are assisted and controlled by a delicate balance of serotonin and norepinephrine, since they also help endorphins lock into antipain receptors in the brain.

Nearly every gland secretes hormones that have been linked to head pain, including the pituitary, thyroid, parathyroid, adrenals, pancreas, and sex glands. However, because they oversee the entire endocrine system, pituitary or hypothalamus disorders are most often linked to chronic headaches.

painlessly asleep. But if you tried to move your fingers without first loosening the cloth, you would find yourself in excruciating pain. This is because exercising causes the release of metabolic wastes that, in this case, have no place to go. Without free circulation, the blood cannot flush out toxins, so they build up in nerve endings and cause pain.

Ischemic pain explains one of the reasons headaches are sometimes linked to a malfunctioning liver. The liver's role is to cleanse the blood, so if it is fed a poor diet and then overworked by too much alcohol, it cannot get the blood flow it needs to thoroughly flush out toxins and waste products, thereby causing a headache.

Psychological Contributors to Head Pain

Until seeing a homeopath, Kathy, a 35-year-old mother of three, had experienced blinding migraines ever since the birth of her first child a decade earlier.

"From the moment of my first migraine, I gave up dancing because I was terrified that the music and the lights would send me into an attack," says Kathy. "But since dance was how I dealt with stress and my tendency to gain weight, I became a wreck. I worried about my next headache, when it was going to come, and how bad it would be. I worried about my weight.

I worried about my kids. The stress from all this fear made my muscles tight and painful as well. I think I even used my headaches as a way to get my husband to take care of the kids."

The biochemical response to constant headache pain is to make the mind and body even more sensitive. The pain nerves become so physically irritated that they react more intensely to smaller and smaller stimuli. This is the point at which psychological factors can heighten headache pain by affecting a sufferer's coping mechanisms.

As in Kathy's case, a person with a headache or who is living in constant fear of one, emotionally withdraws from the world and often feels help-

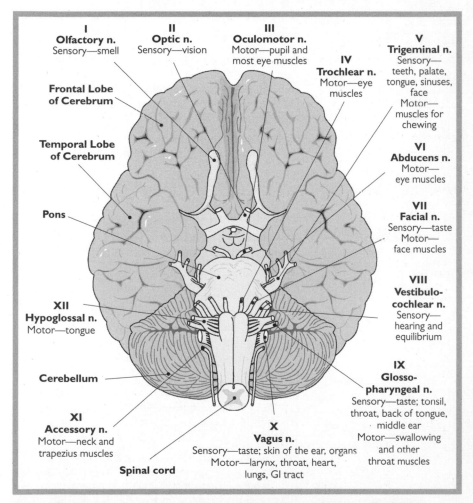

Figure 1.3—The 12 pairs of cranial nerves and their motor and sensory distribution.

less. She refrains from physical activities and "braces" herself against the pain, leading to further muscle tension. She may also get extra care when she has headaches, thereby learning unconsciously to express pain when she wants attention. Although none are the root cause of headache pain, these factors can increase the frequency of headache, adding to a downward spiral that becomes increasingly difficult to break.

Yet, despite growing awareness of the impact of psychological factors, conventional treatments rarely heed them. Kathy saw 5 conventional physicians and took so many drugs that she eventually became intolerant to them.

An Anatomy of the Pains in Your head

PAIN LOCATION	POSSIBLE DYSFUNCTION OR PROBLEM
back of head (occipital)	pelvic organ disease (most important); digestive teeth infection; eye strain; neck muscle pain (cervico-occipital myalgia); emotional tension; middle ear infection; adenoid (lymph gland behind the nose) infection; cerebellar tumor
frontal	digestive dysfunction (most important); constipation; kidney disease; low blood iron (anemia); eye strain; teeth infection; sinus infection
side of head (temporal)	combination of pelvic and digestive dysfunction; small intestinal disturbances; ear infection; teeth infection; tongue disease; brain aneurysm
top of head (vertex)	disease in the ovaries, prostate, bladder, or uterus; anemia; nervous disorders; emotional strain
eyeball region	digestive or pelvic dysfunction; nasal diseases; eye inflammation; 5th cranial nerve pain
sinus area	infection of sinuses or other sinus disorders
upper jaw area	dental pain (infections or amalgam poisoning); blockages of the superior maxillary nerve (upper branch of major nerve that serves the jaw). TMJ; tumors
lower jaw area	dental pain (infections or amalgam poisoning); mumps; blockages of the inferior maxillary nerve (lower branch of major nerve that serves the jaw). TMJ
total head	toxic buildup; hormonal imbalance (particularly estrogen/progesterone ratio in women); liver dysfunction; bacterial growth in bowels; emotional stress

Contraceptives Can Cause Headaches

Recurrent headaches, severe dizziness, depression, difficulty in controlling emotions, brain and nerve abnormalities, and a state of brain cell toxicity are traceable to the use of the Norplant contraceptive, now used by 1 million American women for birth control, reports *Science News*, November 1995.

The "Gate" Theory

First proposed in 1965 by psychologist Ronald Melzack and anatomist Patrick Wall, the "Gate" theory of pain suggests that there is a gating mechanism in the central nervous system that opens and closes, determining whether pain messages reach the brain. The theory holds that although pain is physically felt when the gate is open, it can be mitigated or worsened by psychological factors, such as attention to pain or a sufferer's emotional state.

For example, if a headache comes on while you are proudly watching your child in the school play, your headache will not hurt as much because the brain is preoccupied with more pleasant sensations, causing the gate to close. This phenomenon is similar to that experienced by a football player who gets injured during a play but does not notice the pain until after the game is over.

But if the headache comes on while you are feeling lonely or depressed, you will more likely feel it because such feelings cause the pain gate to open. Some believe that this is one of the reasons headache pain varies in intensity from one attack to another and among different people: the pain may be the same, but the perception of it is different.

In her mind, she had no choice but to listen to a friend who suggested she try an alternative approach.

Like Kathy, you, too, have control over the events that trigger the biochemistry of your headache. The most effective response is sometimes to change the way you live and think. Altering your diet, exercising more, and finding other outlets that make you feel better about yourself and your life may help you respond differently to the cycle of events that produce headache. In and of themselves, these changes may not make your headache go away entirely, but they will restore your ability to feel life more fully.

RECOMMENDED READING

Goleman and Gurin, eds. *Mind Body Medicine*. Mt. Vernon, NY: Consumer Reports Books.

Murphy, Michael *The Future of the Body*. Los Angeles: Jeremy P. Tarcher, 1992.

National Headache Foundation Fact Sheet. Chicago: National Headache Foundation, October 1994.

Office of Scientific and Health Reports, National Institute of Neurological Disorders and Stroke, U.S. Dept. of Health and Human Services Public Health Service, National Institutes of Health. "Chronic Pain—Hope through Recovery." NIH Publication 90-2406 (November 1989), 2.

Rapoport, Alan M., M.D., and Sheftell, Fred D., M.D. *Headache Relief*. New York: Simon & Schuster, 1990.

Rapoport, Alan M., M.D., and Sheftell, Fred D., M.D. *Headache Relief for Women*. New York: Little, Brown and Company, 1995.

Robbins, Lawrence, M.D., and Lang, Susan. *Headache Help*. New York: Houghton Mifflin Company, 1995.

Sternbach, R. Pain: *A Psychophysiological Analysis*. New York: Academic Press, 1968.

Stromfeld, Jan and Weil, Anita. *Free Yourself from Headaches: The Natural Drug-Free Program for Prevention and Relief*. Berkeley , CA: Frog, Ltd. and The Upledger Institute, 1995.

Solomon, Seymour, M.D., and Fraccaro, Steven. *The Headache Book*. Mount Vernon, NY: Consumer Reports Books, 1991.

Chapter 2

What Kind of Headache Do You Have?

More than 70% of Americans take painkillers at least once a month for relief from headaches, 12.5 million Americans get a headache every day, and between 45 and 50 million a year seek medical help for them.

For Peter and millions like him, headaches are a way of life rather than an occasional setback. Ranging from slight discomfort to total disability, headaches are a serious threat to national health in America. It is estimated that more than 70% of Americans take painkillers at least once a month for relief from headaches,[1] 12.5 million Americans get a headache every day, and between 45 and 50 million a year seek medical help for them—and these troubling statistics are on the rise.[2]

Depending upon what you read or hear, you may learn that people suffer from 3 to 300 different types of headaches, each with its own set of causes, symptoms, and points of pain. Some headaches pound, others throb; some sneak up slowly, others hit like a tornado. One or more of these headaches may cause zigzags in your field of vision, crying jags, anger, or aching shoulders; it may occur on the side, top, front, back of your head, or all over.

Even with all the separating, defining, and classifying, it is safe to say that all headaches, no matter what type, are related— because every one of them is a response to a metabolic, structural and/or emotional imbalance.

Why Classify Headaches?

Why are there so many headache types? Primarily because headaches are one of our most complex health problems Only in the past decade or so have researchers realized the need to join together to define common terms.

Uniform classifications have been established as a jumping-off point, resembling the "You Are Here" arrow on a map. When we speak a common language, we can compare notes and discuss treatment ideas. Classification has helped in many ways to elevate headaches to the status of a legitimate biological disorder.

Yet even with all the dividing, defining, and classifying, it is a safe bet to say that all headaches, no matter what type, are related—because every one of them is a response to a metabolic, structural, and/or emotional imbalance. We still do not know exactly why some people respond to such stressors with headaches while others get back pain or stomach ulcers, and determining where you fit into these classifications can be a tricky task if you are not careful. The key to classification, then, is not getting overly concerned with the label or definition but looking at the overall picture.

The Shortcomings of Classification

One doctor we know frequently jokes that the *medley* of headache types and characteristics is what gives people—especially doctors—headaches in the first place. The overlap of symptoms and headache types can cause a lot of confusion and frustration, particularly for those who care more about the cause than whether, for instance, watery eyes suggest a migraine, cluster, trauma, allergy, sinus, eyestrain, or environmental headache. Furthermore, modern headache terminology fails to discern many of the factors and triggers that lead to head pain.

Another major shortcoming of the current classification system is the diagnostic pigeonholing it encourages. Instead of treating people as individuals with specific responses, the patient becomes a set of labels in which the headache is the problem rather than a symptom of an underlying systemic disturbance. Such thinking yields statistics but rarely long-term solutions. Once your doctor has matched your complaint with a group of patterns, you are often left to face your "diagnosis" on your own.

Consider Karen, a 37-year-old school bus driver whose doctor failed to take into account that no 2 headaches are ever alike.

"My family physician told me I was suffering from cluster headaches, and said all he could do to help me was to give me a couple of prescriptions," says Karen. "Since this didn't really help me, I went back a couple of years later, and he suggested I consider surgery. The thought of surgery terrified me so much that I sought the help of an alternative practitioner. Immediately, I saw that he cared more about helping me than he did about figuring what *type* of headache I had."

While a doctor or practitioner may have memorized the details of the classification system, you know more about your headache than anyone. Classification can tell you neither why you got the headache nor how to get better and stay better without drugs.

Conventional vs. Alternative Outlooks

Despite its widespread use, headache classification is still surrounded by confusion. Depending upon which medical text you consult, your headache may be classified as primary (the headache itself being the problem) or secondary (the headache being a symptom of other problems). Some researchers want you to believe that all headaches are tension, migraine, cluster, or "mixed." Others will tell you headaches can be classified into four types: muscle contraction, vascular, traction and inflammatory, and "idiopathic cranial." A third group will tell you headaches are caused by muscular contraction, vascular irregularities, or organic disorders. You will also read that vascular headaches are actually toxin headaches.

The boundaries between these distinctions can seem vague. On the other hand, each classification system is true to some extent. Nearly every headache can be classified as secondary (because few headaches arise spontaneously on their own), and since vascular changes are the primary mechanism of sending pain to the brain and contracted muscles are a universal response to pain, you can assume that all headaches are both vascular- and muscle-related.

Chances are your headache is both simpler and more complicated than any predetermined category defines it. This is why alternative medicine *individualizes* treatment. While most alternative practitioners are familiar with the conventional terminology, some completely reject the notion of headache classification. The body is not merely composed of clearly defined sections and compartments but it is essentially an interrelated, living system much more sophisticated than our intellectual ability to classify. Your best option is to use classification as a way to talk about your headache before delving into its possible causes and solutions.

Headache Types

The most commonly recognized headache types can be distinguished as follows:

- organic headaches
- tension headaches
- migraine headaches
- cluster headaches
- trauma headaches
- allergy/sensitivity headaches (food/chemical/environmental)
- sinus headaches
- TMJ/dental headaches
- eyestrain headaches
- rebound headaches
- exertion headaches

While this list is by no means exhaustive, it provides a practical means of examining the classifications understood and used by most medical practitioners. Each of these 11 types is explored in depth in Chapters 5 through 15. Be aware that there is a great deal of symptom overlap among types. For instance, you may have a migraine headache caused by a food allergy, or a tension headache that feels and acts like a migraine. We recommend that you read two or more chapters to find the most exact expression of your condition.

ORGANIC

Although they constitute only 1 to 2% of all headaches, organic headaches are the most serious headache type and should always be ruled in or out when making any headache diagnosis. Hemorrhages, brain tumors, glaucoma, swollen and diseased blood vessels, concussions, hypertension, and brain infections such as meningitis and encephalitis are all examples of the serious organic disorders that can cause headaches.

Organic headaches are classified in the traction and inflammatory category because the head pain they cause is the result of pulling (or traction) on pain-sensitive brain linings. For the most part, organic headaches begin suddenly, occur daily, and are worsened by exertion and coughing. The sudden onset of a new type of head pain, particularly pain that is not relieved by sleep, that causes waking at night, or that is associated with eye, ear, or nose bleeding, should be investigated immediately by your doctor.

TENSION

Almost everyone gets a tension headache now and then. The muscles in your neck feel like they have been tied in tender knots, and the sky seems to be clamping down on your head. There is a dull pain in your forehead, temples, possibly your entire head. These headaches—also known as muscular contraction headaches—are said to account for approximately 90% of all headaches, although doctors are beginning to believe that this number has been elevated by the overlap of tension and all vascular-related headaches. Tension headaches are caused when the sensitive nerve endings in your head, face, and neck are irritated by excessive muscle tension or spasms.

Headache Symptoms That Signal Danger
Certain headache symptoms may actually be an indication of a serious health condition, such as a brain tumor, infection, stroke, or other life-threatening illness. Symptoms of such conditions include head pain that progressively worsens, projectile vomiting, seizures, changes in speech or personality, and walking difficulties (problems with balance, gait, or coordination). While headaches due to organic disorders are extremely rare, they are very serious. If you are exhibiting any of the above symptoms along with your headache, please consult a physician immediately to ensure proper diagnosis and treatment.

There are two types of tension headaches: chronic, which occur more than 15 times per month, and episodic, which occur less than once or twice a week. For most people, these headaches last for only a few hours, but for some chronic sufferers, the pain never really goes away. Researchers have discovered that tension headaches are similar to migraine headaches, as they appear to be related to constricted blood vessels in the head and/or fluctuations in brain-chemical activity whether or not they are related to tense or irritated muscles.

Tension headaches are triggered by stress, fatigue, depression, digestive disorders, poor posture, or misalignments of the musculoskeletal structures and benefit from therapies associated with dietary changes, musculoskeletal manipulation (such as chiropractic, acupressure, neural therapy, and craniosacral therapy), and relaxation and stress management. Energy machines that produce healing wavelengths, such as ultrasound, diathermy, or the Electro-Acuscope, also provide relief.

MIGRAINE

Affecting nearly 18% of all females and 6% of all males in the United States, migraines, also known as "sick" or bilious headaches, are easily among the most frustrating and debilitating headache types. They account for as many as 64 million days of lost productivity a year, and despite all the research and theories surrounding them, the pain they produce remains a mystery to most doctors and researchers.

Theory suggests that migraines are vascular in nature because the pain they cause seems to be directly linked to the alternating contraction and expansion of blood vessels in the head, which puts pressure on the nearby nerve endings and causes irritation. However, migraines are also associated with rapid fluctuation in neurotransmitters, especially serotonin, the hormone responsible for regulating our perceptions of pain.

Migraine prevalence varies with age, generally beginning in the teenage years, with the highest incidence of migraine occurring in those between 20 and 38 years of age and declining in incidence thereafter. As it is an episodic disorder, recurrence is the key to migraine.

There are two main categories of migraine, common and classic. Both are characterized by a sharp, pounding, blinding pain, the latter preceded by a warning aura consisting of visual disturbances, numbness, or overall weakness which comes on about 30 minutes before onset.

Overall migraine symptoms include lightheadedness, throbbing pain on one side of the head, and frequently nausea, vomiting, dizziness, and hypersensitivity to light, sound, and smells. Migraines appear to be triggered by just about everything but especially by hormonal changes (such as the drop in estrogen level that accompanies a woman's monthly cycle), oral contraceptives, allergies, toxic contamination, hunger, certain trigger foods (including aged cheese, smoked or cured meats, chocolate, alcohol, red wine), bright or flashing lights, changes in altitude or weather, and disturbed sleep patterns.

Contrary to what you may have been told, a migraine is not something you have to learn to live with. You can forget the symptom-controlling drug therapy and learn to prevent migraines from happening. In the majority of cases, if you pay attention and do your home-

QUICK DEFINITION

A **neurotransmitter** is a brain chemical with the specific function of enabling communications to happen between brain cells. Chief among the 100 identified to date are acetylcholine, gamma-aminobutyric acid (GABA), serotonin, dopamine, and norepinephrine. GABA works to stop nerve signals to keep brain firings from getting out of control; serotonin does the same and helps produce sleep, regulate pain, and influence mood, although too much serotonin can produce depression.

Affecting nearly 18% of all females and 6% of all males in the United States, migraines account for as many as 64 million days of lost productivity a year, and despite all the research and theories surrounding them, the pain they produce remains a mystery to most doctors and researchers.

work, you can identify what is causing them, eliminate the trigger from your diet, detoxify and repair your system, and, finally, live migraine free.

CLUSTER

Sometimes called "suicide" headaches because of the intensity of the pain with which they are associated, cluster headaches affect roughly one million Americans, 90% of them male. These vascular-type headaches involve excruciating, knifelike pain behind or near one eye. The strange episodic pain of cluster headaches is accompanied by tearing and reddening of the eye, drooping eyelids, facial flushing, sweating, and nasal congestion. Attacks tend to occur several times daily, always at the same time, for 6 to 8 weeks per year. Typically, they last from 30 minutes to 2 hours, but they rarely go away for more than 3 hours during a cycle.

Other types of cluster headaches include chronic cluster and atypical cluster, also called chronic paroxysmal hemicrania or cluster variant headache. Current theories suggest that cluster headaches may be related to disturbances in the hypothalamus, the part of the brain that affects neurotransmitter levels, and that they are triggered by seasonal or daily biological cycles, particularly since most attacks occur in spring and fall when changes occur in the number of daylight hours. Alcohol, heavy smoking, cold wind, or hot air blowing across the face can trigger an attack, as can dream-filled sleep, trigger foods, and other substances known to dilate blood vessels.

Sometimes called "suicide headaches," due to the intensity of the pain with which they are associated, cluster headaches affect roughly one million Americans, 90% of them male.

Like migraine sufferers, cluster sufferers need not live with pain all their lives. Again, relief is just a matter of determining the cause, eliminating the trigger, and finding the right therapies to cleanse and rebuild the body.

TRAUMA

Trauma headaches, also known as posttraumatic headaches, are usually associated with a head injury, even a minor injury. The pain of trauma headaches can be local or generalized and has been known to last years after the initial injury. These headaches can be confusing because they may occur immediately or develop months after the injury and may cause head pain that bears little relationship to the severity of the initial trauma. Furthermore, they can be hard to pin down because they often mimic migraine or tension headaches.

Once a trauma headache develops, it usually occurs daily and is fairly resistant to treatment. It can be accompanied by dizziness or vertigo (when the patient or the surroundings seem to whirl), mood changes, insomnia, fatigue and a reduced attention span. Trauma headaches tend to benefit most from therapies that work on musculoskeletal structure, such as neural therapy, chiropractic, craniosacral therapy, bodywork, bioenergetic release, acupressure, acupuncture, reflexology, and homeopathy.

≋CAUTION≋

A doctor should be consulted at the first sign of a trauma headache. A trauma headache with drowsiness, especially occurring on the day of the injury, can signify a hematoma, or blood-filled tissue, in the brain. This ruptured blood vessel, a subdural hematoma, requires immediate attention.

ALLERGY/SENSITIVITY HEADACHE (FOOD/CHEMICAL/ENVIRONMENTAL)

Although almost all headaches may be related to allergies or some other sensitivity, certain headaches are more readily attributable to sensitivities than others. Sensitivities vary among individuals, and it is impossible to establish a definitive list of factors that prompt sensitivity headaches. Just about anything you eat, drink, smoke, breathe, use, live next to, and/or wear can, potentially, bring one on.

The offending substance can be anything from diesel fumes to strawberry ice cream. Examples of allergy/sensitivity headaches include MSG headaches, ice cream headaches, nutritional deficiency headaches, constipation headaches, hot dog headaches, carbon monoxide headaches, hypoglycemic headaches, and hangover headaches.

Sensitivity headaches can take many forms, although they usually manifest as dull, aching, generalized pain. Generally, they come on between 4 to 12 hours after contact with or ingestion of the problematic substance. Many doctors classify these headaches as migraines, clusters, or sinus headaches because all of these types can produce similar associated symptoms. Some sensitivity headaches are accompanied by a runny nose, sneezing or a stuffed-up head, but they may not be related to hay fever; milk and milk products may also cause headaches as well as excess mucus.

Allergy/sensitivity headaches are among the easiest to eliminate once the offending substance has been found and removed and the body restored. The healing process may be slow, especially if you have been exposed to the substance for a long time.

SINUS

When pain is experienced in the area of the sinus cavities, people tend to believe they have sinus headaches. However, contrary to what ads on TV suggest, sinus headaches are not that common, and more often than not headaches thought to be sinus headaches are migraine or tension headaches. People with severe sinus infections (sinusitis) rarely get headaches.

A true sinus headache is caused by an infection or allergic reaction and is accompanied by acute inflammation of the sinus itself. The pain tends to be constant and gnawing, and often worsens as the day goes on. Depending upon which of the three sinus groups is affected, the pain can occur between or above the eyebrows or behind the cheekbones. If all sinus groups are affected, varying degrees of pain can be felt in all of these areas. These headaches are quite painful and can be difficult to treat; they usually go away when the sinus condition improves, although there are a number of alternative ways to hasten the recovery.

TMJ/DENTAL

TMJ/dental headaches involve facial pain that is felt most in the jaw and mouth region, especially focused in front of and behind the ear on one or both sides of the jaw. TMJ/dental headaches are caused by muscle spasms associated with dysfunctions of the jaw joint (temporomandibular joint), which is the hinge-like joint attaching the lower jaw to the skull, just in front of the ear canal. Generally, this pain is brought on by jaw misalignments (an uneven bite, TMJ syndrome), stressful movement patterns (jaw clenching, teeth grinding), diseases, dental and mouth problems (faulty bridges, teeth infections), and emotional stress.

Temporomandibular Joint Syndrome (TMJS) is lack of proper function in the jaw joint caused by the misalignment of the teeth and jaw. Symptoms can include pain, clicking, or grating sounds upon opening the mouth, and difficulty opening it very wide. When the teeth and jaw are not aligned properly, the cranium will distort to achieve proper chewing; with the cranium distorted, headaches, neck pain, low-back pain, loss of concentration, insomnia, and even depression, can result.

If your jaw makes popping, clicking or cracking sounds during eating and/or if pain and tenderness arise after eating or yawning (a sign of jaw misalignment), your headache may be related to TMJ syndrome. The pain associated with TMJ/dental headaches is considered less intense than that of migraine or tension headaches; it can express itself, however, in symptoms that mimic either category. These headaches are primarily treated with corrective dentistry and musculoskeletal therapies, although metabolic treatments and emotional/psychological treatments are also key to lasting success.

EYESTRAIN

Eyestrain headaches are described as a mild, steady pain felt in and behind the eyes, forehead, and face, particularly when accompanied by dry and aching eyes. These headaches, like tension headaches, are classified as muscle contraction headaches, and they are mainly triggered by overusing your eyes. They can be brought on by long periods of focused visual work, such as working on a computer or artwork, as well as by reading too long or in poor light, not wearing glasses when needed, or the flickering of computer screens and fluorescent tube lights.

These headaches can also be due to digestive disturbances caused by your diet (especially if associated with burping and belching) and musculoskeletal misalignments. These headaches respond well to behavioral optometry and other musculoskeletal therapies, plus nutritional therapy, relaxation techniques, and behavioral modifications.

REBOUND

Rebound headaches, also called analgesic or painkiller rebound, caffeine withdrawal, and holiday, weekend, or travel headaches, are classified as vascular headaches, but are much less intense than migraine, cluster, and sensitivity headaches. Characterized by dull throbbing pain on both sides of the head, these headaches strike when you miss your daily medication or caffeine "fix."

Overconsumption of or withdrawal from narcotics or caffeine-containing substances, such as over-the-counter pain medications, coffee, and canned sodas, constrict blood vessels, and the subsequent "rebound" dilation can trigger a headache. If taken habitually, any painkiller, whether prescribed or not, can suppress the body's ability to produce its own natural painkillers and result in headaches. Rebound headaches are best treated by gradually removing the rebound-causing substance and by whole natural body detoxification. It often takes a complete lifestyle change to make the shift permanent.

EXERTION

An exertion headache tends to be a brief, throbbing head pain that is experienced during or following physical exertion (such as lifting, running, or sexual intercourse) or passive exertion (like sneezing, coughing, or straining one's bowels). Exertion headaches are vascular in nature, and current theories suggest that their pain comes from exertion-induced swelling in the arteries and veins which in turn makes blood vessels in the head and scalp swell, leading to headache in people who are susceptible, or prone to other headaches.

One example of an exertion headache is the sex headache. The exertion of lovemaking, as well as the contraction of muscles in the neck and head during sexual excitement or orgasm, can cause sudden severe head pain. The pain generally subsides within moments but sometimes can last hours. This pain is sometimes a precursor for migraine or cluster headaches. These headaches are fairly easy to treat with simple lifestyle changes, such as dietary adjustments and relaxation techniques, or structural manipulation.

MASKING THE OBVIOUS

While phrases such as "take a vacation," "get some rest," "try to relax," "find a new job," even "get a new spouse" may issue from a well-meaning doctor, they accomplish little when a patient is sent home with only a prescription for painkillers and a bottle of tranquilizers. Within the field of conventional medicine, headache treatment generally consists of prescribing drugs that help deal with headache pain.

CAUTION

Although exertion headaches are generally harmless, it is wise to have them evaluated by a doctor because they can also signal the presence of a tumor, aneurysm, blood-vessel malformation, respiratory illness, or tooth abscess.

These "treatments" mask what is occurring and cause energy distortions which undermine the healthy functioning of the entire body. With long-term reliance on drugs, even those supposed to be safe, the body becomes more susceptible to secondary complications and other illnesses, both benign and serious. Such treatments, therefore, can often end up producing worse problems than the headache itself.

Another troublesome component of drug therapy is that doctors usually have to tinker with drugs before finding one that will work. The patient is put through repeated visits and alternating prescriptions of adjusted dosages in a strategy that can take months or years. Even then, sufferers often develop tolerance and must start the procedure all over again.

Few people realize that most of the headache research that reaches the mainstream media is funded by the pharmaceutical companies. It is wise to be wary of the suggestion that biochemical imbalances are best solved by ingesting other chemicals, particularly pharmaceuticals. Most of these medications cause side effects. As pointed out by Robert C. Atkins, M.D., these are really "drug effects," the additional effects of drug-based therapy which are as much a part of the action as the effect that brings about symptomatic relief.

Even allegedly worry-free drugs such as aspirin and nonsteroidal anti-inflammatory drugs (NSAIDs), the drugs most commonly used for headache relief, can cause serious trouble. Each year, for example, 10,000 to 20,000 people die as a result of ulcers caused by aspirin and NSAIDs.[3] This danger is compounded by the fact that many Americans have been conditioned to associate headache relief with such drugs, many of which are easy to acquire without a prescription. People can take medications without considering whether they are effective or safe. This is what happens when, for instance, people use over-the-counter decongestants (which often contain caffeine) to treat sinus headaches, even when their problem is a food allergy. This solution seems to work for a while because the headache subsides after a few days. Not realizing that 3 days is the time it takes most headaches to run their course, sufferers keep taking decongestants and actually make themselves worse.

THE TRAPDOOR TO WELLNESS

Each year, Americans consume an estimated 80 billion tablets of aspirin—which means that we as a population take 20 million aspirins a day. It should come as no surprise that headaches are the number-one reason cited for aspirin use. Turn on the TV or pick up a magazine, and somebody will tell you to choose among the 200 brands offering the "safest, fastest, surest, most clinically-proven, doctor-recommended" way to get rid of your headache. In all, $4 billion are spent annually on over-the-counter (OTC) pain relievers alone.

Although downing an OTC painkiller may be a quick way to find relief, those who have traveled this path know that OTC products lose their effectiveness. While it may have initially taken only 2 aspirin to get over your headache, the dose required slowly grows to 3, 4, 5, until you realize that *no* dosage will make your headaches go away in many cases because by

The Most Frequently Prescribed Headache Drugs

All drugs work by blocking an enzymatic pathway the body uses to perform a task. Drugs used for treating headaches serve basic functions. The first is to relieve pain. These drugs go through the central nervous system and block the pathways to keep the pain messengers from reporting to the brain.

The second is to abort an attack in progress. These drugs, which are often mixed with caffeine and other vasoconstrictors, work best for vascular headaches because they shrink the dilated blood vessels.

The third is to prevent an attack from occurring. These drugs, such as antidepressants, beta blockers, and calcium channel blockers, are used to stabilize blood vessels and keep them from contracting and expanding so easily.

SIMPLE ANALGESICS (relief)

work to relieve mild headache pain by numbing the nerve endings in the skin, the tissues, and the blood vessels leading to the brain; they often are combined with caffeine for the added effect of constricting dilated blood vessels.

- acetylsalicylic acid [Aspirin and other over-the-counter (OTC) products]: When taken in high doses or for prolonged periods, aspirin damages tissues in the body, including the lining of the stomach and intestines, laying the groundwork for stomach cramps, heartburn, nausea, and in some cases blood-ridden stools. It damages the immune system, irritates the liver, damages the kidney, and may even lower red blood cell counts and diminish the blood's capacity for clotting. It also causes dependence and rebound headaches.

- acetaminophen (Tylenol and other OTC products): Unlike aspirin, it has no anti-inflammatory effect, so it is often cited as a safer alternative that is gentler on the stomach and does not cause gastrointestinal disturbances. Skin rashes, allergic reactions, and rebound headache are the most common side effects; however, the overuse of acetaminophen, which happens more easily than with aspirin, can lead to liver failure and kidney disease.

NONSTEROIDAL ANTI-INFLAMMATORIES (NSAIDs) (relief and prevention)

generally prescribed for mild headaches; side effects include stomach irritation or bleeding, changes in vision, and fluid retention.

- OTC ibuprofen (Advil, Motrin, Nuprin)
- OTC naproxen sodium (Anaprox)
- indomethacin (Indocin)
- meclofenamate (Meclomen)
- ketorolac (Toradol)

COMBINED ANALGESICS (relief)

for severe headaches, particularly of the vascular variety, combine a simple analgesic, such as aspirin, with barbiturates, narcotics, hydrocodone, and oxycodone hydrochloride. Side effects include drowsiness, dizziness, nausea, constipation, dependency, and rebound headache.

- barbiturates (Fiorinal, Fioricet, Phrenilin, Esgic)
- narcotic (Tylenol #3)
- hydrocodone (Vicodin)
- oxycodone hydrochloride (Percocet)

NARCOTICS (relief)

powerful painkillers that work to relieve severe

head pain, particularly migraines and clusters; side effects include nausea, drowsiness, dizziness, constipation, dependency, and rebound headache.

- codeine
- butorphanol (Stadol): nasal spray or injection
- meperidine (Demerol): a synthetic narcotic

ANTIDEPRESSANTS

(preventive) used for severe headaches, especially migraine and chronic tension, and sometime given to normalize sleep and counter the depression that often goes with reoccurring head pain; side effects include weight gain, dry mouth, fatigue, fluid retention, constipation, blurred vision, insomnia, restlessness, and cardiovascular problems.

- amitriptyline (Elavil)
- nortriptyline (Pamelor)
- doxepin (Sinequan)
- phenelzine (Nardil)
- fluoxetine (Prozac)

ANTIMIGRAINES (relief, abortive) for severe vascular-type headaches, especially migraine and cluster, are often used to stop an attack in progress.

- ergotamine (Bellergal-S, Cafergot, Wigraine):

generally given as ergotamine tartrate, works by constricting the blood vessels of the head, thereby preventing or relieving overly dilated blood vessels. As ergotamine can lead to acute and chronic toxicity, its list of side effects is extensive, including stomach and/or muscle cramps, tingling and swelling in arms and legs, hair loss, tremors, chest pain, dizziness, vomiting, numbness, diarrhea, shortness of breath, changes in heart rate, hallucinations, and convulsions. May also cause dependency and rebound headaches.

- sumatriptan (Imitrex): newest contribution to headache medications, it works by increasing the amount of serotonin in the brain, thereby restoring balance in the tension of the blood vessels; its side effects include increased heart rate, elevated blood pressure, and a feeling of tightness in the chest, jaw, or neck.
- dihydroergotamine (DHE 45): relief for migraines and clusters; side effects include flushing, chest tightness, but less nausea than ergot compounds.
- Ergot compounds

(Ergostat): side effects include dependency, rebound headaches, nausea, cramps, and sometimes agitation.

- isometheptene/dichloralphenazone/acetaminophen (Midrin, Isocom): these sympathomimetic agents offer relief, but their side effects include rebound headaches, drowsiness, and dizziness.

ERGOTAMINE DERIVATIVES (or serotonin blockers) (preventive) effective for vascular-type headaches, including migraine, cluster, sensitivity and some tension headaches, serotonin blockers are believed to work by blocking the direct effect of serotonin on the blood vessels, which inhibits constriction and reduces pain sensitivity; side effects include sleeplessness, stomach pains, hallucinations, problems with blood circulation and the development of scar tissue in the organs, weight gain, and leg cramps.

- methysergide (Sansert)
- methylergonovine (Methergine)
- cyproheptadine (Periactin)

(Continued)

The Most Frequently Prescribed Headache Drugs

BETA BLOCKERS (preventive) used primarily for chronic tension, migraine, exertion, and trauma headaches, beta blockers work by stabilizing serotonin and stopping receptor nerves from dilating blood vessels; side effects include fatigue, depression, weight gain, memory disturbance, faintness, diarrhea, impotence, cold hands and feet, shortness of breath, and lowered pulse; may worsen asthma.

- propranolol (Inderal)
- nadolol (Corgard)
- timolol
- atenolol (Tenormin)
- lopressor

CALCIUM CHANNEL BLOCKERS (preventive) prescribed mainly for migraines and clusters, these are believed to keep blood vessels open by blocking the flow of cellular calcium, a known blood vessel constrictor; not believed to work as well as beta blockers, but produce fewer side effects for asthma sufferers; however, other side effects include constipation and dizziness.

- verapamil (Calan, Isoptin)
- nifedipine (Nimotop)
- diltiazem (Cardizem)
- propanol hydrochloride: prescribed daily to prevent migraine and cluster headaches, has been shown to cause fatigue and weight gain, upset stomach, alter blood pressure, and impair heart functioning.
- cardene

Additional Medications

- OTC antihistamines and decongestants—relief—antihistamines soothe your pain because of their sedative effect, but since they do not affect blood vessels, headaches often reappear as soon as the drug wears off. Decongestants, on the other hand, work by reducing the swelling of blood vessels. Both antihistamines and decongestants are often used by sufferers who mistake their headache as a symptom of a sinus infection because of allergy symptoms. Side effects include increased blood pressure, circulation problems, heart palpitations, anxiety, sleep disturbances, digestive disorders, dehydration, digestive problems, and rebound headaches.

- tranquilizers (Lithium)—preventive—generally prescribed by doctors to ease tension and emotional distress; side effects include drowsiness, weight gain, spaciness, depression, coordination loss, dependence, and addiction.
- steroids (Decadron)—relief and prevention—may cause dependency, stomach irritation, and fluid retention.
- anticonvulsants, such as divalproex sodium or valproic acid (Depakote)—prevention—used for severe migraines and clusters, but must be used in conjunction with other drugs; side effects include nausea, drowsiness, weight gain, tremors, and liver disorders; risky during pregnancy.
- antinauseants (Phenergan, Thorazine, Compazine) to control the side effect of migraines and other drugs with nausea as a side effect, although they themselves cause drowsiness and dizziness.

this point rebound headaches are compounding your existing headache condition.

Sticking to the conventional scenario, once you have exhausted your over-the-counter options, you eventually try the next option and make an appointment with your M.D. Unfortunately, many of these doctors simply give you stronger painkillers, drugs to prevent your headaches, and drugs to keep the first two prescriptions from making you sick, rather than finding out what is causing your headaches.

With all the emphasis on experts, you might decide your doctor isn't sophisticated enough to handle your headaches, so you hop a plane to another state to visit headache clinics. Many of these clinics are following the same regimen as your regular M.D., only on a bigger scale. The clinic puts you through a barrage of tests, and eventually you are told that your headache will not kill you because the test results are negative. Then, with a few words about biofeedback and relaxation, and no mention of dietary connections, individual differences, or prevention, you are given a new prescription and sent on your way.

The American Council for Headache Education (ACHE) claims that most headache clinics are able to cut the frequency of headaches in half and that about 75 to 80% of migraine sufferers improve, 65 to 70% of tension sufferers improve, and almost all cluster sufferers are cured. While this sounds wonderful, these statistics reveal neither the side effects with which these patients now contend nor that they are still suffering from whatever caused the headache symptom.

Remember, a person who is without symptoms and without medications is far healthier than a person who is without symptoms but is on medication. Even if you do not feel side effects from medication, you are exposing your body to risks (including potential kidney failure from overuse) every time you swallow a pill, get an injection, or spray a solution into your nose. Meanwhile, many drugs are so new that all their side effects may not be discovered for years, or the effects may be delayed and you will not detect the cause-and-effect relationship.

CONVENTIONAL TREATMENT OF TENSION HEADACHES

Although they are the most prevalent type of headache, tension headaches

Each year, Americans consume an estimated 80 billion tablets of aspirin—which means that we as a population take 20 million aspirins a day. Headaches are the number-one reason cited for aspirin use. In all, $4 billion are spent annually on these over-the-counter (OTC) pain relievers alone.

are most often shrugged off by conventional doctors. Less dramatic and exotic than other types of headaches, tension headaches tend to be dismissed with little concern. You get a prescription and a couple of lessons in biofeedback, but chances are, until your previously "manageable" headache explodes into a chronic daily problem, you will get little attention from your doctor.

Unfortunately, once tension headaches have become chronic, the typical array of OTC or prescription muscle relaxants, antihistamines, painkillers, and antiinflammatory drugs (the ones that may have made your headache chronic) are rendered practically useless. At this stage, stronger migraine drugs, such as ergotamine, may be prescribed for relief, while so called "prevention" comes in the form of prophylactic drugs, antidepressants, and tranquilizers.

CONVENTIONAL TREATMENT OF MIGRAINE HEADACHES

For conventional doctors, migraines are diagnosed through a process of elimination, then treated with prescription drugs. Time and again, patients report having been told by one or more doctors that they would have to learn to live with their migraines. Some of these patients have also been forced to learn to live with chronic tension headaches that have resulted from the medications prescribed to treat migraines.

Another complaint migraine sufferers share is that they have felt misunderstood or stupid when trying to discuss their condition with a conventional doctor. This observation is substantiated by a Gallup poll conducted in 1995. Out of 1,014 headache patients polled, 54% were migraine sufferers unaware that they had migraines. The study further reveals that, despite having specifically visited their doctors for head pain, significant percentages of sufferers had not even been asked to provide basic information that can lead to correct diagnoses. In fact,

- 44% were not asked about numbness and tingling;
- 38% were not asked about sensitivity to noise;

- 33% were not asked about visual distortions;
- 30% were not asked about light sensitivity;
- 30% were not asked about vomiting;
- 27% said physicians did not ask them about pulsating, throbbing, pain which is the most common migraine symptom;
- 26% were not asked about nausea.[4]

This poll does not reveal whether the misdiagnoses were due to doctor negligence or ignorance. What appears obvious is that despite the proliferation of headache clinics and wonder pharmaceuticals, many migraine patients are not benefiting from conventional medicine.

CONVENTIONAL TREATMENT OF CLUSTER HEADACHES

Like migraines, cluster headaches are elusive and difficult to treat, not because of the headache itself but because of the long road one must take to get to the root problem. Few conventional doctors are equipped to go this route because the prevailing medical model has progressed only far enough to consider the mechanism of clusters and not to see clusters from the whole-body perspective.

Conventional doctors tell patients that cluster headaches are a lifetime syndrome that can be controlled only through the use of prescription drugs, either during the cycle itself, or during remission periods in the hope of buying time between rounds. To stop an attack in progress, doctors sometimes employ a procedure (called a sphenopalatine ganglion block or SBG), in which a probe is used to insert a local anesthetic through the nose into the nerve relay station at the base of the skull. Since the procedure does not prevent future attacks, the cost and time involved in running to the doctor for the brief respite it provides is considered impractical.

In some cases, doctors suggest a procedure (called radiofrequency trigeminal rhizotomy) that seeks to eliminate headaches by deadening the pain fibers in the face, sometimes leaving parts of the face permanently numb.

CONVENTIONAL TREATMENT OF TRAUMA HEADACHES

Medical schools provide so little in-depth training on the musculoskeletal system that problems originating in the head, neck, and spine are often misunderstood or dismissed, leaving conventional doctors no tools but drugs. Unfortunately, not only can drugs make trauma headaches worse by provoking rebound cycles, they can also mask symptoms that would otherwise signal a more serious injury.

Although aspirin and other antiinflammatory medication may increase the tendency to bleed, they are generally given during the first few weeks following trauma. If the headache does not go away with time, conventional doctors progress to more powerful drugs, prescribing those used for tension or migraines depending upon the nature of the symptoms. This includes the range of antiinflammatory drugs, antidepressants, muscle relaxants, calcium blockers, beta blockers, and more powerful migraine inhibitors. As with other headaches, treating a trauma headache through conventional methods often leads to a lifetime of taking pills.

CONVENTIONAL TREATMENT OF ALLERGY/SENSITIVITY HEADACHES

Today, even with the renewed interest in allergy/sensitivity reactions to foods, few conventional physicians are knowledgeable enough to make the connection between food and headaches—due in part to medical training that gives a cursory overview of the relationship between food and immunology. Although conventional allergists outnumber their alternative counterparts 4 to 1, conventional allergy doctors overlook essential connections. For example:

- They focus primarily on Type I reactions, and even these don't account for the new molds and allergy-provoking substances continually being discovered.
- They don't dose patients individually, meaning that everyone who comes in for a test or neutralization gets nearly the same treatment that may use phenol as a preservative. Furthermore, most desensitization doses are too strong, causing a red swelling at the injection site and later worsening of allergy symptoms.
- They don't look for candidiasis or vitamin/mineral deficiencies.
- They ignore the fatty acid connection and rarely discuss the broader implications of diet and its relationship to digestion and allergies.

Again, it is much easier to label someone "psychosomatic" or give them a handful of drugs than it is to figure out what is really wrong.

CONVENTIONAL TREATMENT OF SINUS HEADACHE

You have no doubt seen ads on TV touting the benefits of sinus headache remedies. Lulled by a soothing, authoritative voice explaining scientific-looking diagrams, you are led to believe that any head pain accompanied by a runny nose and watery eyes is called a sinus headache and can be relieved by decongestants.

These medications can make people feel better for a while, so people continue taking them, fooled into believing they are treating headaches caused by sinus problems. It is, however, the caffeine and aspirin, which help most types of headaches, rather than the decongestant, that provides the relief. Eventually, the medication that is taken to prevent a misdiagnosed headache creates a rebound headache as well. Furthermore, decongestants may raise your blood pressure and otherwise impair your circulation, adding further stress to areas that are already problems for headache sufferers. Since most "sinus" headaches are not caused by sinus problems, these side effects are unnecessary.

When people with real sinus headaches start trying OTC decongestants then discover these drugs do nothing for them, they may visit a conventional doctor. The conventional route is to take X rays to confirm the diagnosis and then to treat the underlying infection by prescribing a new regimen of drugs, such as antibiotics, cortisone-based nasal sprays, and stronger de-

Drugs Most Often Prescribed for Cluster Headaches

Prevention

- antidepressants
- antiinflammatories
- antihypertensives
- steroids
- calcium channel blockers
- allergy shots
- lithium carbonate
- methysergide (Sansert)
- verapamil (Calan, Isoptin, Verelan)
- ergotamine tartrate (Cafergot, Bellergal-S)
- divalproex sodium or valproic acid (Depakote)
- ergonovine (Ergotrate), intravenous dihydroergotamine (IV DHE)

To abort an attack

- ergotamine tartrate and ergot compounds (Ergostat, Medihaler ergotamine, DHE)
- intranasal lidocaine or cocaine
- sumatriptan (Imitrex)
- ketorolac injections (Toradol)

To prevent an atypical cluster headache

- indomethacin (Indocin), the antiinflammatory agent most often used for arthritis

congestants. In some cases, reconstructive surgery or surgical draining is prescribed.

CONVENTIONAL TREATMENT OF TMJ/DENTAL HEADACHES

In the world of conventional medicine, tense muscles and pain in the jaw are usually viewed as the result of a headache rather than the cause. By ignoring behavioral patterns, lifestyle, diet, tension, and the strain of repetitive motion, the crucial connection between headaches and TMJ and/or dental problems is missed entirely, and the patient is instead shuffled to neurologists, ear, nose, and throat specialists, and psychologists.

TMJ/dental headaches and the symptoms associated with TMJ syndrome (TMJS) are elusive and wide-reaching and many conventional doctors shrug them off as psychosomatic. In one clinic, in which 300 out of the 350 yearly TMJS patients are women, TMJS sufferers are described as "certain personality types, like the uptight housewife who may or may not have real problems." Oddly, the same clinic performs at least 6 or 7 surgeries each year, treating the rest with a combination of drugs, mouth appliances, dental equilibration (where they grind off tooth surfaces so the teeth meet properly for chewing), and/or mouth appliances.[5]

Incidentally, these same conventional dentists may actually cause or contribute to TMJS, dentistry problems, and the resulting headaches. For example, they may:

- Introduce structural problems, such as dental restorations that don't fit properly, making teeth too high or too low for the jaw.
- Continue to use mercury amalgam fillings, exposing patients to problems of toxic contamination because these fillings are cheaper than gold or silver.
- Make dental appliances the basis of their treatment, ignoring other musculoskeletal, metabolic, and emotional factors that may be involved.
- Inject steroids into the jaw, a technique that can destroy brain tissue and even cause brain abscesses.
- Rely too heavily on pharmaceutical drugs, which mask important symptoms, thus distorting the condition and contributing to impaired immune functioning and other chronic illnesses.

Furthermore, conventional dentists tend to prefer symptomatic control rather than complete removal of symptoms. For example, they may suggest that you limit your intake of food and live on a diet of soft, mushy food for months at a time, or they may tell you to cut up your food into little pieces and avoid foods which require heavy chewing. Some even tell their patients to refrain from opening their mouths except for the narrowest margin when talking, laughing, or yawning. Of course, when looked at from a whole-body perspective, such actions are ludicrous for long-term wellness. It's always better to find the cause and resolve it.

What Can You, the Headache Sufferer, Do?

Sadly, many conventional doctors are not telling their patients about alternatives. As with all new information, mastering alternative treatment requires learning, and many doctors do not take time to learn. This is why you are more likely to find a successful end to your headaches with the natural, holistic approaches of alternative medicine. Alternative practitioners are not taught that there is only one or two sets of tools to apply to headache relief, nor do they believe that headaches are something you have to learn to accept. You only have to learn how to live headache free.

Eventually, the medication that is taken to prevent a misdiagnosed headache creates a rebound headache as well. Furthermore, decongestants may raise your blood pressure and otherwise impair your circulation, adding further stress to areas that are already problems for headache sufferers. Since most "sinus" headaches are not caused by sinus problems, these side effects are unnecessary.

RECOMMENDED READING

Alternative Medicine: The Definitive Guide. Compiled by the Burton Goldberg Group. Tiburon, CA: Future Medicine Publishing, 1994.

"Arthritis Unyielding to Drugs." *Medical Advertising News*. May 1991, 26-27.

Blau, J.N. "Behaviour During a Cluster Headache." *The Lancet*: 342 (September 18, 1993) 723-725.

Braly, James, M.D., and Torbet, Laura. *Dr. Braly's Food Allergy and Nutrition Revolution*. New Canaan, CT: Keats Publishing, Inc., 1992.

Igram, Cass, M.D. *Who Needs Headaches?* Cedar Rapids, IA: Literary Visions Publishing, 1991.

Lipton, Richard B., M.D., Newman, Lawrence C., M.D., and MacLean, Helene, *Migraine, Beating the Odds: The Doctor's Guide to Reducing Your Risk*. Reading, MA: Addison-Wesley Publishing Company, 1992.

Lipton, Richard B., M.D. and Stewart, Walter F., MPH, Ph.D. "Migraine in the United States: A Review of Epidemiology and Health Care Use." *Neurology:* 43, Suppl. 3 (1993), S6-S10.

Nambudripad, Devi S., D.C., L.Ac., R.N., Ph.D. *Say Goodbye to Illness*. Buena Park, CA: Delta Publishing, 1993.

National Headache Foundation Fact Sheet. Chicago: National Headache Foundation, October 1994.

Rapoport, Alan M., M.D., and Sheftell, Fred D., M.D. *Headache Relief*. New York: Simon & Schuster, 1990.

Rapoport, Alan M., M.D., and Sheftell, Fred D., M.D. *Headache Relief for Women*. New York: Little, Brown and Company, 1995.

Robbins, Lawrence, M.D., and Lang, Susan. *Headache Help*. New York: Houghton Mifflin Company, 1995.

Sacks, Oliver, M.D. *Migraine: Understanding a Common Disorder*. Berkeley, CA: University of California Press, 1985.

Solomon, Seymour, M.D. and Fraccaro, Steven. *The Headache Book*. Mount Vernon, NY: Consumer Reports Books, 1991.

Stang, P.E. and Osterhaus, J.T. "Impact of Migraine in the United States: Data from the National Health Interview Survey." *Headache:* 33 (1993), 29-35.

Stromfeld, Jan and Weil, Anita. *Free Yourself from Headaches: The Natural Drug-Free Program for Prevention and Relief*. The Upledger Institute, Frog, Ltd., 1995.

Surgery For Headaches—The Modern Lobotomy

Although much more refined than early surgical attempts, recent surgical approaches to head pain still lean toward the archaic. One patient underwent surgery for cluster headaches that plagued the left side of his head. After doctors attempted to cut off the temporal artery blood flow to the left side of his head by tying off the left temporal artery, the headache merely switched to the right side.

In another case, doctors performed a procedure called a cervical sympathectomy that involved cutting off certain nerves to the neck. When that failed to relieve the pain, they opted for a craniotomy—the surgical opening and exploration of the skull. Unfortunately, this also failed to work, and the poor patient never got rid of his headaches.

The surgery currently heralded as the next cure for headaches, especially cluster, TMJ, and migraine headaches, is called radiofrequency trigeminal rhizotomy, or radiofrequency surgical cauterization. Attributing most head pain to injuries at the site where muscles, ligaments, and tendons attach to the jaw bone and skull, proponents of this procedure promise to revolutionize the standards for relief of head pain with a two-part treatment.

First, while the patient is suffering from a headache, the doctor locates the tender area associated with the injury site and then numbs it with novocaine. If the patient's headache goes away, the source of the injury has been successfully identified, and the second part of the procedure, surgical cauterization, can be performed. In some cases, the novacaine injection itself permanently relieves the pain and no further treatment is needed.

An outpatient procedure that takes between 45 minutes and 1½ hours, the actual cauterization is done by inserting a needle through a small hole at the base of the skull and advancing it to the identified location on the trigeminal nerve. At this point, radio frequency waves are sent through the needle and into the nerve, where they burn a small scar (2mm) in order to destroy the pain-carrying fibers of the trigeminal nerve.

Although it is claimed that temperature is controlled to the extent that pain fibers are "zapped," leaving touch fibers unharmed, this cauterization can leave portions of the face permanently numb. Proponents of the procedure claim to have a 75% success rate, although the "success" of the surgery can mean taking away feelings in the face.

The following requirements are used by the Pain Center in Philadelphia, Pennsylvania, in determining when to refer a patient for surgical cauterization:

1. The patient has undergone at least 2 months of conservative therapy without significant signs of pain reduction.

2. The patient's working diagnosis is "elusive."

3. The patient's pain is inconsistent, without a regularly identifiable pattern.

4. All the therapies tried by the patient provide only temporary pain relief.

5. The patient is developing a dependence on medication.

6. The patient is experiencing emotional difficulties that hinder pain management.

7. The patient is contemplating a major surgery but still feels it is too risky.

8. The patient has undergone a major surgery but is still experiencing pain.

Unlike conventional doctors,

alternative practitioners

are less interested in scientific

theories that seek to explain

the mechanism of headache

than in the underlying

mechanism that makes the

head hurt in the first place.

Most alternative practitioners

agree that headaches can be

caused by almost anything.

Chapter 3

What Causes Your Headache?

To understand why you have headaches, it's helpful to know something about the physiological systems involved in the creation of a headache, including the role of digestion, hormones, the nervous system, your structural condition, and your emotions. There are dozens of possible and interconnected causes for every headache.

B ecause of the millions who suffer from them, headaches are currently regarded as a disease. Unlike other diseases, they do not constitute an "illness," but are instead a symptom of bodily imbalance.

In the world of alternative medicine, you might say that chronic headaches are "welcomed" rather than ignored because they are seen as a plea for help, a plea which, if answered in time, can spare you even more debilitating problems in the future. Like them or not, headaches get your attention, and if you listen carefully, they can reveal systemic weaknesses, health problems, and harmful lifestyle factors that might otherwise go unnoticed.

To help you understand what may be happening in your body when you have a headache, this chapter explains the physiological systems usually involved in the creation of a headache. These include the digestive, endocrine (hormonal), and nervous systems. This information will help you hear what your headaches are telling you—the first step in restoring total body health. It is also necessary groundwork for an understanding of the numerous possible causes of headaches, the focus of the chapter.

INSIGHTS INTO
THE HUMAN ORGANISM

Although the human body is sophisticated in terms of structure and function, all living creatures share basic biological features. No matter what the plant or animal, it must take in energy nutrients (in our case by eating), process the energy (digestion), and excrete the leftovers. Unlike other animals and organisms who rely on only a few food sources for energy, humans are omnivorous.

For the most part, your body does fairly well with what it gets: storing part of its rations as fat for reserves, occasionally rejecting them through diarrhea or vomiting, and taking in the rest, using whatever nutrients it finds to fuel billions of tiny cell engines. To use an analogy, if you feed your high-performance, internal combustion engine low-grade fuel, it will need more fuel to keep its pace and, over time, will begin to sputter, slow down, and finally give out.

Your body needs unadulterated, unprocessed, high-performance "gasoline." Today's world, however, abounds with substances that interfere with the best of our eating intentions. Medications, recreational drugs, alcohol, rancid oils, hormones and antibiotics injected into beef and poultry, spoiled or improperly refrigerated foods, pesticides and other environmental pollutants, and processed, energy-deficient foods are some of the substances draining your overworked "engine."

First Line of Defense—Eating Smart

The primary rule of good health, therefore, is to make a conscious effort not to consume low-grade fuel. If you stuff your body with poor quality foods, you have breached the first level of defense against illness and are forcing your body to rely on internal mechanisms to keep you symptom free. Once you have swallowed a food, your body processes and refines it. Fortunately, protecting and ridding the body of foreign substances is a normal digestive function; it breaks down, however, when the overall system is weakened.

Second Line of Defense—PART 1: Digestion

Your body's fuel refinery is a 30-foot hollow tube called the alimentary canal (see Figure 3.1). Its job is to absorb nutrients while trying to prevent the absorption of abnormal substances. This is accomplished by the coordinated efforts of three processes: (1) the nerve-controlled muscles which push food through the tube; (2) gastric juice secretions by the stomach, pancreas, and liver which allow for the subsequent breakdown of the food; and (3) the absorption of fluids and nutrients by the small and large intestines.

Digestion starts the moment food enters your mouth. As you begin chewing, alkaline enzymes secreted from the salivary and parotid glands set to work on the food to break it down. You can test this by eating a piece of bread: the more you chew, the sweeter it becomes, which is the result of carbohydrates being reduced to sugars.

As you swallow, the food is moved rapidly through the esophagus and lands in the stomach reservoir, where it is stored, liquified and processed

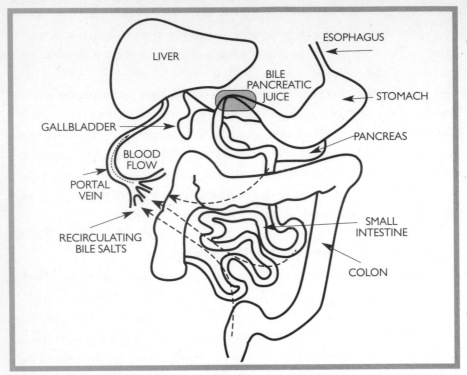

Figure 3.1—The digestive system (the alimentary canal).

by the acidic gastric juices, and eventually emptied into the small intestines. The stomach—under the careful control of the nervous system by way of the vagus nerve and stomach-secreted hormones gastrin and histamine— releases enzymes, namely pepsinogens and hydrochloric acid, to reduce proteins to medium-sized fragments called polypeptides. Once the food is thoroughly broken down into tiny pieces it passes into the small intestine, where it is greeted by an intense secretion of digestive enzymes from the pancreas and bile from the liver.

The intestinal wall of the small intestine is essentially the front-line of the digestive defense because it safeguards against the absorption of toxic molecules. This task is carried out by tiny hairlike fingers (the microvilli) that sift through all partially digested particles and selectively soak up proteins, carbohydrates, fats, vitamins, and minerals as they pass along. Over the ensuing 4 to 6 hours, most of these nutrients are assimilated as the food travels through the first 40 inches of the small intestine, leaving the remaining 20 feet to absorb the leftover water, electrolytes, bile salts, and vitamin B12.

A healthy intestinal wall, one coated primarily with "friend-ly" bacterial microorganisms, provides the protective lining that is necessary to keep damaging substances out of the body's circulation while letting helpful ones in. However, repeated exposure to harmful substances sends the white blood cells living alongside the microvilli into attack mode. Although intended to help, this effort irritates the intestinal lining even more because these white blood cells begin to explode shortly after absorbing the abnormal particles, thus releasing a round of inflammatory hormones, like histamine, with which the intestinal wall must also contend.

At this point, the front line of digestive defense has fallen, and abnormal proteins and toxic particles begin passing through the intestinal membrane into the bloodstream, causing what doctors call "leaky gut syndrome." Now reinforcements, namely the liver, must enter the process.

Second Line of Defense — PART 2: The Liver

The liver, called the "general of the army" by the Chinese, holds a strategic position between the intestinal tract and the general circulation (see Figure 3.1), because nothing enters the bloodstream without first passing through the liver. In a perfect world, this giant blood filter ensures that all useful elements of food undergo interchange, synthesis, oxidation, and storage and that all toxins are metabolized and processed into safe by-products that the kidneys can eliminate.

The liver handles 2 primary facets of detoxification, called "phase 1" and "phase 2" reactions. Phase 1, or oxidation reactions, makes toxins more manageable by directing enzymes to add oxygen to toxins or to subtract electrons from them (the oxidation process). Phase 2, or enzymatic reactions, converts these more manageable, intermediate toxins into water-soluble forms ready for excretion by combining them with amino acids, sulfur, and other compounds (such as sulfate, glycine, glutathione, acetate, glucuronic acid, and cysteine).

As long as these two phases work together, the liver can prevent tox-

Friendly bacteria, or probiotics, refer to beneficial microbes inhabiting the human gastrontestinal tract where they are essential for proper nutrient assimilation. The human body contains an estimated several thousand billion beneficial bacteria comprising over 400 species, all necessary for health. Among the more well known of these are *Lactobacillus acidophilus* and *Bifidobacterium bifidum.* Overly acidic bodily conditions, chronic constipation or diarrhea, dietary imbalances, overly processed foods, and the excessive use of antibiotics and hormonal drugs can interfere with probiotic function and even reduce their numbers, setting up conditions for illness.

A **free radical** is an unstable molecule, including 4 kinds of oxygen, that with an unpaired electron easily combines with other molecules to produce harmful effects. Molecules within body cells react with oxygen (oxidize), producing chemicals called free radicals, which then begin to break down cells. While these are a normal product of metabolism, uncontrolled free radical production plays a major role in the development of degenerative disease, including cancer, heart disease, and aging. Free radicals alter important molecules, such as proteins, enzymes, fats, even DNA. Sources of free radicals include carcinogens, pollution, smoking, alcohol, viruses, infections, allergies, stress, even food and exercise.

ins from damaging the rest of the body. But when the body is repeatedly exposed to pollutants thorough detoxification is no longer guaranteed. Problems such as leaky gut, bacterial overgrowth (dysbiosis), alcoholism, and drug abuse, increase the load on the liver, causing phase 1 reactions to produce intermediate toxins called free radicals faster than phase 2 reactions can process them. This allows free radicals to escape into the bloodstream, and in time, the body goes into "oxidative stress," eventually overloading the system and causing chronic illnesses such as autoimmune diseases, chronic fatigue syndrome, premenstrual syndrome, irritable bowel syndrome, and headaches.

The liver also produces bile, another essential tool of digestive defense. Bile, which is formed by liver cells, performs two important functions. First, it helps to eliminate unfilterable break-down products from the blood (called bilirubin) before they are passed to the kidneys. Second, bile neutralizes stomach acid and eases the intestinal absorption of fats and fat-soluble vitamins. Bile is carried by small ducts into larger canals and finally into the gallbladder. If the liver becomes overloaded with toxins or too much stored glucose, these canals become compressed, which decreases bile flow and impairs digestion.

An overloaded, swollen liver also reduces the flow of blood from the pelvic and abdominal regions. The vein that controls this blood exchange, the portal vein, is 1 of only 2 veins in the body that lacks a valve. So just as it is impossible to blow up a balloon that is already full of air, the back-up pressure of this vein causes the blood to back up and pool in the pelvic areas. This blood pooling may putrefy in time, like stagnant ponds of water, setting the stage for a host of problems including hemorrhoids, bowel irritation, uterine/ovarian or prostate irritation, neck pain and stiffness, and, in severe cases, heart palpitations—all of which can be related to headache.

Once the liver becomes unable to dilute toxins and keep the blood clear, the second line of defense has been exhausted. Now, the body has no choice but to call on its third and final line of defense, the endocrine system.

Third Line of Defense—The Endocrine System

By the time the endocrine glands are forced into high gear, toxins have penetrated the digestive system and have begun irritating organ tissues and other parts of the body. Now the fight is on to see how quickly the en-

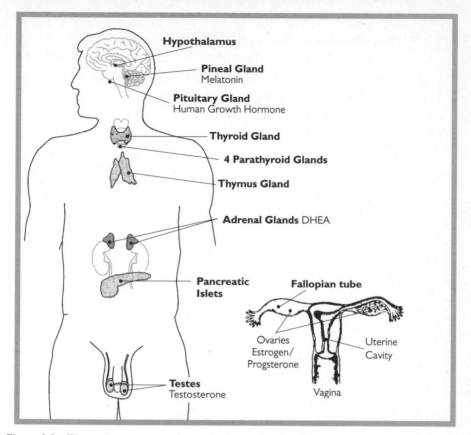

Figure 3.2—The endrocrine system and the key endocrine glands.

docrine system can detoxify and recover before the body gets too weak and damaged.

The endocrine glands include the pituitary, hypothalamus, thyroid, parathyroid, adrenals, pancreas, gonads or sex glands, and other glandular tissue located in the intestines, kidneys, lungs, heart, and blood vessels (see Figure 3.2). Under direct orders from the higher centers of the brain and the nervous system, these glands secrete hormones directly into the bloodstream in an attempt to maintain balance and harmony within the body.

The word "hormone" comes from a Greek work meaning "to set in action," so it should be of no surprise that hormones are powerful electrochemical messengers, even when released in minute amounts. Among other functions, they guide and regulate most of the body's subtle biochemistry, normalize substances that maintain homeostasis, integrate bodily functions, and determine your size, stature, fat and hair distribution, the sound of your voice, your emotions, and the occurrence of head pain. Scientists have identified hundreds of hormones, and new ones are being discovered.

The endocrine glands release their hormones via a complex interplay between higher brain glands (the hypothalamus and the pituitary) and their end-organ glands (the thymus, thyroid, parathyroid, adrenals, pancreas, and the gonads). This process is a sensitive messenger service with individual hormone carriers specially programmed to communicate only with specific hormone receptors.

Endocrine glands, including the testicles, ovaries, pancreas, adrenals, thyroid, parathyroid, and thymus, are central to the regulation and normalization of all the body's complex, interconnected systems, from metabolism and heat production to spermatogenesis and uterine preparations for pregnancy.

Hormones are the chemical messengers of the endocrine system that impose order through an intricate communication system among the body's estimated 50 trillion cells. Examples include the "male" sex hormone, testosterone, the "female" sex hormones estrogen and progesterone, melatonin (pineal), growth hormone (pituitary), and DHEA (adrenal).

THE HYPOTHALAMUS AND PITUITARY

The hypothalamus and the pituitary are the major centers of control, as they govern the release of the body's hormones and set in motion the entire biochemical chain of events. The hypothalamus, which is a section of brain tissue rather than a true gland, exerts direct control over the pituitary by releasing hormones that turn it on. The pituitary then sends special messages, relayed by hormones called gonadotropins, to all the other endocrine glands, telling them what hormones to make and when to make or stop making them.

The pituitary, a pea-sized gland which hangs below the brain and directly behind the eyeballs, is divided into 3 parts, the anterior lobe, the intermediate lobe, and the posterior lobe.

The anterior lobe, or front portion, produces and secretes 6 hormones: (1) prolactin (PRL), which initiates the production of breast milk; (2) adrenocorticotrophin (ACTH), which stimulates the adrenal cortex hormones; (3) thyrotrophin (TSH), which stimulates the production of thyroid hormones (T3 and T4) and regulates the breakdown of fat; (4) somatotrophin (GH), a growth hormone which stimulates all body tissues and fat cells to control the growth of long bones and prevent aging; (5) follicle-stimulating hormone (FSH), which stimulates the maturation of ovarian follicles; and (6) luteinizing hormone (LH), which stimulates the production of estrogen and progesterone in females and testosterone in males.

The intermediate lobe, or middle portion of the pituitary, has cells called melanocytes that produce a hormone, melatonin, which controls skin pigmentation and the tanning process; it also seems to function as an environmental inspector for the blood, as it can detect toxins in the blood and initiate defensive responses to them.

The posterior lobe, or back portion, is an extension of the brain. Rich in specialized nerve cells, it produces 2 hormones: (1) oxytocin, which determines breast milk ejection and smooth muscle contractions in the uterus; and (2) vasopressin, which helps the kidneys and arteries control water reabsorption, controls smooth muscle contraction in the arteries, and aids in circulation.

THE THYMUS

This tiny gland, located in the center of the chest, directly behind the breastbone, is no doubt the most mysterious gland in the endocrine system. All that is known about it is that it is comprised mainly of lymphoid tissue and is a key producer of immune cells, so much so that the Chinese believe it is the place where the body fends off disease and the degenerative effects of aging.

THE THYROID

The thyroid gland is your body's thermostat, the chief pacesetter of your metabolism. Taking the form of 2 separate lobes joined by a tiny islet and situated at the base of the neck just below the voice box, the thyroid is a butterfly-shaped structure that determines the rate your body uses energy. Like the adrenals, it helps run and regulate nearly every organ and system in the body—such as cell reproduction and growth, damaged tissue repair, circulation, heart rate, nerve tissue sensitivity, hair, skin, and nail growth, sex hormone regulation, and both cholesterol and sugar metabolism in the liver.

THE PARATHYROID

The parathyroid glands are small, saucer-shaped knobs that sit on the back and side of each thyroid lobe. These tiny glands secrete a hormone called parahormone that allows more calcium to enter the bloodstream. If the parathyroid malfunctions, calcium levels may fall too low, which can lead to problems in muscles and nerves.

The Metabolic Price of Stress

Whenever you are overexerting or experiencing severe stress, extra proteins are secreted by your glands so that your body can convert them into sugar and use them for instant energy. If this intensity is prolonged for 24 hours or more, your thymus can shrink up to 50% of its normal size, thus severely curtailing the function of a central portion of your immune system.

This stress eventually forces your body to use whatever metabolic resources it has available, which means it takes nutrients and energy from other parts of your body. Chronic bouts of stress also stimulate the overproduction of natural tranquilizers and painkillers, which throws the endocrine system into further imbalance by preventing hormones from sending the proper messages to the brain.

THE PANCREAS

The pancreas, a long, skinny organ that lies atop most of the upper abdomen, performs a hormonal function in addition to a digestive one. As the producer of insulin, this vital gland is responsible for balancing blood sugar (glucose) levels in the body. A sufficient supply of glucose or "blood fuel" to the cells in your body is essential; without this, the cells starve.

THE ADRENALS

With the hypothalamus and the pituitary as the centers of control and the thyroid the master of metabolism, the adrenal glands are the body's energy reserve tank. These 2 triangular-shaped glands perched above the kidneys are responsible for overall health and vitality, since they supervise all hormone functioning. Each of these glands is divided into 2 parts, an inner section called the medulla and an outer layer called the cortex.

The adrenal medulla produces a set of hormones called catecholamines—which include the stress hormone adrenaline (also known as epinephrine), nonadrenaline (or norepinephrine), and dopamine, all of which have been shown to vary during the vascular changes that occur during some headaches. All of these hormones play an important role in the way you deal with danger, intense emotion, low blood sugar, extreme temperatures, oxygen shortages, low blood pressure, and stress.

The adrenal cortex manufactures steroidal hormones. These are divided into 3 categories: the mineralocorticoids, which help control the body's fluid balance by regulating the kidney's reabsorption of sodium and potassium; the glucocorticoids, which affect the metabolism of carbohydrates, proteins, sugar, and fats, maintain blood pressure, and enable the body to respond to physical stress; and the sex hormones, androgens and estrogens, which are responsible for male and female characteristics.

The chemistry of life depends on the adrenals' ability to control the internal fire: If there is too little oxidation, the internal fire will not burn, yet too much will cause burnout. Therefore, the adrenals must constantly monitor glandular activity, nerve energy, physical energy, and oxidation throughout the entire body. In addition, the adrenals support immunity, determine red and white blood cell counts, aid in blood clotting, and control voluntary muscles, bodily strength, the heart muscles used in circulation, blood pressure, uterine tone, and involuntary muscle contractions in tubular organs (peristalsis).

THE GONADS

The sex glands, the ovary and testes, are the most difficult glands to regulate. Sex hormones, such as estrogen, progesterone, DHEA, and testosterone, have a delicate function and require constant fluctuations in the glandular balance to stay in tune. For proper coordination between the sex glands and the sex hormones, the pituitary must be doing its job exactly as it should. If this fails to occur, the biofeedback mechanism by which the ovaries or testes self-regulate, the hypothalamus, and the pituitary are knocked out of kilter, and the entire system is thrown off balance.

The Nervous System: The Central Control Center

Your body is controlled by two interrelated systems, the endocrine system and the nervous system. The nervous system is comprised of the brain, the spinal cord, the nerve fibers, plus all the chemical messengers that ensure communication throughout the body.

The billions of cells that make up your brain are housed in the cerebellum and in 2 large lobes called the left hemisphere and right hemisphere. These hemispheres float in a pool of cerebrospinal fluid and are further safeguarded against outside danger by the skull (cranium) and by the meninges, protective coverings that rest just above the wrinkled layer of brain, called the cerebral cortex, nearest the skull. The brain itself sits on a pillar of tissue known as the brain stem. The oldest part of the brain, the brain stem controls the basic functions of the human body, including consciousness, heart beat, blood pressure, and breathing.

The brain stem descends through an opening in the skull and connects

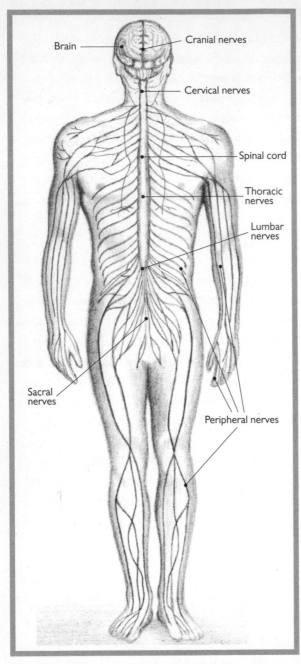

Figure 3.3—The nervous system.

Brain

Cranial nerves

Cervical nerves

Spinal cord

Thoracic nerves

Lumbar nerves

Sacral nerves

Peripheral nerves

to the bundle of nerves known as the spinal cord. Besides being protected by the vertebrae, the spinal cord, like the brain, is covered by meninges and surrounded by cerebrospinal fluid. Two types of nerves are believed to pass between the spinal cord and the brain: large bundled nerve fibers carrying the sense of touch and the smaller bundles carrying sensations of pain.

The brain and the nerves speak to each other, nerve cell by nerve cell, via a distinctive group of chemicals called neurotransmitters. Neurotransmitters are the doorway to a functioning nervous system; they facilitate sensory perception, muscle contraction, emotions, thoughts, and the awareness of pain. Most neurotransmitters carry out multiple tasks throughout the brain and nervous system. They are like words whose meanings change to suit the needs of their users.

Two crucial neurotransmitters involved in the perception of pain are serotonin, which also regulates the diameter of blood vessels, digestion, smooth muscle tissue operations, mood and stress reactions, and relaxation, as well as other functions; and endorphins, which lessen pain and affect message transmission between nerves. Other key neurotransmitters include dopamine, norepinephrine, and acetylcholine, all of which play some role in the way you perceive your head pain.

Your Ache Is More Than a Pain in the Head

Now that you have a basic understanding of how your body works and the vital role the digestive, endocrine, and nervous systems play in your overall health, we can turn to how and why these systems malfunction and how headaches are produced as a result. With this information, you can choose the treatments that will be most effective for your particular type of headache and address the underlying imbalances as well.

QUICK DEFINITION

A **neurotransmitter** is a brain chemical with the specific function of enabling communications to happen between brain cells. Chief among the 100 identified to date are acetylcholine, gamma-aminobutyric acid (GABA), serotonin (5-hydroxytryptamine), dopamine, and norepinephrine. GABA works to stop nerve signals to keep brain firings from getting out of control; serotonin does the same and helps produce sleep, regulate pain, and influence mood, although too much serotonin can produce depression.

Just as there are many different types of headaches and headache patterns, there are a variety of theories as to why people get headaches, most of them unproven. While conventional medicine ignores the bigger picture by focusing on isolated theories that tend to separate the head from the body, alternative medicine looks for systemic, underlying disturbances.

Most headaches are caused by an interplay of conditions in which many factors interact with and exacerbate one another. For example, a woman's migraine may be caused by a hormonal imbalance resulting from a yeast overgrowth (candidiasis), which in turn contributes to food allergies; her mother may have suffered from migraines as well. Someone else's headaches could be linked to a back problem that has compromised digestion. The order of causes listed in these examples could be reversed with the same result. Causation theories can be likened in many ways to the chicken and the egg: we don't know which came first, but there they both are.

These days nearly everything is blamed for nonorganic headaches: serotonin, genes, hormones, overcooked food, the environment, blood clotting, chemicals, nitrates, tyramine, cigarettes, fumes, circulation, allergies, preservatives, weather changes, blocked energy, sleep disruptions, repressed emotions, spinal misalignments, alcohol, stress, vitamin, mineral and/or enzyme deficiencies or overloads, teeth grinding, pollution, hypertension, aftershave, perfume, constipation, trauma, life's challenges, muscle spasms,

> **When both parents suffer from migraines, there is a 75% chance that their child will also suffer from them; if one parent has migraines, the child has a 50% chance of getting migraines, and if a distant relative is prone to migraines, there is a 20% chance of getting them.**

fatigue, bright lights, noise, fever, anemia, and crowds. The list could fill pages.

Conventional medicine tends to rely on a much smaller list of causes, such as serotonin levels, genetic influences, and hormonal imbalances. Alternative medicine, considers the spectrum of possible causes and triggers. As understanding the prevailing causation theories can help get your search for healing underway, each of the major theories is discussed in this chapter and then briefly reviewed in discussions of different headache types in Chapters 5 through 15.

It is our intent to draw your attention to the likelihood that it is not one but *many* factors at once that are causing your head pain. With this insight, you will be able to identify the major causes of your headache and choose the alternative treatments most suited to your particular condition.

Conventional Medical Theories of What Triggers Headaches

The groundwork for the Western understanding of nonorganic headaches came during the late nineteenth and early twentieth centuries, but it was not until the 1930s and '40s that researchers discovered that head pain resides in the tissues between the skull and brain, rather than in the brain itself. Between 1950 and 1970, the biochemical mechanisms of the headache became the focus of scientific attention.

By the 1980s, due in large part to advances in technology, researchers began to integrate the biochemical, vascular, and neurological concepts that serve as the bases of current headache theories. These theories and scientific advances do little more, however, than describe the mechanism of headaches, without explaining the causes that make the head hurt.

VASCULAR IRREGULARITIES

Vascular theories (based on changes in blood vessels) hold that headaches, especially migraines, begin in the cortex, the wrinkled layer of brain nearest to the skull. In response to certain triggers, the cortex sets off an electrical ripple, causing a wave of nerve cells to fire and then go quiet. This creates a reaction in the brain's major nerve, the trigeminal nerve, releasing chemicals that inflame or constrict the nearby blood vessels, the main mechanism of head pain.

Scientists have advanced our modern understanding of headaches with research into the relationship between vascular change—the constriction and dilation of blood vessels—and headaches. While vascular changes are an important aspect of a headache attack, they are not the whole story nor the root cause.

SEROTONIN FLUCTUATIONS

Since research into vascular irregularities uncovered the existence of the brain chemical serotonin, researchers have been attempting to prove that head pain signals start deep in the brain, in areas deficient of this important pain-regulating hormone. Founded on the premise that low serotonin levels make people more vulnerable to headaches, the serotonin receptor hypothesis first swept through the medical community about 35 years ago, causing excitement within the field of headache research. Reduced levels of serotonin are believed to make you more susceptible to most other triggers as well and lower your threshold for pain.

Unfortunately, serotonin theories do not extend to the reasons why a person might have low levels of serotonin, except to suggest that it may be an inherited tendency. Instead, serotonin theories have become a stepping stone for pharmaceutical companies looking to develop headache medications. Since the release of the serotonin-enhancing headache drug Sumatriptan, low serotonin has been widely touted as a cause of headaches.

However, other research suggests that increased serotonin levels are linked to the onset of headaches. In addition, little attention is paid to the relationship between serotonin and diet or serotonin and stress, even though serotonin levels have been shown to increase in response to allergic reactions to food and the biochemical reactions to stress.

GENETIC PREDISPOSITION

There is a growing agreement among conventional headache researchers that heredity plays a significant role in one's susceptibility to headaches, especially in the case of serotonin-related migraines. According to data re-

Physiological and Psychological Factors That Can Affect Serotonin Levels

- hormonal shifts
- climatic changes
- caffeine withdrawal
- alcohol
- sensitivities and allergic responses to certain foods, beverages, and additives
- sensitivities and allergic reactions to one's environment, such as air pollutants, perfumes, cleansers, and bright or flashing lights
- changes in routine, such as sleeping more or less than usual, going to bed or rising at a different time, and excessive hunger caused by skipped meals,
- stress, which includes negative stress, such as overwork, as well as stress over a positive event such as a birthday party or wedding

leased by the National Headache Foundation, when both parents suffer from migraines, there is a 75% chance that their child will also suffer from them; if one parent has migraines, the child has a 50% chance of getting migraines, and if a distant relative is prone to migraines, there is a 20% chance of getting them.[1] In addition, researchers in Paris have discovered a link between a locus on chromosome 19 and familial hemiplegic migraine.[2] Other studies suggest that those who suffer from dietary-related migraines have a genetically determined inability to produce adequate amounts of the monoamine oxidase group of enzymes that normally helps to detoxify food.

A family history of migraine or other headaches does not necessarily mean that you will get headaches. It only suggests that you may be more *susceptible* to the various factors that trigger headache attacks. The way you respond to these triggering factors depends more on your actions than your genes, which means a genetic predisposition does not doom you to headaches for the rest of your life.

Even when genetically predisposed, among some individuals, headaches occur only after constant exposure to a triggering factor, such as sitting next to a heavily perfumed coworker. Triggering factors also may vary from one family member to another. For example, a mother and daughter might both suffer from migraines, but the mother's attacks may come on after she eats dairy products, while the daughter can eat dairy with no problem but gets headaches whenever she sits in front of the computer screen for more than an hour.

PSYCHOSOMATIC SYNDROME

When all the testing and guessing arrives at nothing and your headache fits no existing set of criteria, you may be told that your headache is all in your head (or emotions). Conventional medicine has always preferred to blame conditions on psychosomatic illness than to surrender to ignorance. In fact, during the last century, an estimated 50 to 80% of headache patients have come home from their doctors with a diagnosis of hypochondriasis, neurosis, and/or psychosomatic illnesses. Shifting the onus to the sufferer obscures the fact that the doctor may not know what to do next.[3]

Alternative Theories of What Triggers Headaches

Unlike conventional doctors, alternative practitioners are less interested in theories that seek to explain the mechanism of headache than in the underlying factors that make the head hurt in the first place. Most alternative practitioners agree that headaches can be caused by almost anything. All of the alternative causes and theories listed below involve the way your body adapts and draws upon its resources to keep itself functioning and free of disease. Although we have loosely divided these causes into 3 categories—metabolic/bioenergetic/biochemical imbalances, structural imbalances, and emotional/psychological factors—keep in mind that all are related and imbalances in one system cause imbalances in others.

A family history of migraine or other headaches does not necessarily mean that you will get headaches. It only suggests that you may be more **susceptible** *to the various factors that trigger headache attacks. The way you respond to these triggering factors depends more on your actions than your genes.*

METABOLIC/BIOENERGETIC/ BIOCHEMICAL IMBALANCES

Metabolic imbalances arise from illness or dysfunctions that interfere with the normal workings of your digestive, endocrine, respiratory, or central nervous systems. Because the number of conditions that can contribute to such imbalances are too numerous to list in their entirety, we focus in this chapter on those that are known to be a factor in causing or triggering the mechanism of headaches.

BLOOD CLOTTING

One cause of headaches, particularly migraines, relates to blood clotting,

General Adaptation Syndrome (GAS) Model

Developed by the physiologist Hans Selye, M.D., the General Adaptation Syndrome (GAS) model offers an explanation as to how and why headaches and other symptoms of illness develop. The model breaks the body's process of illness into 3 stages: the alarm stage, the resistance stage, and the exhaustion stage.

THE ALARM STAGE: The alarm stage is the initial acute reaction to any irritant or stress factor. For example, say you jogged 3 miles in one workout session, although you usually don't jog. By the next day, you will undoubtedly be stiff and sore, maybe even inflamed. If you are healthy, these symptoms will pass quickly, and your muscle will return to normal as the self-regulating, balancing mechanisms of your body do their work.

However, if you continue to overwork your injured muscle, or if your body is also struggling with other stressors, such as inadequate nutrition or a grouchy boss, your muscles must adapt to accommodate the repetitive stress, and, eventually, the whole body is forced to adjust and compensate in order to keep functioning.

THE RESISTANCE STAGE: Once this whole body compensation occurs, your body enters the resistance stage, the period when your body is trying to repair itself. Your muscles, while not as sore, will become increasingly less elastic and more fibrous, placing stress on the points where they are anchored to the bone. This stage often passes without major symptoms; it can last for as many years as your body's resources and reserves will allow, a time factor which is determined by your overall health and constitution.

If you are constantly overwhelmed by deadlines, eat junk food, or load up on painkillers, your ability to adapt and resist illness will be much lower than that of someone who eats a balanced diet, sleeps soundly every night, and has plenty of ways to reduce stress. This explains why people respond differently even when faced with identical health challenges.

THE EXHAUSTION STAGE: Exhaustion occurs at the end of the resistance stage, when the adaptive mechanisms stop working. This is the stage of chronic disease. No longer able to cope with repetitive and/or multiple stress factors, your body begins to constrict the pathways that bring blood to the brain, which, among other things, leads to headaches.

also known as platelet aggregation or clustering. When the body becomes either physically or emotionally stressed, it reacts by tightening. According to research conducted by James R. Privitera, M.D., of Covina, California, the blood, like the mind and the body, also tightens in response to stress, creating little knots in the bloodstream.

These knots are called blood clots, and come about because excess prostaglandin (allergy-related) and adrenaline (stress-related) hormones cause platelets to stick together. As it thickens blood, this clotting constricts the arteries and reduces the blood supply to the brain, thereby causing the blood vessels to dilate, leading to headaches. Furthermore, platelets, which

A Quick Look at Headache Causes

TYPE OF DYSFUNCTION	LIST OF POSSIBLE CAUSES
Conventional medicine views headaches as the dysfunction	vascular irregularity, serotonin fluctuation, genetic predisposition, hormonal imbalance, psychosomatic syndrome
Alternative medicine views headaches as a symptom of an imbalance in one or more of the following areas:	
Metabolic/Bioenergetic/ Biochemical	blood clotting, *Candida*, chemical and environmental sensitivity, constipation and other digestive disturbances, chronic fatigue syndrome, food allergies and sensitivities, Hashimoto's autoimmune thyroiditis (HAIT), hypoglycemia, leaky gut syndrome, loud noises, nutritional deficiencies, sleeping patterns, strong light, weather and altitude changes
Structural	dental problems, musculoskeletal misalignment, poor posture
Emotional/ Psychological	stress, anxiety, depression, repressed emotions

contain nearly all of the blood's serotonin, tend to release their contents during clotting, triggering further serotonin abnormalities and adding yet another reason for the head to throb.

In his practice, Dr. Privitera looks for the evidence of blood clotting in headache sufferers by examining live blood cells under a darkfield microscope (a special microscopic viewing device that allows researchers to examine blood cells while they are still alive). In one study, 95% of the headache sufferers Dr. Privitera tested had significant clotting. Clinical evidence has shown that patients with clotting tend to respond well to alternative medicines such as chelation, nutritional, and herbal therapies, especially the use of essential fatty acids (EPA, primrose oil), vitamin C, vitamin E, vitamin B6, magnesium, garlic oil, *Ginkgo biloba*, and ginger.

Conventional physicians rarely test for clotting when they examine their patients, despite the fact that blood clots suppress the immune system and contribute to heart attacks, strokes, arthritis, and other degenerative diseases.[4]

QUICK DEFINITION

A **platelet** (also called thrombocyte) is a disc-shaped or irregularly-shaped cell produced in bone cell marrow, then released into the blood where it is essential for clotting. In a healthy individual, an estimated 200,000-300,000 platelets are found in 1 cubic millimeter (mm) of blood.

93

CANDIDIASIS

Candidiasis or systemic yeast overgrowth can cause headaches. In healthy individuals, the form of yeast known as *Candida albicans* is present in the body and confined to the skin, vagina, and lower bowel. This yeast is usually harmless and kept in check by "friendly" (digestion-enhancing) bacteria called *Bifidobacteria* and *Acidophilus*.

However, if the intestinal environment is altered, by immune-suppressing factors such as processed or chemicalized foods, steroids, the birth control pill, mercury (especially from dental amalgams), heavy metals, and the overreliance on antibiotics and other drugs, the healthy *Candida* begins to grow out of control, becoming an aggressive fungus that wipes out the entire ecosystem of the gut. Eventually, the *Candida* begins to proliferate in other body tissues, and in some cases, begins to outnumber every other cell in the body.

QUICK DEFINITION

Darkfield microscopy is a way of studying living whole blood cells under a specially adapted microscope that projects the dynamic image onto a video screen. The skilled physician can detect early signs of illness in the form of known disease-producing microorganisms. Also the amount of time the blood cell stays viable and alive indicates the overall health of the individual.

Commonly overlooked by conventional physicians, despite being on the rise, *Candida* can cause many disorders, ranging from headaches, allergies, vaginitis, and thrush (a whitish fungus in the mouth or vagina) to genitourinary tract, eye, liver, heart, and central nervous system diseases. *Candida* also causes many of the symptoms associated with headaches, including chronic fatigue, depression, digestive problems, lightheadedness, severe PMS, memory loss, and mood swings.

Other symptoms include rectal itching, coughing, wheezing, earaches, recurrent fungal infections, and reduced sex drive. All of these symptoms tend to worsen in moldy places (such as a basement), damp climates, and after consuming high-sugar foods. As is the case in other serious conditions, attempts to alleviate your headache without addressing the underlying condition of *Candida* will prove futile, possibly harmful, in the long term.

CHEMICAL AND ENVIRONMENTAL SENSITIVITIES

Like the world around you, you are 100% chemicals, which is why it is wrong to assume that all chemicals are toxic or harmful or that all things natural are safe. When we speak of environmental factors that trigger headaches, we are referring to any of the tens of thousands of chemicals which are part of today's environment.

As a citizen of the industrialized world, you have little option but to live in regular contact with inhalants (substances that pass through your nose, throat, and bronchial tubes) and contaminants (substances that produce a reaction through direct skin contact). Would you believe that over 2 billion pounds of pesticides were dumped on U.S. crop lands, lawns, fields, and forests in 1989 alone?[5] And that is just one category of pollutant. Whether it be pollen, mold, phenolic substances, hydrocarbons, formaldehyde, radioactive fallout, or carbon monoxide, many substances in the air are creating a crisis in our bodies in the form of allergies, digestive problems, cancer, and headaches, to name a few.

Why have we become so allergic? Probably because we have been polluting our environment for only 80 years or so, meaning both we and the planet are still struggling to adapt to such sudden environmental changes. Like overly porous organisms, people with headaches have a tendency to take in more pollutants than others, making them even more susceptible.

Contactants: Molds, Dust, and Pollens—Although seemingly innocent, petting the cat, talking a springtime walk in the woods, or using a new body lotion can bring on a serious headache for the sensitive or allergic person. Environmental inhalants and contactants such as molds, dust, pollens, mites, grasses, spores, flowers, poison oak and ivy, and animal dander, as well as manufactured substances (synthetic or otherwise) such as cosmetics, hair dyes, detergents, nail polish, woolens and other fabrics, rubbing alcohol, and powders, are proven sources of allergies, and can trigger headaches and a host of other symptoms.

Headaches associated with natural environmental substances tend to be linked to hay fever-like symptoms, including runny nose, itchy eyes, congested head, and skin reactions such as hives and rashes. Headaches related to manufactured substances tend to be associated with more subtle reactions that are harder to correlate with head pain, such as asthma, joint pains, constipation, stomach aches, mood swings, and body swelling.

Smoking—Cigarette smoke inhalation, including exposure to secondhand smoke, is another evoker of headaches. First the nicotine in cigarettes constricts the blood vessels, then the carbon monoxide overly expands them. The rapid back-and-forth motion of constriction and expansion creates an ideal condition for triggering headache attacks, particularly among those who are already prone to vascular irregularities (such as those with high serotonin levels or inherited tendencies to headaches). Smoking

Healthy Alternatives for Your Household

One way to eliminate the effects of chemical sensitivity is to replace toxic products with ingredients that are cheaper and more earth-friendly.

- Soaps and dishwashing liquids made with vegetable or coconut oil biodegrade quickly and are much less toxic than other products.
- BORAX disinfects and deodorizes.
- WHITE VINEGAR inhibits mold growth, cuts grease, dissolves mineral accumulation, and freshens the air.
- BAKING SODA acts as a mild abrasive and deodorizer.
- SALT contains bacteria-inhibiting properties and works as an excellent nonscratching abrasive cleanser.
- LEMON JUICE breaks down mineral and tarnish buildup, cuts grease, and freshens the air.

Here are some commonly used products and suggestions on how to replace them with more natural ingredients:

- AMMONIA-BASED CLEANERS: apply undiluted white vinegar in a spray bottle and use as you would any cleaner.
- BLEACH LAUNDRY ADDITIVES: whiten laundry by adding ½ cup white vinegar, baking soda, or borax to each load.
- DRAIN CLEANERS: pour ½ cup baking soda into the drain and immediately follow with ½ cup of vinegar; let sit for 15 minutes, then pour boiling water down the drain; follow with plumbing snake or plunger.
- HOUSE AND GARDEN INSECTICIDES: mix 2 tbsp. oil-based dishwashing liquid to 2 cups of water; pour into a spray bottle and spray on leaves when needed.
- RUG AND UPHOLSTERY CLEANERS: add baking soda paste directly to stains, let it dry, then vacuum up.[6]

also disrupts the nutritional balance of the body, which in turn can affect digestion and lead to headaches.

One study published in the journal *Headache* looked at the link between headache occurrence and cigarette smoking, and showed that smokers had more intense headaches, higher levels of depression, and more associated symptoms. Furthermore, those who smoked cigarettes with higher nicotine content reported more headaches than those who smoked milder cigarettes.[7]

Carbon Monoxide and Other Chemical Pollutants—Whether you realize it or not, there is a good chance that you will encounter as many as 10,000 different manufactured chemicals in your lifetime. Products you may take for granted—such as cleaners, paint thinners, perfumes, shampoos, aftershaves, cosmetics, propellants—contain scores of chemicals, flavorings, colorings, preservatives, pesticides, deodorizers, and antibacterials, none of which are good for your health.

You also breathe smoggy air, car exhaust, secondhand cigarette smoke, and inhale fumes caused by formaldehyde, plastics, ethanols, phenols, alcohols, natural gas, hydrocarbons, benzene, bromine, carbon tetrachloride, chlorine (or its gas), dioxin, fluoride, industrial cleaners, kerosene, paints, PCBs, and solvents.

Every one of these substances can cause pain and allergy symptoms among sensitive people. Problems caused by these chemicals include neurological disorders, tissue and nerve irritation, respiratory and circulation difficulties, and inflammation. Chemical fumes such as formaldehyde, car exhaust, diesel, and secondhand cigarette smoke, are especially devastating to the headache-prone because they gain direct access to the brain through the nose.

Exposure to environmental pollutants is compounded by modern construction methods. Having learned how to tighten up buildings and conserve energy, we give our lungs less air from outside. While in the past the air in a home or office building would replenish itself every 2 to 4 hours, now, thanks to vinyl siding, insulation, vapor barriers, paneling, and caulking, this process can take up to 2 days.

The by-products of heaters, air conditioning systems, gas appliances, kerosene heaters, and wood stoves, plus chemicals in materials used to build and furnish the house, such as particleboard reinforcements, carpeting, laminates, glues, mattresses, and books, circulate inside, making a hypersensitive person even more sensitized.

Carbon monoxide (CO) is a highly toxic, potentially lethal gas. Because it is missing an oxygen molecule (unlike its cousin, carbon dioxide, CO_2), when it enters the bloodstream it looks for oxygen with which to bond. Red blood cells are its favorite mate because they contain hemoglobin, a natural carrier of oxygen.

Thus, every time a molecule of CO is inhaled, a red blood cell is neutralized, depleting the body's store of oxygen. According to research, the CO bond is irreversible once it is made, which is why carbon monoxide is so deadly. One breath of contaminated air from your gas stove, furnace, or car, and millions of your red blood cells are unable to absorb oxygen as they pass by the lungs on their route through your body. Since the brain is your number-one oxygen consumer, your head suffers first.

Heavy Metals—As the industrial revolution swept our world, industrial chimneys began venting heavy toxic metals into the environment. Defined as the combustion product of fossil fuels, heavy metals are some of the oldest toxins known to man, but human exposure to heavy metals—a primary symptom of which is headaches—has increased several hundred percent in the last century. Along with it the incidence of liver and kidney damage, high

Is Your Brain Polluted?

Many people experience the subtle symptoms of toxic overload without realizing it. To see if you are one of the growing legion of the chemically sensitive, ask yourself the following questions:

- Does your nose pick up smells that others don't notice?
- Do you sometimes feel spacey or foggy when you walk inside stores or buildings?
- Do strong smells from, for instance, perfumes, cleansers, even restaurants, make you feel queasy or bothered in some way?
- Do you feel clear and happy one day and muddled and terrible the next for no apparent reason?
- Does alcohol make you sick?
- Do some drugs and medications, even vitamins, make you feel worse?
- Does driving in city traffic cut down your ability to react quickly and clearly (especially compared to rural driving)?
- Does your mind wander for no apparent reason, more than usual?

If you answered yes to 3 or more of these questions, you may be suffering from chemical poisoning.

blood pressure, anemia, and cancer have also increased.

The most commonly recognized instigators of heavy metal toxicity include cadmium (emitted by cars, industrial exhaust, and cigarettes); aluminum (emitted with industrial exhaust and by cookware, food cans, antacids, and deodorant); arsenic (in pesticides and cigarette smoke); lead (paint, hair dyes, auto and industrial exhaust); nickel (paint, exhaust); sulfuric acid (pesticides); asbestos (installation, exhaust); and mercury (car and industrial exhaust, dental amalgams, and tooth powders).

Copper, lead, and mercury toxicity causes headache most often, because all three metals have a chemical component that is drawn to nerve tissues. This means exposure to them usually disrupts the way nerve impulses are received by the brain and nervous system. All heavy metals, however, leach and displace minerals, such as iron, zinc, and magnesium, and disrupt normal enzymatic functioning—all of which can cause headaches as a by-product. Because these metals accumulate over long periods, many people do not realize that they are being poisoned until the body quits fighting.

Dental mercury fillings are a common source of heavy metal sensitivity. Metals used in fillings, such as mercury, tin, copper, silver, and sometimes zinc, can corrode or disassociate into metallic ions (charged reactions) that migrate into other parts of the body and disrupt nerve reactions in the central nervous system.

This is especially problematic in dental fillings made of two different types of metal. The result is like having a nickel cadmium battery in the mouth: electrons flow between the metals and mix with saliva, creating an unhealthy electromagnetic field. Called electrogalvanism, this charge can disturb the body, producing chemical toxins, influencing the release of hormones and neurotransmitters, like estrogen and serotonin, and throw the system out of balance. Occasionally, so much metal accumulates in the mouth, that it acts like an antenna, picking up and amplifying the "sea" of electromagnetic pollution that has now become a fact of life.

The television program "60 Minutes" first brought national attention to the plight of those affected by mercury poisoning by airing a segment on the dangers of mercury amalgams. DAMS (Dental Amalgam Mercury Syndrome), Inc., has furthered this awareness with a campaign requiring dentists to have patients' signed consent before having their teeth filled with mercury amalgam.

In Germany, the federal department of health (BGA) has issued advisories against mercury amalgam use; the first in 1987, warning against its use in pregnant women, a second in 1994, warning against its use in all women of childbearing age. In addition, Germany's largest manufacturer of dental amalgam announced in 1993 that it would no longer manufacture it.[8]

David Kennedy, D.D.S., of San Diego, California, former president of DAMS, Inc., reports that in Sweden, the government picks up 50% of the cost of removing mercury amalgams and 100% if a physician finds evidence of mercury toxicity in the person's body. Dr. Kennedy also reports that 10% of U.S. dentists refuse to use mercury amalgams. As he puts it, "If 10% of U.S. pilots refused to fly 747s, would you feel safe flying on one?"

> *"I don't feel comfortable using a substance designated by the Environmental Protection Agency to be a waste disposal hazard. I can't throw it in the trash, bury it in the ground, or put it in a landfill, but they say it's okay to put it in people's mouths. That doesn't make sense."*
>
> —Richard D. Fischer, D.D.S.

For more information about mercury amalgams and their toxicity, contact: DAMS, Inc., 6025 Osuna Blvd. NE, Suite B, Albuquerque, NM 87109; tel: 505-888-0111; fax: 505-888-4554.

Despite the fact that the EPA considers mercury amalgam a hazardous material and warns dentists not to touch it when placing it in patients' mouths, the American Dental Association and the Food and Drug Administration refuse to ban its use, denying that mercury can actually leach from the mouth into tissues, brain, and nervous system.

Silver Mercury Amalgams

Silver mercury fillings (which are 50% mercury and 25% silver) are by far the most dangerous type of dental amalgam. Declared a poison in the 1500s and more toxic than arsenic, mercury is still being inserted into countless mouths by conventional dentists. These fillings are particularly insidious in that mercury is a cumulative poison, the effects of which are not always seen right away but develop over time. According to DAMS (Dental Amalgam Mercury Syndrome), Inc., a nonprofit organization dedicated to ending dental amalgam syndrome, many people suffer from mysterious bouts of headaches, infertility, muscle spasms, depression, menstrual disorders, allergies, fatigue, candidiasis, and other chronic illnesses without any inkling that they may be caused by mercury amalgam poisoning.

> **However, 2-3 bowel movements per day is a measure of true health.**

CONSTIPATION AND OTHER DIGESTIVE DISTURBANCES

If you take a trip to your local drugstore, you can't help noticing based on the number of drugs for it, that constipation is a major problem in the United States. Constipation, or the inability to move one's bowels and eliminate wastes, is a potentially serious condition that contributes to a variety of health problems, headaches among them. Constipation is particularly harmful because it allows toxins to stay in the body and be reabsorbed back into the system until, in chronic cases, it undermines the entire bodily system, affecting digestion and the absorption of nutrients.

Conventional and alternative physicians disagree as to what constitutes regular bowel movements. Alternative doctors say at least 1 (preferably 2-3) bowel movement a day is necessary, while conventional doctors generally do not, but both agree that waste elimination may be related to body type and biochemical make-up and that poor diet, stress, and the misuse of laxatives are the most common contributors to sluggish bowels. Alternative doctors believe that side effects from prescription and nonprescription drugs, as well as pollution and other chemical and environmental toxins, are also to blame.

One theory on the relationship of constipation to headaches is built on the concept of referred pain. The intestinal reflexes and the head are intimately connected by the vagus nerve, which provides a direct line to the stomach, intestines, liver, pancreas and colon. Although not a pain nerve per se, the vagus is capable of carrying messages when irritated. A plugged-up bowel can lead to headaches by increasing pressure on the colonic nerves,

The **vagus nerve** is the 10th and largest cranial nerve (out of 12) that coordinates swallowing, speech, breathing, and heart rate. It runs down both sides of the body, passing through the ear, jaw, larynx, heart muscles, stomach, intestines, and the mucous membranes of the lungs, kidneys, and digestive tract.

which then send pain along the most direct route, which is straight for the head. This is why constipation headaches usually go away after a healthy bowel movement. However, 2-3 bowel movements per day is a measure of true health.

Diet-related headaches may not be due to constipation, but instead reflect some kind of internal disturbance in the digestive tract. A bowl of popcorn or a piece of cold pizza late at night, for instance, can interfere with your digestion, making it work overtime; too much of one type of food may throw your liver into overdrive, making it swell and strain the gallbladder.

In Chinese medicine, the head is seen as a compact representation of the digestive system, so head pain always points to a corresponding location in the digestive system. The forehead, for instance, is related to the intestines, the side of head to the liver, galbladder, and circulation, and the back of head to the liver and kidneys. Because of how the head is structured, overconsumption of expansive foods, such as sugar, alcohol, caffeine, and fruit juices, is believed to result in pain in the forehead or over the eyes, while a dull, constant pain in the back or side of the head is believed to result from the overconsumption of contractive foods, such as meat, eggs, and salt.

In Germany, the use of mercury amalgam fillings has been restricted since 1992; for example, use in children or pregnant or nursing women is not allowed. In Sweden, the government picks up 50% of the cost of removing mercury amalgams and 100% if a physician finds evidence of mercury toxicity in the person's body.

CHRONIC FATIGUE SYNDROME

Once known as Epstein-Barr virus, chronic fatigue syndrome (CFS) is a long-term, whole-body immune dysfunction, the origin of which medicine has yet to identify, although some alternative practitioners believe it is caused by rampant allergies. Its most recognizable symptom is abnormal fatigue lasting 6 months or longer. Other symptoms include headache, low-grade fever, sore throat, muscle and joint pain, confusion, mood swings, and depression. According to ACHE statistics, about 50% of CFS sufferers get headaches. Headaches associated with CFS are some of the most difficult to treat.

Signs of a Malfunctioning Digestive System

GENERAL AREA OF SYMPTOM	SYMPTOM	POSSIBLE ROOT CAUSE
SKIN	yellow skin	liver dysfunction
	brownish spots on face and hands	liver dysfunction
	red nose	liver dysfunction
	cracked, calloused feet	pancreatic dysfunction
EYES	flashing lights	liver dysfunction
	vision problems	liver dysfunction
NOSE	nasal congestion and discharge	colon (large intestinal) dysfunction
MOUTH	dry and sticky, sometimes with tongue coated yellowish white	liver dysfunction
	cracked lips	stomach or small intestine irritation; impaired ability to metabolize salt
	bitter, metallic taste	liver dysfunction
	canker sores	gastric and/or small intestine irritation (due to food sensitivity, internal toxicity, stress or nutrient/zinc, B12, folic acid, or iron deficiency)
THROAT	throat spasm	sensitivity or allergic reaction to food
	sore throat/tonsillitis	lymphatic blockage (due to impaired liver function)
	esophagus spasm	ingestion of allergic food
STOMACH	heartburn and/or belching	stomach dysfunction; food reaction or insufficient production and secretion of liver bile

FOOD ALLERGIES AND SENSITIVITIES

People today live on foods that used to be regarded as luxuries and seldom consider how unnatural the year-round availability of non-native, nonseasonal foods is. Americans consume 3,000 synthetic substances and over 10,000 other chemicals not intended for consumption. Artificial flavorings,

STOMACH (cont.)

	nausea	liver dysfunction
	belching, bloating, overfull sensation, indigestion, and/or nausea	stomach not secreting enough stomach acid
	bloating and gas formation	pancreatic dysfunction (pancreas not secreting enough pancreatic juice into small intestine, causing malabsorption of fats and fat-soluble vitamins or of carbohydrates and proteins)
LARGE INTESTINE	intestinal pain and spasms, flatulence	insufficient bile production in the liver, which may lead to intestinal bacterial over-growth, parasites, intestinal inflammation, colitis
	rectal itching	worms, intestinal dysfermentation, or low production of stomach acid
	hemorrhoids	swollen liver backing up into the colon and pelvic areas
	constipation	liver dysfunction
	appendicitis	insufficient or poor quality bile
NON-SPECIFIC SYMPTOMS	dizziness, blind spells, mental fatigue, and/or depression, poor appetite, difficulty sleeping, and/or unusual or disproportionate anger	possible symptoms of liver/digestive dysfunction
	difficulty climbing stairs (esp. after meals), excessive mucus, bacterial overgrowth, leaky gut syndrome, nutritional deficiencies	possible symptoms of dysfunction in small intestine

colorings, flavor enhancers, preservatives, extenders, blenders, bleachers, anticaking and antifoaming agents, antifungal drugs, antibacterial agents, and hormones are just some of the substances commonly found in many foods today.

The body, unprepared and overwhelmed, is being forced to deal with

Circulating Immune Complex

When a food is not digested properly, it becomes an allergen. The immune system attacks this allergen and creates what is called a circulating immune complex, or CIC. These CICs, rather than the actual food particles, pass through the intestinal walls and get into the bloodstream. Once in the body, CICs situate themselves in the various organs and systems. Many kinds of illnesses can result from CICs because they tend to gravitate toward weak areas in the body.

these dietary changes as best it can—and it isn't having an easy time of it. People are becoming immunized against the foods they eat for nourishment, forcing their bodies into a chain of reactions that causes many conditions, including headaches. Many of these reactions are not allergic reactions per se, but events that are triggered when indigestible substances escape undigested into the bloodstream.

One of the reasons allergic reactions produce throbbing headaches is because they increase serotonin levels, and thereby put your blood vessels on the painful roller coaster of constriction and expansion. Further, many allergy-producing foods produce a double effect because they contain substances which behave like serotonin when they hit the bloodstream. Remember, there is no such thing as a predefined allergic response. Everybody reacts differently. The pages that follow list some of the substances most frequently implicated in triggering headaches.

Dairy—Forget what the billboards tell you, milk isn't Nature's perfect food. In fact, cow's milk and other dairy products have been linked to a host of abdominal and intestinal problems, food allergies foremost among them. Besides creating excess secretions of phlegm and mucus, milk contains more than 60 different proteins, 31 of which have been linked to allergic reactions in humans and 150 also implicated as a cause of diabetes.

Studies report that milk reactions hit the brain and nervous system the hardest, which explains why dairy-allergy headaches are accompanied by depression, fatigue, and irritability. Further, your body cannot fully assimilate the calcium in milk. Try leafy green vegetables, grains, nuts, and supplements instead.

Salt—Found in nearly everything we eat, from canned soup to potato chips to cookies, salt is another common headache trigger. The overconsumption of or sensitivity to salt can make blood vessels hypersensitive to the other foods you eat, especially when consumed at the end of the day on an empty stomach. Evidence suggests that when coming in contact with too much salt, the stomach lining sets off a reflex action that increases the absorption of salt, and since salt is present in every cell of the body, this overload can trigger an allergic reaction.

In one study, John B. Brainard, M.D., of St. Paul, Minnesota, legitimized the link between salt and migraine by asking a dozen lifetime migrainers to record their incidence of attack for a year, 6 months before giving up salt and 6 months afterwards. Avoidance of salt markedly reduced the incidence of migraine in 10 out of 12 people.[9]

One way to tell if you are having a problem with salt is to look for excess water retention and puffiness around the chin, face, and eyes. If retaining fluid, you may want to limit your sodium intake to under 3 grams a day, which is about 1 to 1 ½ teaspoons of salt. Season with herbs and other salt-free combinations, and when you do use salt, use sea salt because it offers more nutrients.

Sugar—Those sugar blues: the headachy crash you feel shortly after the euphoric energy rush of cookies or pastry, often hold the key to a headache sufferer's woes. Particularly linked to hypoglycemia (low blood sugar) and its related symptoms, sugar is a powerful drug, whose effects, like coffee, often go unnoticed and unhindered.

Although sensitivities to sugar, especially to refined cane and beet sugar and high fructose corn syrup, have been documented since the 1920s, many people are still unaware of the negative effects of this substance—particularly now that sugar has gone from being an occasional luxury to a daily staple.

Amines—The Greek philosopher Plinius was not far off when he identified dates as the source of headaches. Today we know dates contain proteins that have an amine (an organic compound containing nitrogen) in their structure. Recognized for their headache-causing properties, amines trick the body into releasing vasoconstricting substances like serotonin, setting blood vessels up for later dilation and the headache throb.

Tyramine, phenylethylamine, histamine, and octopamine are the amines most often implicated in food allergy/sensitivity headaches. Tyramine is the most common of these amines, found in alcoholic beverages, especially red wine; in dairy products such as sour cream, yogurt, and aged and hard cheeses; canned or pickled meats and fish such as herring; in fruits such as figs, dates, and raisins; fermented products such as sauerkraut, soy sauce, and pickles; and yeast products, particularly fresh baked breads and cakes. Phenylethylamine is found in chocolate and cheese; histamine in fish, cheese, and beer; and octopamine in citrus fruits such as oranges, grapefruit, and lemons.

Alcohol—The most obvious alcohol-related headache is the kind that comes from overindulgence, but even a sip can bring one. Although most doctors agree that amines and genetic sensitivities are involved in the headache-triggering process, they disagree as to the exact reason why some people get a headache from alcohol while others do not.

Causes have been linked to the fermentation process, impurities, sulfates, and other preservatives in alcohol, and the by-products produced by the body as it attempts to metabolize it. Some experts say alcohol itself is a vasodilator; others contend that, because of its high sugar content, alcohol causes blood sugar instability, and thus leads to hypoglycemic swings and headaches. Alcohol-induced headaches are related to all these factors.

In a study, 9 out of 11 migraine sufferers came down with a full-blown headache within 3 hours of ingesting red wine, while those who drank vodka remained headache free. Men who consume more than 2 cups of coffee a day (240 mg caffeine), have a 30% greater chance of having headaches than men who drink 2 cups or less. Avoidance of salt for 6 months markedly reduced the incidence of migraine in 10 out of 12 people who were lifetime migrainers.

While all alcoholic drinks can lead to headache, some beverages are more threatening than others. Vodka ranks low on the trigger list, red wine high, with port, champagne, and bourbon right behind it. Red wine is potent because it contains twice or three times the amount of tyramine, and is also rich in secondary components which include tyramine-containing grape substances, aldehydes from the distilling process, and sulfites. (For more on sulfites, see Preservatives below.)

In a study conducted at the Princess Margaret Migraine Clinic in London, England, 9 out of 11 migraine sufferers came down with a full-blown headache within 3 hours of ingesting red wine; those who drank vodka remained headache free.

Caffeine—Caffeine is the headache paradox. A powerful vasoconstrictor with painkilling properties likened to acetaminophen, caffeine can stop a headache dead in its tracks. This is why it is used in many pharmaceutical headache remedies. This

What Else Is in That Bottle?

Generally, when you order a drink from a bar, you don't think twice about what's in it—unless, of course, you have allergy/sensitivity headaches. Here are the main ingredients in some of the most popular alcoholic beverages—all of which can be allergenic.

Wine	grapes, yeast, other fruits (such as pineapple, plum, or apple), sugar, sulfites, and clarifiers (such as egg whites, fish glue)
Beer	malted barley, corn, wheat, rice, hops, yeast, gelatin, salt, ascorbic acid, dextrin, and clarifiers
Brandy and distilled wines	grapes (sometimes flavored with other fruits, such as plums and apricots), sugar, caramel, yeast, flavorings, clarifiers
Whisky	corn, barley, and other cereal grains, yeast, malt enzymes, caramel, flavorings
Gin	wheat (English gin), corn (American gin), malt wine (Dutch gin), sugar, juniper berries
Rum	sugar cane, molasses, yeast, flavorings
Sake	fermented rice, sugar
Tequila	maguey (Mexican plant), sugar
Liqueurs	usually made from whisky, brandy, or a neutral spirit, fruit products, and flavorings, herbs, and spices. [10]

cure only works, however, when used *sparingly* because when consumed in excess caffeine causes a rebound expansion of blood vessels as it wears off, triggering the rebound headache.

Like alcohol, tolerance to caffeine varies tremendously, some individuals being extremely sensitive and others drinking a pot a day without obvious symptoms. On the other hand,

See Chapter 14, Rebound Headaches, for more information about the side effects of caffeine.

studies have shown that men who consume more than 2 cups of coffee a day (240 mg caffeine) have a 30% greater chance of having headaches than men who drink 2 cups or less; females in the same category increase their risk by 20%.

In addition, caffeine has been shown to increase blood pressure, raise cholesterol levels, heighten PMS, cause food sensitivities/allergies, worsen stress and anxiety, bring on insomnia, and interfere with healthy digestion—essentially not a substance you want in large amounts in your body.

Preservatives—Preservatives are both a boon and a bane. Our foods last longer, taste better, and are more convenient—yet is this worth the price we pay in health? While the FDA still claims preservatives are safe, many researchers and dietitians are claiming otherwise. For the most part, the long-term effects remain largely unknown, although theories abound regarding the immuno-supressing effects of preservatives and the cancers they cause. One effect that has been documented is the link of preservatives to headaches.

In a University of Florida study, the incidence of migraine doubled for the majority of participants when they took aspartame, and their headaches lasted longer and were marked by increased signs of shakiness and diminished vision.

The best known of these headaches may be the "hot dog" headache, or the headache caused by nitrates or sodium nitrates, the chemicals added to meats to preserve their freshness. Nitrate-containing meats are easy to recognize; they are the ones with an artificial red color, such as hot dogs, bologna, salami, bacon, and sausage. Hot dog headaches get their name from two University of California neurologists, Neil H. Raskin, M.D., and William R. Henderson, M.D. They studied a 58-year-old, hot dog-loving headache sufferer and discovered that he got headaches 8 out of 13 times when he drank a nitrate solution (similar to that found in hot dogs) and zero times when he drank the placebo.

Sulfites, the preservatives used in wines, dried fruits, fast food french fries, and salad bars, are another known headache trigger. Salt derivatives of sulfuric acid, sulfites are used to maintain freshness and flavor or at least to extend the appearance of such. With sulfites, vegetables can sit uncovered in air all day and look like they came fresh from the refrigerator.

Other preservatives, such as tartrazine, food colorings such as FD&C Yellow No. 5, which is frequently added to margarine and orange soda, and benzoic acid are also known headache triggers.

Excitotoxins: Aspartame and MSG— A number of chemicals scientifically proven to damage the nervous system have been nicknamed excitotoxins. When neurons are exposed to these substances, they begin firing impulses, until they die several hours later, as if they had been excited to death.

Some excitotoxins are industrially-made and used only for research purposes, but others are actually amino acid compounds borrowed from Nature, including aspartate, the primary ingredient in aspartame, and glutamate, the active ingredient of monosodium glutamate (MSG).

Developed as flavor-enhancers, aspartame and MSG were specifically designed to stimulate taste buds and thereby fool one into thinking that such otherwise flavorless products as processed soups and fat-free cookies taste good. Many dysfunctions of the nervous system, strokes, hypoglycemia, seizures, and headaches are linked to the build-up of excitotoxins in the brain. These substances are believed to affect sensitive people by directly dilating the blood vessels, which also causes headaches.

The chemical sweetener aspartame known popularly by the brand names NutraSweet and Equal, manages to reconcile two irreconcilable things: sweetness and slimness. As a result, aspartame is in diet colas, wine coolers, chewing gum, cookies, cakes, ice cream, candy, and even multivitamins and laxatives.

Unfortunately, like other excitotoxins, this food ranks among the leading triggers of headaches. In a University of Florida study, the incidence of migraine *doubled* for the majority of participants when they took aspartame, and their headaches lasted longer and were marked by increased signs of shakiness and diminished vision. Headaches are the most common side effect cited by those who consume aspartame-containing products.

MSG has a similar, though longer history. For thousands of years, Chinese and Japanese cooks have been using a special seaweed ingredient to highlight the flavor of their dishes. It was not until the 1950s that manufacturers were able to isolate this special property and turn it into a multi-million-dollar product: MSG.

Initially, this seemingly safe and natural ingredient was embraced as the answer to mediocre cooks everywhere. Cookbooks listed MSG as an important spice, and major companies added it to everything from soup to nuts to baby food. After all, it was only an amino acid. But by the late 1960s, research began to tell another story. Rats and other animals fed MSG in doses equal to what was being added to baby food were developing brain lesions and suffering from toxic complications impossible to ignore.

However, as is currently happening with NutraSweet, the FDA did

QUICK DEFINITION

Aspartame is an artificial sweetener made from 2 amino acids, aspartic acid and phenylalanine. It was discovered in 1965 and approved by the FDA in 1981. Today it is found in over 5,000 food products and generates annual sales of $1 billion. Aspartame is 200 times sweeter than cane sugar. The phenylalanine content is a health hazard to those suffering from phenylketonuria (1 out of 15,000 people), which is sensitivity to excess phenylalanine. Critics claim that this substance can elevate blood pressure, produce insomnia, render one more sensitive to pain, increase the desire for food, contribute to eye degeneration and possibly mental illnesses, and perhaps worsen Parkinson's.

ignore them, until one of the researchers, John W. Olney, M.D., a neuroscientist at the Department of Psychiatry at Washington University in St. Louis, testified before a Congressional committee and demanded that MSG at least be removed from baby food. Yet not only is MSG still sold in obvious form, it is also added to seasonings and meat tenderizers, canned meats, packaged soups, and potato chips, often camouflaged under names such as natural flavorings, kombu extract, hydrolyzed vegetable protein (HVP), hydrolyzed plant protein (HPP), autolyzed yeast, calcium caseinate, and sodium caseinate.

Chemical Residue in Produce—Some people are known as "multiple fruit sensitives" because they are allergic to nearly all fruits, regardless of family. This condition, however, suggests a sensitivity not to the food itself but to chemical and/or pesticide residue. This correlation was first proposed in the 1950s by Theron Randolph, M.D., of Chicago, who pioneered the concept of chemical allergy when one of his fruit-sensitive patients didn't react when he ate an unsprayed apple.

Strawberries laced with arsenic and spinach ridden with DDT are two examples of the poisons encountered in supermarket. Unless you buy organically-grown products, nearly every fruit and vegetable for sale today has traces of fungicides, herbicides, fumigants, or pesticides. Over 400 of these substances are currently licensed in the United States for use on produce.

Bananas are ripened with ethylene gas, coffee is roasted over a gas flame, and cucumbers, peppers, and apples are often coated with paraffin wax derived from petroleum. Pesticides reside in the crevices of leafy vegetables such as lettuce, spinach, cabbage, broccoli, cauliflower, and Brussels sprouts—and also penetrate the whole body of fruits—such as grapes, cherries, pears, apples, and berries.

One of the best ways to determine whether your headache is being triggered by chemical and pesticide processes is to eat organically grown produce to see if it brings on the same effects.

OTHER FACTORS INVOLVED IN FOOD ALLERGY/SENSITIVITY

Too Much Food—Research suggests that the average diet contains between 500 and 1,000 calories *more* than the body needs. The sheer weight of all this food passing through the digestive system never gives it a chance

Foods Most Likely to Trigger Headaches

To avoid headaches, avoid these commonly known trigger foods or eat them in small amounts or only on special occasions:

MEAT AND FISH: hard sausage, bologna, salami, pepperoni, hot dogs, ham, spam, pork, organ meats, pickled herring, sardines, cod, herring, game meats

DAIRY PRODUCTS: cow's milk, ripened cheese (blue, brick, Brie, Camembert, cheddar, Colby, Emmenthaler, Gouda, Gruyere, mozzarella, most Stilton, Parmesan, provolone, Romano, Roquefort), cottage cheese, sour cream, yogurt, eggs

FRUITS AND VEGETABLES: all overripe fruits, avocados, bananas, citrus fruits (oranges, grapefruit, lemons, limes, kumquats, tangerines), pineapples, red plums, raspberries, figs, dates, raisins, onions, asparagus, eggplant, tomatoes, pea pods, beans (broad, fava, lima, navy), nuts, peanut butter, seeds (pumpkin, sunflower, sesame), anything pickled, fermented or marinated (sauerkraut, pickles)

BREADS AND GRAINS: corn (very common trigger), popcorn, wheat, wheat germ, rye, yeast baked goods (especially when hot and fresh from the oven), sourdough bread, donuts, yeast extracts

DRINKS AND BEVERAGES: anything with caffeine (black or green tea, cola, coffee), alcoholic beverages (especially beer, red wine, and champagne)

OTHER FOODS: anything containing preservatives (especially benzoic acid and tartrazine), MSG, aspartame, high amounts of refined sugar, salt, vinegar (except white vinegar), chutneys, chocolate (except white chocolate which contains cocoa butter, not chocolate liquor, a source of tyramine), commercial gravies, and meat extracts.

to rest and repair.

Food Addiction—Eating the same food compulsively can cause allergies over time. There is also a link between binge eating and food addictions.

Limited Diet—A national survey discovered that, despite our opportunity to select from among hundreds of foods year-round, Americans chose to consume almost 80% of their calories from only 11 foods. Like a food addiction, eating the same foods, especially for those who are sensitive or prone to leaky gut syndrome, causes the body to rebel and to react to them as allergens.

One out of 4 public water systems in America has violated federal standards for tap water, and according to the Environmental Protection Agency, the tap water supplied to 30 million people in America contains potentially hazardous levels of lead.

Drugs—Many drugs that start out seemingly harmless can become dangerous over time as the body slowly builds up an immunity, until it eventually no longer accepts the drug. Cortisone, Indocin, aspirin, Tylenol, Cardiazem, Coumadin, and Hydralazine have been implicated in drug-induced headaches.

Antibiotics also bring on headaches because they are usually taken when the body is in a weakened state, which can alter intestinal bacteria, providing an ample breeding ground for *Candida*. Antibiotics also are so often overprescribed, that they end up presenting further difficulties to an already distressed immune system.

Other drugs that can trigger headaches include caffeine-containing drugs (responsible for rebound headaches); birth control pills (which not only bring on headaches but also aggravate existing conditions like PMS); hormone replacement drugs (which upset blood sugar equilibrium); blood pressure medications (which reduce blood flow to the brain); and diuretics (which reduce blood flow and suppress the assimilation of minerals such as potassium, calcium, and magnesium).

Water—Unless you live on a remote mountaintop, chances are you do not draw your water from a fresh running spring. Instead, you turn on your faucet and hope that city officials were not lying when they said the water was safe to drink. Unfortunately, even with a filter, tap water is not the safest to drink, especially if you are headache-prone.

One out of 4 public water systems in America has violated federal standards for tap water,[11] and according to the Environmental Protection Agency, the tap water supplied to 30 million people in America contains potentially hazardous levels of lead.[12] With every cup of tap water you swallow, you increase your risk of being exposed to heavy metal and/or chemical toxins, especially if you fill your glass during the times the water districts add any of the 700 chemicals available for use in water supply.

Studies are being published monthly about the contaminants that are finding their way into the water system, either through evaporation and reabsorption, runoff, or by seeping into underground wells. These contaminants include chlorine, fluoride, chemical solvents, disease-causing bacteria, pesticides, the ammonia by-products of livestock urine, cesspool spills, and acid rain.

If you suspect your water is chemically contaminated, call your local water agency and ask to have it tested. Even if it passes and you are advised that your water is safe to drink, try boiling it for 8 minutes or more before drinking, or, better yet, use filtered spring water for a week or two and see if you notice a difference.

In a survey conducted in a small western Illinois community whose drinking water had been contaminated by the industrial chemical solvent trichloroethylene (TCE), 54% of the 106 respondents reported severe or frequent headaches. Some people are so sensitive that they only have to shower in the water to be affected by it.

HASHIMOTO'S AUTOIMMUNE THYROIDITIS (HAIT)

An autoimmune illness in which the body produces antibodies that attack the thyroid as if it were a foreign enemy, HAIT is a mysterious illness that often goes unnoticed. Studies have shown that 3% of the population is afflicted with HAIT, the majority being women who have a family member with the disorder.[15]

Besides headaches, the symptoms of HAIT include deep fatigue, allergy/sensitivity problems, digestive disorders, depression, anxiety, sleep disturbances, memory loss, heart palpitations, muscle and joint pains, PMS, weight gain, and swallowing difficulties. Like other disorders, HAIT is often so intertwined with these conditions that it is difficult to distinguish one from the other. But studies show that it may be closely linked to systemic candidiasis and/or chronic fatigue syndrome.

One reason HAIT is not recognized by conventional medical doctors is that the routine tests used to detect thyroid disease do not note blood level changes in antithyroid antibodies. If your symptoms lead you to suspect HAIT, make sure to have your physician perform a specialized blood test, called an antithyroid antibody panel. Keep in mind that, despite what conventional doctors may suggest, even minor elevations in antithyroid an-

See this chapter, Third Line of Defense—The Endocrine System, on page 80 for more information on hormones.

Hormones are the chemical messengers of the endocrine system that impose order through an integrated communication system among the body's estimated 50 trillion cells. Examples include the "male" sex hormone, testosterone, the "female" sex hormones estrogen and progesterone, melatonin (pineal), growth hormone (pituitary), and DHEA (adrenal).

tibodies may be significant and warrant attention.

In addition to natural thyroid medication, HAIT responds well to a well-balanced diet of whole, nutrient-rich foods and nutritional supplements, especially essential fatty acids (GLA, EPA), vitamin C, and vitamin B complex. HAIT may be hereditary, so all family members who are exhibiting possible symptoms should be checked for the disorder.

HORMONAL IMBALANCES

As they function in a way similar to neurotransmitters, hormones play a major role in headache pain. Although the sex hormones estrogen and progesterone are most commonly associated with headaches, other hormones have been linked to headaches. These include pituitary hormones (such as FSH, LH, ACTH, TSH, vasopressin, and prolactin); thyroidal hormones (triiodothyronine and thyroxine); pancreatic hormones (insulin, glucagon, and somatostatin, which are responsible for balancing blood sugar); and adrenal hormones (stress hormones adrenaline and noradrenaline and steroids such as cortisol and cortisone).

In fact, all the major endocrine glands initiate hormonal events that, if prolonged, throw hormone levels out of balance, which can result in head pain. For example, when you become emotionally stressed or your blood sugar drops, hormonal and endocrine changes are triggered throughout the body. This in turn stimulates excess neurotransmitters, such as serotonin. These reactions are designed to handle a temporary threat only. If you keep the body in this state, the immune system will eventually be compromised, increasing your susceptibility to illness.

A faulty diet, particularly one resulting in rapid drops in blood sugar, also interferes with hormone functioning and the immune system, paving the way for headaches. Foods high in sugar and refined carbohydrates are poison to the adrenal glands and can create a big problem considering that the adrenal gland is responsible for the synthesis of 45 hormones.

Histamine is another hormone that makes headaches worse. It is produced in the tissues rather than in a gland, and has been linked to vascular-type headaches, especially migraines, clusters, and other headaches related to allergies or sensitivities, because it is one of the prostaglandins that helps to control the inflammatory responses of the body.

Signs of Malfunctioning Endocrine Glands

GLAND	SIGNS AND SYMPTOMS
ADRENAL GLANDS	low energy and fatigue
	dizziness and lightheadedness upon rising
	tired feet and weak ankles
	dehydration
	water retention and swollen extremities
	excessive body hair (women)
	enlarged breasts (men)
	excess fatigue and depression during menopause
	postpartum depression
	hypoglycemia
	indigestion (caused by malabsorption of nutrients)
	joint inflammation and arthritis
	allergies
	increased skin pigmentation and brown spots
THYROID GLAND	headaches worse in morning, better in the afternoon
	low ambition and motivation
	restlessness and irritability
	easy or excessive weight gain
	low body temperature
	high cholesterol and triglicerides
	hypersensitivity to changes in weather
	light sensitivity
	dry, chapped, and flaky skin
	cracked heels
	brittle finger nails
	hair loss
	constipation
	shortwindedness
	sluggish energy and fatigue
	proneness to crying under pressure, depression
	easy distraction due to low concentration levels
	memory loss
	mood swings
THYROID	hypoglycemia
	puffy upper eyelids and swollen skin
	loss of outer edge of eyebrows
	carpal tunnel syndrome
	iron deficiency anemia
SEX GLANDS	decreased sex drive
	decreased pubic hair
	premenstrual breast tenderness, heavy menstrual flow, short menstrual cycle, water retention (caused by excessive estrogen)
	late menses, short and light menses, small breasts (caused by low estrogen)
	late menses, scant blood flow, small breasts (caused by excessive progesterone)
	painful periods, early menses, long flow, pelvic pain (caused by low progesterone)

Histamine and Your Headache

Histamine is a natural substance found in the mast cells, large connective tissue cells which produce allergic responses in our body. These cells are found throughout the body's tissues, but are particularly concentrated in the skin, nose, and lung linings, gastrointestinal tract, and reproductive organs. When antibodies sense an allergen (a substance perceived as foreign to the body), they trigger the mast cells to release histamine and 28 other chemicals, and the allergic response flares.

Histamine is what gives us runny noses, red, itchy eyes, hot, tender, or swollen body parts, flushing, and the other symptoms associated with allergic reactions. Histamine causes the blood vessels to widen, enabling more fluid to pass into body tissues, resulting in swelling. It also triggers the contraction of the smooth involuntary muscles in the lungs, blood vessels, heart, stomach, intestines, and bladder which, if prolonged, becomes muscle spasm. These reponses are the body's attempt to heal itself from the effect of the allergen, although in the process they can make us feel miserable.

If histamine and related biochemicals are released in the chest, you may experience coughing or asthma-like symptoms; if they are released through the skin, the symptoms may be hives or eczema; if in the intestines, the allergic response may be diarrhea; and if in the brain, the result may be a migraine headache.

In response to an allergen, the immune system releases histamine. Again, this is designed as a temporary measure. If the body is kept in a state of allergic response, too much histamine is released, causing overexpansion of blood vessels and increased secretion of stomach acid, which in turn produces a headache. It may also produce allergy-like symptoms such as sneezing, flushing, skin itching, diarrhea, and shortness of breath.

HYPOGLYCEMIA (LOW BLOOD SUGAR)

Not to be confused with primary hypoglycemia, a rare condition which is generally related to an insulin-secreting tumor, hypoglycemia (known officially as secondary hypoglycemia) is a common metabolic blood sugar disturbance—and one of medicine's most controversial topics. If you talk to a conventional physician, you will probably hear that hypoglycemia is an overemphasized and rare disorder that has little to do with headaches. You will be told that your headaches, mood swings, fatigue, bloating, and overall malaise are due more to nerves and worry than to blood sugar abnormalities, even though there is ample documented evidence that headache sufferers dramatically improve when placed on special diets designed for the regulation of blood sugar.

Hypoglycemia occurs when there is a lower than normal amount of blood sugar, or glucose, in the blood; this usually results from there being too much insulin (the pancreatic enzyme that regulates blood sugar levels), or simply from not having eaten enough for the calorie expenditure the body in putting out. Symptoms typically include headaches, weakness, anxiety, irritability, a tendency to faint, even temporary personality changes.

Since many organs are involved in blood sugar control, it is impossible to attribute hypoglycemia to a single cause, although an overstimulated pancreas is usually a factor. Other causes, such as too much coffee, infrequent or missed meals, too many carbohydrates or refined sugars, food allergies, nutritional deficiencies, emotional stress, lack of exercise, hormonal imbalances, thyroid or ovarian problems, and weak adrenal glands, are also involved in this disorder.

LEAKY GUT SYNDROME

Leaky gut syndrome occurs when, unequipped to deal with this overload, the digestive system is forced to respond in any way possible. This means breaking down whatever substances it can and changing the permeability of the intestinal barrier, allowing toxins, chemicals, and partially digested foods into the bloodstream. This leads to a host of digestive and allergic reactions, including the release of inflammatory hormones which dilate the blood vessels and cause headaches.

LOUD NOISES

Whether it be the jet overhead, the shouts of children, or the groans of a dishwasher, loud noise is a headache trigger. Japanese researcher Hiroshi Sakamota, M.D., performed extensive research on the adverse effects of noise and discovered that noise can upset the body's endocrine function, especially the pituitary-gonadal functions, which affect secretions of serotonin. One of Dr. Sakamota's studies took place in a Japanese village near a jet airfield. He discovered that more than half of the citizens of the village complained of headache, fatigue, palpitations, shoulder aches and pains, insomnia, digestive disorders, and decreased sex drive.[14]

NUTRITIONAL DEFICIENCIES

The typical American diet, although plentiful, leaves a lot to be desired. When you give up quality for convenience, it takes a toll. People can find a ready-made hamburger within minutes or drive to the corner for chips and coke, but how many stop to think about what these foods are doing to

American Eating Trends

A U.S. Department of Agriculture survey of what Americans ate in 1994 shows that Americans consumed 33% of their calories from fat, down from 40% in 1977, but that 30% of Americans are overweight, up from 22%. They eat 6% more calories per day and 22 pounds of salty snacks per year compared to 17.5 pounds in 1977. Children aged 5-16 drank 23% more soft drinks than in 1977.

their bodies?

One hundred years ago, only 10% of the American diet was refined or processed; by 1950, the figure had grown to 25%. Today, the United States is in the midst of a dietary crisis, with refined or processed foods constituting almost 90% of the average daily diet. Containing too little fiber, nutrients, fresh foods, and complex carbohydrates, most American diets contain too many highly processed foods and chemical additives and too much sugar, salt, and saturated fat.

Faulty diet can create a host of health problems, including headaches. When the cells do not get good food, the blood becomes unbalanced, digestion and nutrient absorption become difficult, oxygen does not get transported properly, hormones cannot do their job, histamines leak into the tissues, the brain suffers, and nerves swell.

SLEEPING PATTERNS

Adequate rest is essential to any health-care regimen, particularly since too little of it makes you a prime candidate for headaches. The brain chemicals that govern sleeping and waking cycles are the same ones that have been linked to headaches: serotonin and norepinephrine. A balanced relationship between serotonin and norepinephrine is necessary for a good night's sleep. Changes in your sleeping patterns or a missed night of sleep can disturb this balance and increase your chances of getting a headache. Keep in mind that many sleep disturbances are caused by an underlying dysfunction in the digestive system and liver detoxification pathways.

Research has shown that headaches, particularly clusters and migraines, tend to come on between the hours of 6 A.M. and noon, which for most people are the hours when they are either waking up or most fully awake. Rapid eye movement (REM) sleep, the period of sleep when dreams occur, has also been linked to headaches, cluster and migraines occurring immediately before or after REM sleep, and atypical cluster headaches coming on during the REM stage itself. People with headaches are also prone to other sleep irregularities, such as sleepwalking, nightmares, bedwetting, and nighttime teeth grinding.

STRONG LIGHT

The glare of direct sunlight reflected off snow, sand, or the windshield, computer screen or TV, oncoming headlights, fluorescent lights, camera flashes, or flickering lights can be all it takes to set off your headache. These headaches may involve a combination of both vascular and muscle tension responses, as the heat from the sun or bright lights can dilate blood vessels and the act of squinting can strain muscles. Thus, while most commonly linked to migraine and tension headaches, strong light can contribute to any type of headache, since all have some degree of vascular or muscular response.

This trigger is easy to avoid with reasonable attention and appropriate precaution. Wearing dark sunglasses, looking away from the camera flash, using a good computer monitor, watching less TV, tinting your car windows, and switching to full-spectrum lighting are just a few of the measures that prevent your headache from being triggered by strong light.

WEATHER AND ALTITUDE CHANGES

In the mind of a headache sufferer, a full moon, hot gusts of wind, and a threatening thunderstorm do not always conjure up images of sweet romance and a cozy fire. Instead, to those who are weather-sensitive, these conditions are more likely to mean a broken date, a darkened room, and painkillers. This is because various weather changes fill the air with positive ions (molecules that are missing electrons and carry a positive charge). In hundreds of experiments in Europe and elsewhere, researchers have re-

Dangers of the Modern Diet

The process of refining and preserving removes the nutrients from foods which cannot be adequately replaced by so-called "enrichment," despite the claims made by advertisers.

- Refining, preserving, and processing often changes the remaining nutrients into forms unrecognizable or unusable by the body.

- Processing foods removes much of their valuable fiber (the substance that bulks up the stool and eases elimination), causing further reabsorption of the wrong foods by compromising the body's ability to remove toxins and other indigestible matter.

- Refining, preserving, and processing creates foods that are capable of passing immediately into the bloodstream before getting the opportunity to be broken down into useful properties.

- Refined sugars (especially white sugar) inhibit the protective effects of white blood cells and stress the pancreas and adrenal glands.

- Excessive salt intake brings about an imbalance or deficiency in other minerals, such as calcium, magnesium and potassium.

- Saturated fats inhibit the metabolism and slow down the digestive system, increasing the odds of allergies, heart disease, and obesity.

peatedly shown that air heavy with positive ions, described by some as "dead" air, can trigger the release of serotonin and bring about respiratory problems, irritability, aggression, depression, stress, aches and pains, and headaches.

Positive ions are released by certain barometric pressure fluctuations, such as the lull before the storm, gray days, dry winds, approaching cold or warm fronts, and pollution alerts. Negative ions, on the other hand, are associated with steady weather, clear, cloudless skies, sunshine, heavy rainshowers, waterfalls, and clean-air days, weather conditions which, data shows, are related to well-being, lowered blood pressure, and greater productivity. Some sufferers are so sensitive to weather that they can predict a storm before there is a cloud in the sky.

Like weather, changes in altitude can bring about a headache in sensitive individuals unacclimated to high altitudes. Researchers believe that these headaches, sometimes accompanied by nausea and vomiting, are linked to the reduction of oxygen at higher elevations, which causes the blood vessels to dilate.

There are steps you can take to build up your resistance to positive ions and oxygen-poor environments. First, since weather is only a trigger and not a cause of headaches, you can eliminate other triggering factors and thus reduce your oversensitivity. Second, you can enhance your self-care practices whenever you travel or notice weather patterns shifting.

STRUCTURAL IMBALANCES

DENTAL PROBLEMS

Care of the mouth is crucial to overall health. Infections in and around the teeth and jaw, root canals, allergy or toxicity from dental restoration materials, electrogalvanism, mercury fillings, and TMJ syndrome can cause problems in the body and lead to headaches.

Since most dentists are trained only in rudimentary diagnostic methods and treatment, they deal mainly with the superficial health of the mouth, leaving less obvious problems undetected. For example, X rays do not always pick up pockets of infection underneath the teeth, and root canals and tooth extractions often leave behind infectious residues. As a result, the patient's health can continue to deteriorate, and chronic illnesses such as chronic fatigue syndrome, TMJ syndrome, allergies, digestive disorders,

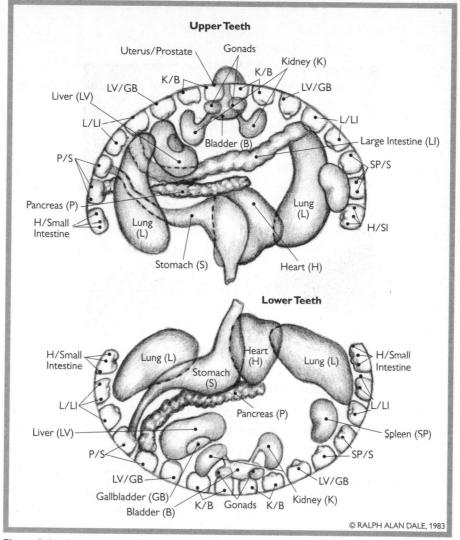

Figure 3.4—Organ and teeth correspondences on acupuncture meridians in the mouth.

toxicity, or headaches can follow.

Dysfunctions in the mouth can weaken the organs and overall bodily systems through the following mechanisms:

- Infected teeth and gums can cause toxins to leak out and compromise other body functions, especially the immune system.
- Each tooth in the mouth corresponds to a specific energy pathway as described by acupuncture, so infections, sensitivities/allergies to

121

specific restoration materials, or other mouth dysfunctions can block energy pathways and lead to problems within related organs and systems.

- Electrogalvanism occurs when differing dental restoration materials mix with saliva and create an electrical response. This creates a battery in the mouth and causes toxic materials in fillings to erode and leak into other areas of the body.

- The silver mercury used in dental fillings can release heavy metals into the system and cause toxicity. People with silver mercury amalgams often are unaware of the problem, which could explain their "mystery" illnesses. (See pages 98-100 in this chapter for more information on mercury amalgam fillings.)

- Without being aware of it, many people have developed an uneven bite, or malocclusion. Whether due to previous dental work or an inherited trait, the biting surfaces do not align properly and cause the muscle on one side of the jaw to become stressed, creating tension in the cranium, neck, and back, or TMJ syndrome. Over time, this creates serious craniosacral misalignments that can lead to the weakening of other organs and body systems.

MUSCULOSKELETAL MISALIGNMENTS

A sound musculoskeletal structure is vital for optimum health and without it you are prone to a wide range of health problems, including headaches. Although musculoskeletal misalignments are usually associated with external factors such as prolonged stress, poor posture, ill-fitting shoes, or a traumatic injury, they can also come about due to internal dysfunctions, such as allergy/sensitivity problems, digestive disturbances, and hormonal imbalances.

Just about everyone carries some stress in the muscles of the face, skull, upper shoulders, or back at some point in life. If this stress continues over time, it can lead to chronically contracted muscles, which cause the underlying structure of the body to pull and contract. Many people are walking around today with one side of their body longer than the other or their head tilted to one side.

Generally, the musculoskeletal system has a cause-and-effect relationship with the entire body. When the spine and musculature are misaligned, the blood supply and the nervous system signals cannot circulate freely to all parts of the body. This forces the spine and muscles to further compensate for the reduced energy in ways for which they were not designed.

A good example of this mechanism is seen when looking at musculoskeletal imbalances originating in the head and neck. As the most mobile part of your spine, the head and neck affect the way your weight comes through your feet, so that head and neck misalignments may throw off your hips and force you to compensate with your spine. The shoulder muscles that run upward along the base of the skull may be forced to shorten, the back tissues of the neck may become overstretched, and the jaw may become retracted, all of which pinch or place increased pressure on the nerves running through the base of the skull, down the neck and shoulders, and at the juncture where the jaw and skull meet.

Over time, your neck and head become like the pole that tightrope walkers use to keep their balance, struggling against all these other holding patterns, blocking energy and causing further muscle strain, blood vessel restriction, nerve irritation, and headache. This can compromise other functions of the body, bringing about chronic disturbances such as increased emotional tension, digestive disturbances, hormonal imbalances, and toxicity.

Other results of unhealthy structure include tightness or restriction in cranial bone movement or in the membrane surrounding the brain and spinal cord (the dura); imbalances in cerebrospinal fluid pressure; fibrosis (a disorder in which fibrous connective tissue replaces normal tissue in the muscles or organs); scar tissue formation in the region where the top of the neck meets the base of the skull (called the suboccipital area); and restrictions in the movement of the back of the skull and the first 2 cervical vertebrae (called the atlas and axis).

If your neck is out of alignment due to poor posture or trauma, the brain can actually go into partial asphyxiation as the oxygen level decreases and the carbon dioxide level increases. Headaches, especially tension headaches, are symptoms of this occurrence. The trapezius muscle is one of the major muscles associated with headaches arising from bad posture.

Not only can musculoskeletal misalignment influence the tone of the muscles that attach to the neck and head, but it can also shut off blood supply to the brain. This is because 30% of the blood that gets delivered to the

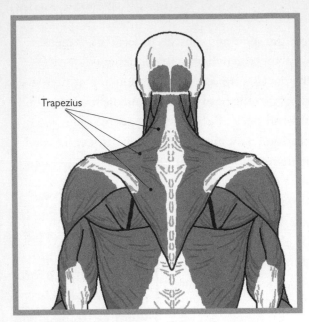

Figure 3.5—The trapezius muscle.

brain comes through the vertebral artery. If your neck is out of alignment due to poor posture or trauma, the brain can actually go into partial asphyxiation as the oxygen level decreases and the carbon dioxide level increases. Headaches, especially tension headaches, are symptoms of this occurrence.

POOR POSTURE

Hunching over your desk, slouching on the couch, and wearing ill-fitting shoes all put undue pressure on the spinal column, pinching nerves and muscles, and leading to head pain. The trapezius muscle, the triangular-shaped muscle that covers your shoulder blades, is one of the major muscles associated with headaches arising from bad posture.

Tense, burdened, or just plain tired people tend to roll their shoulders forward, contracting the trapezius, pulling on the pain sensors in the muscle tissue, causing these muscles to pull and strain the scalp, which in turn jams the cranial bones and puts extra pressure on the artery that runs up the back of the skull, reducing blood circulation to the brain and resulting in chronic headaches.

Poor posture is closely related to digestive function. Eating poorly, for instance, favoring devitalized, processed foods, decreases digestive function, and the resulting drop in energy can cause difficulty in keeping good posture.

EMOTIONAL/PSYCHOLOGICAL FACTORS

STRESS, ANXIETY, DEPRESSION, AND REPRESSED EMOTIONS

Emotions, especially chronic stress and anxiety, are powerful triggers of headaches; unchecked, they can have a disastrous effect on your body, both chemically and structurally. They can make you tired, deplete your oxygen, and set off the release of pain-stimulating chemicals. They can cause your shoulders to tighten, your stomach to hurt, and your estrogen to soar— all of which may contribute to your headaches. Furthermore, since your body responds differently when you are depressed than when you are happy and relaxed, it may be your emotional state when you encounter a stressor, rather than the condition or trigger itself, that brings on your headache.

Christiane Northrup, M.D., internationally acclaimed physician, writer, and speaker on issues concerning women's health and healing, observes that unexamined or repressed emotions are toxic emotions. In her view, "toxic emotions" are the underlying cause of many maladies, including headaches. She also notes the existence of "toxic people" (from your work, family, or past, who bring emotional pain and turmoil into your life), toxic thoughts and attitudes (negative and self-critical thoughts that undermine your well-being), and "toxic ideas" (disempowering beliefs perpetuated by society, such as that drugs are the only way to physical well-being). "Your mind and your body are intimately connected. What your mind thinks," your body feels, states Dr. Northrup."[15]

Unfortunately, many suppress rather than express their emotions. We learn to "keep a stiff upper lip," "grin and bear it," "grit our teeth," "look the other way." But buried emotions eventually find other ways to communicate, and since it is the mind that keeps us from them, what better way to get our attention than to create a pain in the head?

Furthermore, some headache sufferers have what is called the "headache personality." This is the style of the hard-driving perfectionist who censors emotions and internalizes stress. People who fit this profile prefer taking medicines, putting off finding out what is really wrong, because they are afraid of a headache interfering with their daily performance. Even those who are intelligent, health-conscious people, delay the inevitable, convinced that the right opportunity will come along, as long as it isn't "right now"—that is, until "right now" hits them like a flash flood.

Take the case of Tom, a successful real estate agent in his forties. Tom was a hard worker, a perfectionist who prided himself on his 12-hour work days and frequent sales. As he brought home more money, he was too emotionally and physically exhausted to spend time with his wife and son. Eventually,

Somatization

Somatization is the technical term for the process that occurs when mental anguish is not acknowledged consciously and expresses itself as a physical problem. Studies have shown that somatization happens more frequently to those who are unable to express their feelings, possibly because such individuals find it easier to accept a physical complaint than a psychological one.

Tom began to wake up in the morning with dull, throbbing headaches which worsened as the day wore on, making him feel like his head was being squeezed by a vise. Tom told no one about his headaches, however, because he wanted to avoid being labeled a hypochondriac or weakling. So he inadvertently added two more emotional stressors to his list: the shame of having headaches and the worry about when the next one was going to strike.

A major misconception about headache sufferers is that they are weak and unable to cope with the stresses of everyday life. The classic stereotype of a headache is that it is somehow the sufferer's fault and therefore not to be taken seriously. So, rather than support and compassion, people often offer a pat on the back and a lecture about being uptight and stressed out and what to do to change. Little do they realize that the headache is physically real and that the physical reality makes the sufferer uptight, not the other way around.

The expression "It's all in your head" stigmatizes the headache sufferers, making them wonder if a personal defect is causing the problem. It is important to understand that, yes, emotions can and do lead to headaches, but other factors, such as digestive and metabolic dysfunction, may be the underlying cause of the problem. In other words, stress, anxiety, and emotions can make headaches hurt more. Even when healthy coping mechanisms are in place, the fear of your next headache is enough to make you anxious and stressful. This pattern is one of the many vicious cycles associated with chronic headache conditions.

HEADACHES AND THE FEMALE CYCLE

According to Greek myth, Zeus developed his first and only headache when he discovered that his wife Hera conceived a child without help from him or any other male. Midwives diagnosed this headache as pregnancy, so, paving the way for modern Caesarean section, his head was split with an ax and out popped Athena. An active imagination (particularly if it belongs to a sufferer of hormonal headaches) might suggest that the real reason behind the preponderance of headaches among women is the revenge of Zeus.

If only this were true, women might have some way to offer appeasement to their angry heads. As it is, more than 20% of the women in America suffer from some type of headache around the time of menstruation, and the majority of them are migraines. However, since little research has been done on the connection between hormones and headaches (what has been done having focused primarily on migraines), it is important to remember that hormones undoubtedly play a role in *all* headache types.

Hormone fluctuation has been proven to cause a change in serotonin levels, which means that imbalances in estrogen or progesterone, either too little or too much, can either cause headaches or trigger them in women who are already predisposed to headaches. These headaches tend to come before, during, or after flow times (when estrogen drops off), but they can just as easily strike when a woman is ovulating (when estrogen is at its highest).

In a study of 300 women conducted by Lee Kudrow, M.D., Director of the California Medical Clinic for Headache in Encino, California, estrogen-containing preparations were shown not only to increase the frequency of migraine attack but also to induce headaches in women who had

Are You Stressed Out?

If you answer yes to more than 5 of the questions below, you definitely are stressed out and could benefit from some of the techniques and Emotional/Psychological therapies listed in Chapter 4. In parentheses are some underlying metabolic considerations which may be playing a role.

- Do you often grind your teeth? (digestive dysfunction—parasites)
- Is your breath shallow and irregular? (metabolic low energy—food allergy/sensitivity)
- Are your hands and feet cold? (hormonal imbalance—adrenal/thyroid weakness)
- Do you have trouble sleeping or tend to wake up tired? (liver dysfunction, food allergy/sensitivity)
- Do you often have an upset stomach? (food allergy/sensitivity)
- Do you get mad or irritated easily? (liver dysfunction)
- Do you feel worthless? (low energy, chronic fatigue)
- Do you constantly worry? (food allergy/sensitivity, hormone imbalances)
- Do you have problems concentrating and articulating your thoughts? (low energy, digestive, hormonal imbalances)
- Do you frequently fidget, chew your fingers, or bite your nails? (food allergy/sensitivity, digestive disturbances)
- Do you have high blood pressure? (food allergy/sensitivity, digestive disturbances)
- Do you eat, drink, or smoke excessively? (low energy—poor food quality)
- Do you sometimes turn to recreational drugs just to get away? (the need for stimulants is a sign of low energy—poor food quality)

127

> *In a study of 300 women, estrogen-containing preparations were shown not only to increase the frequency of migraine attack, but also to induce headaches in women who had not previously had them. When these women were taken off the estrogen, the frequency of their headaches declined dramatically.*

not previously had them. When these women were taken off the estrogen, the frequency of their headaches declined dramatically. [16]

Research suggests that estrogen has a potent effect on brain chemistry, influencing serotonin levels as well as the functions of other important hormones, including those that regulate the perception of pain, blood vessel dilation and constriction, water retention, and blood pressure. This suggests many reasons why headaches arise during times when estrogen levels change. In addition, prolactin, the pituitary hormone that regulates the production of breast milk in nursing mothers, appears in higher than normal levels in the blood of some women experiencing a migraine attack.

In seeking medical help for their headaches, women often face an additional burden. Medications generally affect women differently than men, a fact frequently ignored by doctors prescribing in doses determined by data gathered through research conducted mainly with male subjects. In addition, physicians are more apt to label women than men as hysterical, or imagining symptoms. Given the sometimes elusive nature of headache causes, women can be more frustrated than helped by consulting a doctor. Fortunately for women, alternative practitioners who see beyond the conventional misconceptions and research prejudices realize that hormonal imbalances, whether the cause or result of physiological and psychological stress, can be corrected.

What makes hormone-related headaches so frustrating is their apparent inconsistency. Some women's headaches end when they get pregnant, while other women experience headaches for the first time during pregnancy. The same can be said for women going through menopause, undergoing hysterectomies, or taking birth control pills or hormone replacements.

Menarche (onset of menstruation)—Until puberty, boys and girls generally get headaches with equal frequency, yet after age 12, when a girl's menstrual cycle begins, the incidence of headache among females rises dramatically, with girls becoming 2 to 3 times more headache prone.

Menstruation—Current studies show that 75% of all migraine sufferers are women, 65% of them experiencing migraines immediately before, during, or after menstruation or ovulation. Headaches that occur before the onset of menstruation are called PMS headaches because they tend to be part of the overall premenstrual syndrome, which includes back pain, breast tenderness and swelling, nausea, mood swings, and general irritability. Those that occur during menstruation, on the other hand, are more often accompanied by abdominal cramping and tend to be classified as menstrual migraines or tension-type headaches.

Oral contraceptives—Oral contraceptives, including the birth control pill and the morning-after pill, as well as the estraderm patch, have been shown to worsen headaches in half of the women who already suffered from them. According to National Headache Foundation (NHF) data, 70% of the women who developed headaches after they began using oral contraceptives found that their headaches disappeared after they stopped taking them.

Hormone replacement therapy—Most alternative doctors agree that synthetic hormone replacement therapy is not safe. Estrogen especially has serious side effects, including the suppression of the disease-fighting part of our immune system. According to NHF research, estrogen replacement pills are a known headache trigger and 58% of migraine cases have been shown to improve once hormone replacement was reduced or stopped.

Pregnancy—Although some women may experience more migraines during the first trimester, most report relief during the third month—and some even report that this is the first relief in their lives. Researchers believe that the higher estrogen levels during pregnancy or the additional endorphins that are produced during the later stages of pregnancy are responsible for headache relief. Even so, some women experience migraines for the first time in their life within days of delivery, which is attributed to the dramatic reduction in estrogen and metabolic changes affecting blood vessels following childbirth.

Menopause—The experience of migraines varies from woman to woman in the same way the experience of menopause does. There is no way to predict how an individual woman will react to her body's dwindling supply of estrogen. For some women, headaches vanish, while others feel

The B.A.D. Headache

One type of headache that is experienced almost exclusively by women (by as many as 15 million in America every year) is attributed to a non-life-threatening heart defect rather than hormones. It is called a benign autonomic dysfunction (B.A.D.) headache and occurs when one of the valves of the heart does not close all the way because of what is called a mitral valve prolapse.

This headache is generally accompanied by chest pain, rapid heartbeat, and blood pressure changes and is more prevalent in women who tend to break out in red blotches during times of stress and/or have unusually large pupils. Although they sound terrifying and final, these headaches are not linked to actual heart disease or any other serious disorder, and respond to alternative treatments.

them more intensely, perhaps due less to hormone shifts than to the stress associated with this transitional time. However, research suggests that the majority of those with headaches experience a worsening as they enter menopause, with a gradual tapering off afterward.

Hysterectomy—Like pregnancy and menopause, total hysterectomy tends to have inconsistent effects on headaches. Although it more often produces a worsening of symptoms, this may be related to hormone replacement therapy as well as the hysterectomy itself.

THE ROLE OF HORMONES IN THE FEMALE CYCLE

A good way to understand sex hormone function is to examine how a woman's menstrual cycle is controlled by the relationships among the hypothalamus, the pituitary, and the ovaries—the two almond-sized glands in a woman's pelvis.

During the first 14 days of a normal 28-day cycle, the hypothalamus produces a gonadotropin-releasing hormone and sends it to the anterior pituitary, stimulating the release of a follicle-stimulating hormone (FSH). The FSH increases the flow of estrogen and induces the ovaries to produce a mature egg. At midcycle, just before ovulation, the hypothalamus prompts the anterior pituitary to release a luteinizing hormone (LH), which increases the production of progesterone and stimulates one of the ovarian follicles to release a ripened egg. LH also ensures that the uterine lining (endometrium) has sufficient blood supply for the egg to establish itself in the uterus if it is fertilized.

If the egg is not fertilized, estrogen continues to rise for about one week and then tapers off. At the start of menstruation, when the uterine lining begins to slough off, the estrogen level plummets, eventually returning to the original baseline level, where it remains until the next cycle.

Although it may seem like it, this process is far from simple. Every hormonal relationship depends on the hypothalamus secreting its releasing hormones in a perfectly timed, intermittent manner. If this fails to happen, the pituitary cannot respond with the right proportion of FSH and/or LH, meaning the crucial estrogen/progesterone ratio will be off and the entire system thrown into confusion. Furthermore, poor functioning of the liver, small and large intestine, and thyroid, as well as allergy problems, can disrupt a normal menstrual cycle by inhibiting the ability to balance overproduction of estrogen and/or progesterone—which may explain why many women's cycle-related headaches begin on the first day of menstruation.

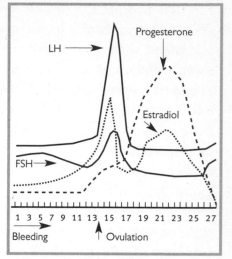

Figure 3.6—Hormone levels during the menstrual cycle.

Children and Headaches

Contrary to popular belief, children also suffer from the undiscriminating plague of headaches. Head pain is the cause of more than 4.2 lost school days per child (K-12) every year, and 40% of all children have had at least one headache by age 7.

Although most of these headaches are tension headaches, studies indicate that 7 to 18% of all U.S. children also suffer from migraines, with some sufferers as young as 2 years old. Some researchers believe this number may actually be higher because many children's migraines are misdiagnosed as a symptom of a flu or cold. Before the age of 12, boys are more likely to be afflicted with migraines, but after the onset of puberty, migraines become far more common in adolescent girls.

Like adults, children can be hit by the frustrating and complex range of conditions of which headaches are a symptom. Digestive disturbances, improper diets, allergies/sensitivities, environment, birth trauma, accidents, TMJ syndrome, eye problems, emotions, and having a parent with a headache condition are just some of the problems that can bring about a child's headache.

Studies indicate that 7 to 18% of all U.S. children suffer from migraines, with some sufferers as young as 2 years old. Some researchers believe this number may actually be higher because many children's migraines are misdiagnosed as a symptom of a flu or cold. Before the age of 12, boys are more likely to be afflicted with migraines, but after the onset of puberty, migraines become far more common in adolescent girls.

Children's headaches are more difficult to classify in adult terms because a child's pain tends to take on different forms. Head pain in a child may occur all over rather than in one spot, or, in the case of a migraine, there may be no head pain at all but, instead, symptoms of nausea, confusion, or dizziness. A child's headache may not last as long as an adult's, and it often is accompanied by diarrhea and abdominal pain, no matter what type. Some children are just too young and lack the words to describe how their headache feels.

If you are the parent of a child with a headache, you need to be especially sensitive, addressing your child's experience with love and sympathy while also giving him or her enough room to develop individual coping mechanisms. Above all, try not to focus on the problem so much that you worsen it by increasing a child's tension and fear. There are many things you can do to understand and prevent the underlying condition that is causing your child's head pain. These measures include the following:

■ Keep a record of your child's headache in a headache diary, including a note of any activities or emotions your child experienced around the time of the headache.

■ Watch your child's diet carefully and eliminate trigger foods and substances that cause sensitivities, especially refined sugar. Also, try to avoid feeding your child too much of the same food, such as wheat, as repetition can bring on headaches and other allergic reactions, although this may not happen until your children are adults.

■ Do not expose your child to cigarette smoke.

■ Ensure that your child eats and sleeps regularly and consistently.

■ Feed your child allergy/sensitivity-free foods. (See the list of common food triggers in this chapter.)

■ Try giving your child a back or foot rub or an herbal bath, since this can release tension and help an upset child feel nurtured and specially cared for.

- Encourage your child's enjoyment of outdoor exercise because breathing fresh air is important to health. Support your child's ability to relax and appreciate quiet activities, such as reading and drawing.
- Foster your child's ability to express whatever thoughts and emotions he or she may be having, since repressing or ignoring them creates additional stress and tension.

Paying attention to the factors listed above can do a lot to help your child. Children respond especially well to nondrug treatments once the triggers of their headaches are discovered and eliminated. You may also find that your child experiences fewer headaches and headaches of less severity when she or he realizes that headaches are not serious abnormalities.

However, if your child is experiencing headaches more than once a month or devoloping severe symptoms such as a high fever, vomiting, confusion, or extreme fatigue, you need to consult a physician to make sure these are not symptoms of a more serious condition, such as meningitis or encephalitis. Generally, only about 1 in 20 children suffer from headaches that are caused by neurological illness or other serious disorder.

The Elderly and Headaches

Headaches are common in elderly people, most of them benign, tension-type headaches. Yet as people age, headaches can also signal a more serious problem, especially in those who have not experienced headaches before. The elderly are particularly susceptible to organic conditions such as temporal arteritis, hypertension, cervical arthritis, neuralgia, glaucoma, strokes, and brain inflammations. Since they often take medication, the elderly are also more likely to experience complications and side effects that could include headaches.

Another common cause of headaches among the elderly is cerebrovascular disease, which is a condition that causes temporary blockage within an artery (blood clot) that reduces blood flow to the brain. Headaches caused by cerebrovascular disease typically occur with other signs of poor brain functioning, such as weakness, numbness, impaired senses, confusion, dizziness, poor memory, and lack of balance. These headaches are

See Chapter 4, Why Alternative Medicine Is Your Best Strategy, for more information on starting a headache diary.

Smoking, Migraines, and Stroke Risk

French doctors found in a study of 212 women that those under the age of 45 with a previous history of migraines had a significantly higher risk factor for stroke; if they smoked cigarettes, the risk was even higher. However, men of all ages and women older than 45 were not more likely to have stroke if they had migraines, according to research reported in the *British Medical Journal*, July 31, 1993.

usually experienced as throbbing pain in the front, back, or side of head, depending upon which artery (the front, carotid, or the back, vertebrobasilar) is affected. The potential for a serious health condition to be the cause of headaches among the elderly make it essential, particularly if you do not normally get headaches, to consult a medical professional in order to rule out the possibility of an organic disorder.

RECOMMENDED READING

Ashford, N.A. and Miller, C.S. *Chemical Exposures: Low Levels and High Stakes.* New York: Van Nostrand Reinhold, 1990.

Blaylock, Russell L., M.D. *Excitotoxins: The Taste That Kills.* Santa Fe, New Mexico: Health Press, 1994.

"Dental Amalgam: A Scientific Review and Recommended Public Health Service Strategy for Research, Education, and Regulation." Final Report of the Subcommittee on Risk Management of the Committee to Coordinate Environmental Health and Related Programs. Public Health Service, January 1993.

Diamond, Seymour, M.D. *The Hormone Headache.* New York: Macmillan, 1995.

Donovan, P. "Bowel Toxemia, Permeability and Disease—New Information to Support an Old Concept." *A Textbook of Natural Medicine*, eds. J.E. Pizzorno and M.T. Murray. Seattle, WA: John Bastyr College Publications, 1989.

Ecobichon, D.J. and Joy, R.M., eds. *Pesticides and Neurological Diseases.* Boca Raton, FL: CRC Press, Inc., 1982.

Frazier, Claude A., M.D. *Coping with Food Allergy.* New York: Quadrangle/The New York Times Book Company, 1974, 318-319.

"Headache in Children." Chicago: National Headache Foundation, 1994.

"Hormones and Migraines." *National Headache Foundation Fact Sheet.* Chicago: National Headache Foundation 1994.

Igram, Cass, M.D. *Who Needs Headaches?* Cedar Rapids, Iowa: Literary Visions Publishing, 1991.

Lahiri, Asok K., M.D. "Headaches in the Elderly." *National Headache Foundation Newsletter* 87, Winter 1993, 6-8.

Leviton, Richard. *Brain Builders!* New York: Simon & Schuster, 1995.

Littlewood, J.T., et al, "Red Wine as a Cause of Migraine." *Lancet:* 1, March 12, 1988, 558-559.

National Headache Foundation Fact Sheet. Chicago: National Headache Foundation, October 1994.

"Pesticides and Groundwater: A Health Concern for the Midwest." Navarre, MN: Proceedings of the Freshwater Foundation Conference, Oct 16-17, 1986.

Price, W.A. *Dental Infections* Volume 1: Oral and Systemic. Cleveland, OH: Benton Publishing, 1973.

Privitera, James R., M.D. "Clots: Life's Biggest Killer." *Health Freedom News,* September 1993, 22-23.

Remmes, Anne, M.D. "Headaches and Sleep." *National Headache Foundation Quarterly:* 87, Winter 1993.

Robbins, Lawrence, M.D. and Lang, Susan S., *Headache Help.* New York: Houghton Mifflin Company, 1995.

Rogers, Sherry A., M.D. *The EI Syndrome.* New York: Prestige Publishing, 1986.

Rudolph, C.J., D.O., Ph.D. et al, "An Observation of the Effect of EDTA Chelation and Supportive Multivitamin Trace Mineral Supplementation of Blood Platelet Volume: A Brief Communication." *Journal of Advancement in Medicine:* 3, 3, Fall 1990.

Vliet, Elizabeth Lee, M.D. *Screaming to Be Heard: Hormonal Connections Women Suspect and Doctors Ignore.* New York: M. Evans and Company, Inc., 1995.

Yudkin, Marcia. "The Forecast for Tomorrow Is Headaches." *Natural Health,* January/February 1993, 40-41.

The American Council for Headache Education (ACHE) claims that most headache clinics are able to cut the frequency of headaches in half and that about 75 to 80% of migraine sufferers improve, 65 to 70% of tension sufferers improve, and almost all cluster sufferers are cured. While this sounds wonderful, these statistics reveal neither the side effects with which these patients now contend or that they are still suffering from whatever caused the headache symptom.

Why Alternative Medicine is Your Best Strategy

It was so easy. To think of all those years I spent in pain, bouncing from one prescription to another, when all I had to do was stop eating sugar and dairy products. If I'd only known, maybe I would have noticed my children growing older.

—Susan, a former migrainer

Humans have been searching for an end to headaches since prehistoric days. Archeological digs have uncovered skulls dating from Neolithic times and the Bronze Age, with holes drilled in them, causing much speculation on early attempts to free headache sufferers from the "demons" of head pain. Happily, treatment strategies, especially those employed by alternative practitioners, have evolved considerably since these early attempts, and today, whether your headache is related to allergies/sensitivities, nutritional deficiencies, hormones, or any of the other causes listed in Chapter 3, there is a treatment strategy that is right for you.

This chapter introduces some important aspects of diagnosis, factors to consider in selecting a course of treatment, and what to expect from an alternative medicine practitioner.

When to Seek Medical Attention

Before exploring the spectrum of alternative strategies, keep in mind that, although not usually the case, some headaches are a sign of a more serious condition. Even if you have been experiencing headaches for years, you should consult a physician immediately if any of the following describes your headaches:

- severe pain that comes on suddenly
- head pain accompanied by high fever
- head pain that worsens progressively over time, especially if it follows a head injury
- head pain that is accompanied by mental confusion, seizures, mood swings, or other serious neurological symptoms
- head pain that occurs after physical exertion, straining, coughing, or sexual activity
- head pain that first appears after the age of 55
- head pain that is chronic or diminishing your quality of life.

For information on specific treatment of individual headache types using the various alternative medicine modalities, see Chapters 5 through 15. Chapters 16 and 17 offer detailed explanations of these techniques.

Although most often not the case, headaches can be a sign of a more serious health condition. It is advisable to consult your physician to eliminate this possibility.

Since only 1 to 1.5% of all headaches (this includes all types and levels of severity) are caused by life-threatening illnesses, the primary benefit of having your headache evaluated by a medical practitioner may be simple reassurance, although if something is seriously wrong, you will more likely have a good outcome if you seek early treatment.

One of the problems with headaches is that it is often difficult to tell the difference between ordinary, benign headaches and those that are symptomatic of a major disease. Medical tests simply rule out the possibility that your headache is as serious as it is painful. In any case, good sense, a concept referred to by the medical establishment as "clinical judgment," by both you and your doctor, is essential when deciding whether to put yourself through a series of tests. If you will feel better, by all means do everything necessary to establish that your symptoms are not harbingers of disaster.

What an Alternative Practitioner Will Do

Even with its confounding variety of causes and triggers, the headache must be approached like any other problem: find the cause and fix it. A good mechanic wouldn't dream of touching your car until he figured out why you brought it to him in the first place. Nor should you expect to get help from a system of medicine that starts tinkering around with your head without listening to how your body runs. If you have already heard, "There's noth-

ests Practitioners May Use to Determine the Cause of Your Headache

- Tests to rule out the possibility of serious causes: Computed Tomography (CT, formerly CAT scan), Magnetic Resonance Imaging (MRI), brain scan, electro-encephalography (EEG), spinal tap (lumbar puncture), or angiography and other X rays

- Tests to determine the possibility of allergy: NAET, elimination diet, or specialized blood testing

- Tests to detect vitamin or mineral deficiencies: blood, hair, or urine analysis, gut permeability, and Phase I/Phase II liver detoxification

- Tests to look at digestive functioning: blood, urine, and stool analysis

- Tests to check out hormonal levels and gland functioning: high-tech blood, saliva, and urine analysis

- Tests to detect toxic metal contamination: analyzing hair or tissue samples or in some cases blood and urine

- Tests to determine body electromagnetic energy fields and related blocks and dysfunctions: biodigital O-Ring test, electrodermal screening, or applied kinesiology.[1]

ing more we can do for you," don't despair. You have the opportunity to work with an alternative medical practitioner and find real healing.

This is not to suggest that an alternative physician will always be able to figure out what is wrong with your head on the first consultation. Instead, on your initial—as well as subsequent—visits, the physician will ask questions to gather clues, and the two of you will join together as a team, piecing the bits of information together until you get a clear, recognizable picture. Alternative practitioners regard you as a *whole* person; they want to know who you are, what kind of constitution you have, and the situations affecting your life.

As you talk about yourself, the physician will usually be studying your face, skin, hair, body, and mannerisms to get additional information regarding your overall state of health. This time is for both you and the practitioner because talking about yourself in the context of your headache is an essential step in the healing process, one that gives you the chance to unravel parallels and relationships that you may not have thought about previously.

On your first visit, you and the practitioner will go over such information as:

- your family headache history (to uncover genetic links)
- the details of your first headache (to understand the exact nature of your personal headache expression)
- warning signs of an approaching headache (to differentiate different types of headache)

- the onset, frequency, and duration of your headache (to further understand your headache)
- the symptoms associated with your headache (to link up other physiological systems)
- the type of pain you experience and its location (to differentiate underlying causes)
- the foods you eat, especially likely triggers (to search for allergy/sensitivity clues)
- your sleeping patterns (to link physiology, especially liver function, with emotional stressors)
- your lifestyle and job (to understand your stressors)
- additional stresses in your life (to help you understand and communicate your fears and worries)
- known allergies and sensitivities (to make your practitioner's job easier)
- the relationship of your headache to your menstrual cycle (to link hormonal dysfunction, if applicable)
- your goals, dreams, and ambitions (to better understand you as an individual)
- The doctors you have seen and what they told you (to consider previous opinion);
- the results of previous medical tests (to ensure appropriate tests have been taken to rule out organic causes)
- the medications you have taken or are taking (to evaluate the results and the toxic side effects of their use)
- any other medical conditions of which you are aware (to understand overall health and how it relates to the subsequent

Acute and Gradual Onset in New or Different Headaches

What doctors want to rule out in acute headaches:

BLEEDING INTO THE BRAIN
- subcranial bleeding—subdural hematoma
- intracranial bleeding—stroke

BRAIN INFECTION
- meningitis
- encephalitis

CIRCULATORY PROBLEMS
- arteriosclerosis/ischemia
- decreased blood flow (leading to stroke)

What doctors want to rule out in gradual onset (subacute) headaches:

- temporal arteritis (inflammation of the temporal artery)
- intracranial hypertension or pseudotumor (increased pressure in head)
- cluster headaches
- trigeminal neuralagia
- eye pseudotumor
- brain tumors
- body tumors (especially adrenal tumors)

Although alternative practitioners will guide and correct your process, they maintain that you are the center of control and that you do not need an expert to ride in on a white horse and rescue you from your pain. Alternative medicine is seen as a tool for empowerment, for ultimately you are responsible for whether your body becomes strong and healthy.

development of your head pain).

Compassion, a willingness to understand, professional competence, and scientific understanding are all important tools in the world of headache treatment. A good practitioner works with you to create the blueprint you need to plan and build a healthy body and mind.

Although alternative practitioners will guide and correct your process, they maintain that you are the center of control and that you do not need an expert to ride in on a white horse and rescue you from your pain. Alternative medicine is seen as a tool for empowerment, for ultimately you are responsible for whether your body becomes strong and healthy. Only you have the power over your ability to heal. You do not need an M.D. or a Ph.D. to understand your body; you live in it.

What an Alternative Practitioner Will Not Do

As a headache sufferer in America, you face a double dilemma. On one hand, you do not want your headache to be the sign of some serious organic disorder; yet on the other, once you realize you are among the 98.5 to 99% of the population whose headaches are not life-threatening, you are stuck with a prevailing medical system that does not know how to help you. This is not much consolation when it means a life in pain or on prescription drugs.

Conventional medical doctors are certainly not engaged in a conspiracy to keep you in pain. Instead, schooled in a system that does not treat the body as a whole, they may try to make you (and themselves) feel better by handing you an official definition of your headache and answering your questions with classification terminology that leaves you wondering just what it was you asked.

Others may stab wildly in the dark, ordering test after test, trying different medications, hoping to stumble on what will finally help you; when this does not happen, they may bounce you from neurologist to dentist to optometrist, what doctors call punting, hoping somebody else will be able

Your Route to Headache Relief

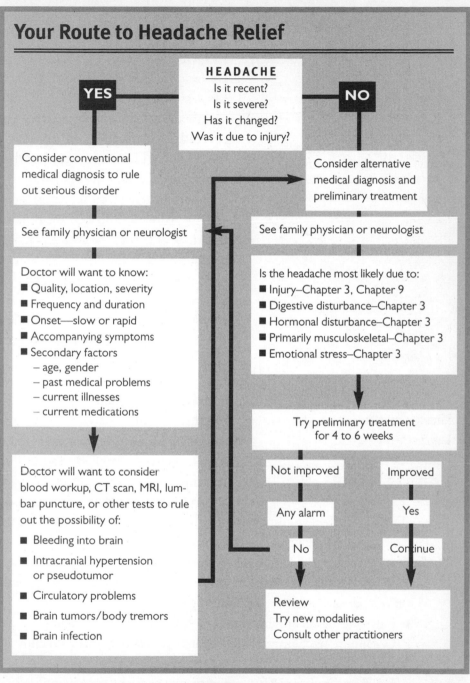

HEADACHE
Is it recent?
Is it severe?
Has it changed?
Was it due to injury?

YES

NO

Consider conventional medical diagnosis to rule out serious disorder

Consider alternative medical diagnosis and preliminary treatment

See family physician or neurologist

See family physician or neurologist

Doctor will want to know:
- Quality, location, severity
- Frequency and duration
- Onset—slow or rapid
- Accompanying symptoms
- Secondary factors
  - age, gender
  - past medical problems
  - current illnesses
  - current medications

Is the headache most likely due to:
- Injury–Chapter 3, Chapter 9
- Digestive disturbance–Chapter 3
- Hormonal disturbance–Chapter 3
- Primarily musculoskeletal–Chapter 3
- Emotional stress–Chapter 3

Try preliminary treatment for 4 to 6 weeks

Doctor will want to consider blood workup, CT scan, MRI, lumbar puncture, or other tests to rule out the possibility of:
- Bleeding into brain
- Intracranial hypertension or pseudotumor
- Circulatory problems
- Brain tumors/body tremors
- Brain infection

Not improved

Improved

Any alarm

Yes

No

Continue

Review
Try new modalities
Consult other practitioners

You can use the chart above to help you figure out how to proceed with getting treatment for your headaches. Begin by asking yourself the 4 questions in the box at the top. If you answer *yes* to any of the questions, go to the left of the chart and consider following the route suggested in the boxes under "yes." If you answer *no* to the questions, the route directed by the boxes under "no" will probably be more helpful for you in eliminating your headaches.

The Many (Treatment) Roads To Rome

Alternative medicine offers a wide variety of treatment options. Some of these, such as chiropractic, osteopathy, craniosacral therapy, and the various systems of bodywork, address structural imbalances within the body. Others focus on maintaining the body's biochemical balance of hormones, enzymes, and nutrients, in order to maintain proper cellular function. These include diet, nutritional supplements, herbal medicine, and enzyme therapy. Still others seek to restore mental and emotional balance, including mind/body medicine, biofeedback training, meditation, hypnotherapy, guided imagery, and neuro-linguistic programming. Finally, systems such as acupuncture, homeopathy, energy medicine, magnetic field therapy, and neural therapy address the energetic levels of the body.

— BURTON GOLDBERG

Source—*Alternative Medicine: The Definitive Guide*, compiled by the Burton Goldberg Group. Tiburon, CA: Future Medicine Publishing, 1994.

to provide the answer they cannot.

A few conventional medical doctors will even attempt to transfer their confusion to you by suggesting you take a look at your personal problems or emotional issues. As many of you have discovered, such escapades are not only a waste of your time and money, but they also cost you many hours of pain.

Alternative medical practitioners, on the other hand, will treat your headache as part of the whole complex system which is your body. They tend to look for imbalances in that system which may be producing the headache. By addressing the imbalance, rather than treating the symptom, they can help you eliminate your headaches.

Finding the Right Practitioner

Although there are thousands out there, it is not always easy to find an alternative practitioner. It is difficult to trust yourself to both a treatment you have never tried before and a therapist whom you have never met. Furthermore, the field of alternative medicine is rapidly growing and expanding, which means there are more practitioners and healing methods to choose from. So then, what do you do when you want to go see an alternative practitioner, but do not have a personal recommendation to go by?

- Call some of the numbers listed in Appendix A under "Helpful Organizations." These are established professional membership organizations and training programs that demand high standards and a uniform level of quality among members. Many provide referrals, either to a practitioner in your area or to another professional organization closer to your home.
- Check your local phone book for professional organizations or

schools that provide training in the modality that interests you. Chances are they will be able to refer you to someone in your area.

■ Visit your local health food store, therapy center, or yoga school and start asking people if they know of any qualified practitioners of the modality you are seeking. Very likely you will be able to gather a number of business cards as you begin the selection process.

■ If you have access to an on-line computer service, this can be another useful way of finding a practitioner near you. You could post a notice in an alternative (also called holistic or complementary medicine) users group, posting your location, the type of modality you are looking for, and a request for local recommendations. You will probably get numbers and a chance to hear from others who have had direct experience with the treatment you are researching.

■ Finally, you can go through the phone book directly, checking for practitioners by looking up the modality itself (if it is there), or you can visit your local library for other directories.

For a listing of alternative medicine practitioners, see Future Medicine Publishing's *Alternative Medicine Yellow Pages.*

For more information about types of alternative medicine and patient stories of individual practitioners, see Future Medicine Publishing's *Alternative Medicine: The Definitive Guide.*

Now that you have a list of names, the next step is to choose the one that will be a good match for you. You can do this in a number of ways. One is by trusting your intuition. If this does not steer you, you can try calling or visiting the various offices and getting a feel for the practice by talking to the receptionist and the practitioner. Be sure to ask pointed questions, such as whether the practitioner is certified by an established organization, what kind of certification program it was, how many years he or she has been practicing, what kind of success rate he or she has had with headaches and their underlying conditions, how many treatments has it generally taken to treat these conditions, and what you do if relief is not found. Also, be sure to go over the price, payment schedule, and the treatment procedure to make sure it is acceptable.

Once you find the right therapist and make an appointment, remember, you are there for yourself. This means that you can ask as many questions as you want as long as they are appropriately associated with your condition. If for some reason you feel that the practitioner is not listening or seems perturbed by your queries, communicate your feelings. If you still do not feel heard, look for another practitioner who is more sensitive to your individual needs. Also keep in mind that it is unethical for a practitioner to ask for fees in advance of treatment; similarly, watch out for practitioners who promise you a miracle cure. Good practitioners who have had experiences of spontaneous healing possess a certain reverence for the process and tend to talk about their healing abilities in an understated yet confident manner.

Headaches tend to happen when too many things are stimulated at the same time, meaning that not just one but several, even as many as 20, factors can trigger biochemical changes that result in head pain.

Headache Diary

To help you understand the nature of your headache and assist your practitioner in figuring out its underlying cause, it is a good idea to begin keeping a written record of your headache experiences before you visit an alternative practitioner. Called a headache diary, this record will allow you to observe your headaches over time, by which you can get a better idea of the how, what, when, and where—factors that may have played a role in triggering them. Because headache triggers differ from person to person, be aware that it may take some dedicated detective work for you to determine the underlying cause of your headache and its specific triggers.

Headaches tend to happen when too many things are stimulated at the same time, meaning that not just one but several, even as many as 20, factors can trigger biochemical changes that result in head pain. Imagine the phenomenon as the overflow that happens when you add water to an already full glass. For example, when Shirley eats a chocolate bar on a good day of the month, nothing happens, but, if she is premenstrual, there is a full moon, it just stopped raining, she is stressed about her job, and she eats a chocolate bar, chances are she will experience a headache.

Keep in mind that some foods may need to be in combination to trigger your headaches. For instance, if cheese by itself is no problem, it could be when combined with nitrate-containing sausage in a pizza. These and other elusive triggers must be identified before you can manage them, another reason why headache diaries are important.

Headache Diary Guidelines

Record the magnitude of the headache using a scale from 0-10, 0 denoting associated symptoms with no head pain, 10 denoting the worst possible pain. Make your record as complete as possible, recording exact times, the ingredients consumed in meals and snacks, the chemicals, smells, lights, and/or sounds to which you had been exposed, emotions, sleep times, where in menstrual cycle, and so on. Do so by answering the following questions:

- What did the pain feel like (sharp, throbbing, dull, squeezing, pressing, etc.)?

- Where do you experience the pain (temples, forehead, behind the eye, back of the head, neck, etc.)?

- Is it localized or generalized?

- What time of day did your headache come on?

- How long did it last?

- How many days between this headache and your last?

- Did you have any symptoms before the onset of your headache?

- What symptoms accompanied or followed your headache (dizziness, vomiting, light sensitivity, etc.)?

- What events were happening in your life before or around the onset of your headache and how were you feeling about them (both emotionally and physically)?

- What medications, either prescription or OTC, were you taking before headache? What dosage(s)?

- What foods had you eaten (including the contents of all the meals you had eaten within a 96-hour period)?

- What environments were you in before your headache attack (exposed to bright lights, perfumes, cigarette smoke, pollution, fumes)?

- Did the weather change?

- Did your lifestyle patterns change (more or less sleep, overwork, irregular eating, stress, depression, fatigue, etc.)?

- What physical activities did you engage in during the 12 hours preceding your headache (sports, sexual activity, medical tests, injuries, etc.)?

- If you are a woman, where are you in your cycle? Are you pregnant? Are you going through menopause? Are you taking birth control pills or undergoing hormone replacement therapy? (It is helpful to mark down the day of your menstrual cycle in your diary; the first day of menses should be noted as day one.)

You'll need to pay attention to a number of factors, these include: the date and time of each headache, what you sense when you get the first inklings of onset, when it becomes full-blown, when it ends, the associated symptoms (such as nausea, teary eyes, or light patterns), where the pain is located (such as left side, temple, or forehead), the general character of the pain (such as throbbing, squeezing, or dull), its intensity (whether you had to stop what you were doing and lie down or if you could continue working), duration,

I used to take 7 different medications for my migraines and chronic daily headaches. Some were for pain, others for depression, and I had to take additional drugs just to deal with the acne and nausea caused by the other prescriptions. I always felt doped up and run down. I stopped driving because I was afraid I wouldn't be able to react quickly enough if someone cut me off. Basically, I was imprisoned in my own pain-ridden body. Then I saw an advertisement in the newspaper and decided to give acupuncture a try. I went to a naturopath who not only treated me with needles and herbs but also taught me how to eat. Although it was hard at first, I stuck with it, and today, 3 years later, I am off all of my medications, my figure is back, and my headaches are a memory from the past.

—Maggie, a housewife in her late 40s

triggers (such as red wine or ice cream), aggravating factors (such as noise, bright lights, or stress), what treatment you tried (such as ice, OTCs, acupressure, or herbs) and whether or not it was successful.

Keep in mind that there is generally a 3- to 12-hour lag period between when a food is consumed and the onset of your headache (but sometimes it can take up to a week). As soon as your headache comes on, write down everything you ate in recent hours plus any other possible stimuli whether it be emotional, hormonal, and/or environmental. You may notice your headache intensifies on the weekend, when you do not have your daily cup of coffee, or when your in-laws are over. Once you have identified possible triggers, eliminate as many as you can. This may be enough to end your headaches, but, if not, rest assured that your time was not spent in vain; when you go to see a practitioner, this preliminary work will give you both a head start in your detective work.

Treat the Whole Body, Not Just the Head

Unlike one-time ailments that can be treated and forgotten, chronic headaches require a constant commitment. If you fall off the wagon and go on a chocolate binge, for example, chances are your headache will reappear. On the other hand, armed with the knowledge of the consequences of such a binge, you need only get back up and try again. Finding a treatment method that works, establishing long-lasting wellness, requires a sustained look at the big picture and multiple approaches that often include changes in diet, lifestyle, and exercise habits.

Optimum health depends on the proper functioning of 3 interconnected systems in your body. The first is the metabolic process, which involves the absorption and utilization of nutrients, as well as the elimination of wastes, and all the complicated biochemical relationships that are necessary for proper cellular function. The second system is the musculoskeletal structure, which includes all the muscles, bones, ligaments, nerves, blood vessels, and organs, as well as their various functions. The third system is made up of your mind, emotions, and spiritual outlook.

Since headaches are most often the result of multiple causes, one therapy modality alone will not be as effective in eliminating your headache as a combination of therapies addressing the different causes.

The first system, your biochemistry or metabolism, is directed by the interactions of your hormonal, circulatory, and digestive systems. When they are functioning smoothly, your entire body benefits; when they are at odds, the rest of your organism suffers. Food allergies and toxic contaminants interfere with proper metabolism, and detoxification, allergy elimination, proper nutrition, vitamins, enzymes, and minerals are essential to good health.

The second system, your musculoskeletal system, is the building in which you live; your tissues, muscles, ligaments, tendons, and bones are like the steel, wood, brick, concrete, and glass building materials. If you are to withstand the storms and earthquakes of your life, you must have a firm foundation. It needs to be maintained and strengthened through healthy choices and habits, like exercise, stretching, and good posture, otherwise structural imbalances occur and health problems follow.

The third system includes your emotions, personality, lifestyle, psychological condition, and spiritual outlook. The body and mind directly affect one another; stress and conflict in the mind will most certainly produce tensions in the body. Headaches are not just in your head. Dealing with your emotions, for example, can have a positive impact on your health.

A balanced energetic interplay among these 3 systems is essential to effective and comprehensive headache treatment. If one is imbalanced, the others cannot thrive, which leads the way to ill health.

Useful Short-term Strategies for Decreasing and Eliminating Your Pain

(See Chapters 16 and 17 for details on the techniques below.)

- acupuncture/acupressure
- detoxification therapy
- elimination diet
- flower essences
- herbal medicine
- homeopathy
- neural therapy
- structural realignment (osteopathy/chiropractic/alphabiotics/craniosacral therapy)

Determining the Most Effective Therapy

When your body is weakened, it often needs a jump-start to set in motion its capacity to heal itself. Alternative therapies provide this and remove obstacles to your overall healing process. No matter what its underlying cause, each headache can be treated in at least 5 different ways. Don't be tricked into thinking that one remedy is the answer; it often takes a combination of therapies to resolve the condition that has caused your headaches.

Many alternative physicians specialize in more than one modality (such as the naturopath who uses homeopathy, herbs, and massage), and those who do not often work closely with specialists in other alternative health-care fields. This is good news for headache sufferers, because headaches respond well to combination therapies, especially a mix of metabolic, structural, and psychological/emotional treatments.

METABOLIC/BIOCHEMICAL/ BIOENERGETIC-BASED THERAPIES

The alternative treatments in this category work particularly well for vascular-type headaches, as well as for headaches stemming from underlying conditions such as hormonal imbalances, digestive disorders, blood clotting, immune deficiencies, allergies/sensitivities, systemic toxicity, circulation problems, nutritional deficiencies, and overall body stress.

STRUCTURALLY ORIENTED THERAPIES

Poor vertebral alignment can reduce blood flow to the brain, and chronic dysfunction can throw off the body's structure, making structurally oriented therapies an important tool for headache relief and prevention. Besides keeping you from unnecessary surgery (only 1% of head or neck pain sufferers for whom surgery is recommended actually require it[2]), these therapies can be combined with other therapies to reduce stress, mitigate pain, and provide both short- and long-term relief for all types of headaches.

PSYCHO/EMOTIONAL THERAPIES

Scientific studies document the fact that positive feelings and attitudes bolster the immune system, while negative ones tear it down. Your attitude toward and response to stressful emotions affects your headaches for better or worse. Headaches can be an opportunity for you to find a healthy way to release your negative or unexpressed feelings. Many modalities are designed to help you accomplish this and heal the psychological and emotional components of your headache. It is important to remember that while others can help you, ultimately, it is you who must change if you want to heal.

Long-term Strategies to Eliminate Headaches

Determine and eliminate your exposure to headache trigger(s).

- allergy testing
- elimination diet
- headache diary
- nutritional and hormonal analysis

Modify your response to any reaction-causing foods and/or substances.

- acupuncture
- allergy desensitization
- homeopathic desensitization
- Nambudripad allergy elimination technique

Detoxify your system.

- acupuncture
- Ayurvedic medicine
- bodywork
- detoxification therapy
- herbal therapy
- homeopathy
- naturopathy

- nutritional therapy
- traditional Chinese medicine

Repair your system metabolically, structurally, emotionally.

- **metabolic/bioenergetic repair**
  —acupuncture
  —Ayurvedic medicine
  —energy medicine
  —environmental medicine
  —herbal medicine
  —homeopathy
  —nutritional therapy
  —neural therapy
  —oxygen therapy
  —traditional Chinese medicine
- **structural repair**
  —alphabiotics
  —bodywork
  —biological dentistry
  —chiropractic
  —craniosacral therapy
  —neural therapy
  —osteopathy
- **emotional repair**
  —aromatherapy
  —biofeedback
  —flower essence therapy
  —hypnotherapy
  —psychotherapy (many methods)
- **self-care**
  —affirmations/autosuggestions
  —breathing exercises
  —creative visualization
  —dietary changes/vitamin supplementation
  —exercise
  —folk remedies

—ice and heat

—journal writing

—lifestyle changes

—massage

—meditation

—relaxation exercises

—headache support groups

RECOMMENDED READING

Alternative Medicine: The Definitive Guide. Compiled by the Burton Goldberg Group. Tiburon, CA: Future Medicine Publishing, 1994.

"Arthritis Unyielding to Drugs." *Medical Advertising News* (May 1991): 26-27.

Braly, James, M.D., and Torbet, Laura. *Dr. Braly's Food Allergy and Nutrition Revolution*. New Canaan, CT: Keats Publishing, Inc., 1992.

Clark, Linda, M.A. *A Handbook of Natural Remedies for Common Ailments*. Greenwich, CT: The Devin-Adair Company, 1976.

Faber, William J., D.O. *Pain, Pain Go Away*. San Jose, CA: ISHI Press International, 1990.

Herzberg, Eileen. *Migraine: A Comprehensive Guide to Gentle, Safe & Effective Treatment*, Rockport, MA: Element Inc, 1994.

Hills, Hilda Cherry. *Good Food to Fight Migraine*. New Canaan, CT: Keats Publishing, Inc., 1979.

Igram, Cass, M.D. *Who Needs Headaches?* Cedar Rapids, IA: Literary Visions Publishing, 1991.

Jensen, Bernard, D.C., Ph.D. *Tissue Cleansing through Bowel Management*, 10th ed. Escondido, CA: Bernard Jensen Publishing, 1981.

Lipton, Richard B., M.D., Newman, Lawrence C., M.D., and MacLean, Helene. *Migraine/Beating the Odds: The Doctor's Guide to Reducing Your Risk*. Reading, MA: Addison-Wesley Publishing Company, 1992.

Nambudripad, Devi S., D.C., L.Ac., R.N., Ph.D. *Say Goodbye to Illness*. Buena Park, CA: Delta Publishing, 1993.

National Headache Foundation Fact Sheet. Chicago: National Headache Foundation, October 1994.

Rapoport, Alan M., M.D. and Sheftell, Fred D., M.D. *Headache Relief*. New York: Simon & Schuster, 1990.

Rapoport, Alan M., M.D. and Sheftell, Fred D., M.D. *Headache Relief for Women*. New York: Little, Brown and Company, 1995.

Robbins, Lawrence, M.D. and Lang, Susan. *Headache Help*. New York: Houghton Mifflin Company, 1995.

Sacks, Oliver, M.D. *Migraine: Understanding a Common Disorder.*, Berkeley, CA: University of California Press, 1985.

Simpson, Kristine, et al., eds. *The Experts Speak 1996: The Role of Nutrition in Medicine*. Sacramento, CA: Kirk Hamilton PA-C, 1996.

Solomon, Seymour, M.D., and Fraccaro, Steven. *The Headache Book*. Mount Vernon, NY: Consumer Reports Books, 1991.

Stang, P.E. and Osterhaus, J.T. "Impact of Migraine in the United States: Data from the National Health Interview Survey." *Headache* 33 (1993), 29-35.

Stromfeld, Jan and Weil, Anita. *Free Yourself from Headaches: The Natural Drug-Free Program for Prevention and Relief*. Palm Beach Gardens, FL: The Upledger Institute, Frog, Ltd., 1995.

Part Two

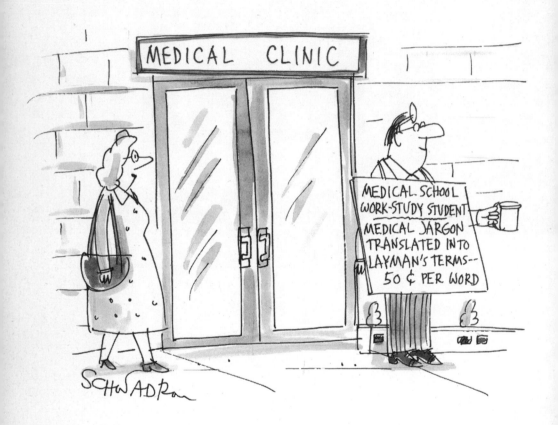

Chapter 5

Organic Headaches

Organic headaches result from causes such as a brain tumor or hemorrhage. Conventional medicine emergency procedures are normally required to respond to the urgency of the condition, but once the crisis is over, alternative medicine can help rebuild health.

Although all headaches are organic in nature, the term "organic headaches" denotes headaches that are signs of more serious, or even life-threatening, medical conditions. While only 10% of severe headaches (1 to 1.5% of *all* headaches) are expressions of serious problems, they warrant discussion, especially because organic headaches serve as a loud warning that must be heeded immediately if the sufferer wishes to be successfully treated.

Most, but not all, organic headaches are marked by excruciating pain that appears suddenly, with little or no warning. The onset of an organic headache may be the first time the sufferer has ever felt such intense pain. With time, these headaches become increasingly persistent, until it is impossible to ignore them. Organic headaches can disguise themselves in rare instances as other types of headaches, especially migraines, so any headache that fits the symptoms described below should be discussed immediately with a medical professional. Tests such

Organic Headaches at a Glance

The following conditions produce headaches that are considered "organic" in nature and may have serious health implications.

- Brain tumor
- Meningitis
- Aneurysm
- Trigeminal neuralgia
- Occipital neuralgia
- Temporal arteritis
- Glaucoma
- Subdural hematoma
- Hemicrania continua
- High blood pressure
- Spinal tap

MRI, or magnetic resonance imaging, is a scanning test which uses radiofrequency radiation to produce a high resolution picture of the body part under scanning. This test can pick up abnormalities in the body that are not visible in an X ray. **CT** (computed tomography) scan, formerly CAT scan, is an X-ray technique that provides a detailed cross-section view of tissue structure in the part of the body being scanned; it is useful for detecting tumors, fluid accumulations, and bone dislocations. **EEG** refers to electro-encephalogram, which is a map or graph of electrical activity in the brain, as measured in brain waves. Brain wave activity varies considerably during the day from sleep to heightened alertness; generally, faster states indicate intellectual activity or anxiety while slower states indicate relaxation or sleep.

as MRIs, CT scans, X rays, EEGs, and blood tests can all be used to determine the nature of these headaches.

More than 300 conditions are believed to be responsible for organic headaches. The most common of these headaches include brain tumor headaches, meningitis headaches, encephalitis headaches, brain hemorrhage (or aneurysm) headaches, cranial arteritis headaches, temporal arteritis headaches, glaucoma headaches, concussion headaches, and severe hypertension headaches. Many of these conditions do not cause headaches right away but instead lead to a gradual worsening, until the condition begins to occupy so much space that it stretches brain membranes or the pain-sensitive blood vessels at the base of the brain. Some of the most common types of organic headaches are described below.

> *The term "organic headaches" is used to denote headaches that are signs of more serious, or even life-threatening medical conditions. While only 10% of severe headaches (1 to 1.5% of all headaches) are expressions of serious problems, they warrant discussion, especially because organic headaches serve as a loud warning.*

BRAIN TUMOR HEADACHE

Affecting only 1% of headache sufferers, headaches that arise in conjunction with a brain tumor are caused by a tumor growing and pressing against the meninges, the major arteries or sinuses in the skull. Since a brain tumor must grow rather large before it actually reaches a place with pain-sensitive nerves, these headaches are usually a sign of a brain tumor in its advanced stages.

It must be noted, however, that not all brain tumors cause head pain; those that do result in headaches that either come on slowly as an intermittent, generalized pain gradually becoming more frequent and severe over time or strike suddenly and grow progressively worse in a very short period of time.

Symptom Chart—Organic Headaches

SYMPTOMS	HEADACHE TYPE	PAIN LOCATION
Description: intermittent, generalized pain that gradually becomes more frequent and severe; worse with head movement, stooping over, coughing, and/or straining; more pronounced in the morning (Note: brain tumors are not always accompanied by headaches.) **Other Symptoms:** mood swings; speech and personality changes; concentration difficulties; visual and other sensory disturbances; problems with balance, gait, and/or coordination; unexplained drowsiness; convulsions; fainting; vomiting; weakness or numbness in one part of body **Duration:** relatively recent in origin **Frequency:** tends to increase in severity, duration, and frequency until continuous	**BRAIN TUMOR HEADACHE**	near or around tumor site, usually one-sided
Description: intense, generalized headache of sudden onset, often with considerable eye pain **Other Symptoms:** high fever; light sensitivity; mental confusion; drowsiness; vomiting; stiff neck; causes overall sickness and total disability	**MENINGITIS HEADACHE**	total head pain
Description: early symptoms similar to migraine or cluster headache **Symptoms of Small Rupture:** persistent neck pain and stiffness followed by mental confusion and pain in back and legs **Symptoms of Burst Vessel:** (leading to stroke) sudden unbearable headache, double vision, neck rigidity, and loss of consciousness	**ANEURYSM HEADACHE**	varies according to occurrence of clot or ruptured vessel
Description: intense stabbing pain that lasts from seconds to minutes; mainly in middle to old age	**TRIGEMINAL NEURALGIA HEADACHE**	facial area, especially mouth and jaw
Description: jabbing pain like icepick stabs in back of the head; generally accompanied by neck and shoulder tenderness; mainly in middle to old age	**OCCIPITAL NEURALGIA HEADACHE**	back of head and neck

UNDERLYING CAUSES AND TRIGGERS	PRIMARY AND SECONDARY TREATMENTS	SELF-CARE TREATMENTS	WHERE IN THE BOOK PAGE #
Causes: unknown	see medical doctor; can be supplemented by: ■ acupuncture ■ herbal medicine ■ homeopathy ■ neural therapy ■ nutritional therapy ■ traditional Chinese medicine	■ aromatherapy ■ affirmations ■ biofeedback ■ breathing exercises ■ creative visualization ■ exercise ■ flower remedies ■ herbal supplements ■ folk remedies ■ ice and heat ■ journal writing ■ lifestyle changes ■ meditation ■ massage ■ nutritional therapy ■ support groups ■ relaxation techniques	Page 159
Causes: inflammation of brain membranes brought on by bacterial or viral infection	see medical doctor		Page 164
Causes: rupturing or bursting of blood vessel **Triggers:** high blood pressure, heart disease, physical exertion	see medical doctor		Page 165
Causes: unknown nerve disorder	see medical doctor		Page 165
Causes: unknown nerve disorder	see medical doctor		Page 166

Symptom Chart—Organic Headaches (continued)

SYMPTOMS	HEADACHE TYPE	PAIN LOCATION
Description: piercing, burning, or jabbing pain, especially when chewing or opening mouth **Other Symptoms:** weight loss, weakness, body aches, low-grade fever, vision disturbances (which can lead to blindness if not treated); mainly among people over 50	TEMPORAL ARTERITIS HEADACHE	temples, around ears, and on side of the jaw
Description: throbbing pain, reddened eyes; seeing halos or rings around lights	GLAUCOMA HEADACHE	around or behind eye or in forehead
Description: localized or generalized pain after severe head injury; can mimic migraine or cluster headache symptoms **Other Symptoms:** visual disturbances, impairment of speech and/or other sensory and intellectual functions; fatigue, mood swings, concentration difficulties, memory loss; drowsiness, especially within minutes or hours of injury **Frequency:** once it starts, occurs daily and is frequently resistant to treatment	SUBDURAL HEMATOMA HEADACHE	at site of injury or total head pain
Description: dull, throbbing pain interspersed with brief but intense jabs of pain; pain can last 5 minutes to an hour and recur up to 5 times in 24 hours; accompanied by migraine-like symptoms	HEMICRANIA CONTINUA HEADACHE	on one side of the head
Description: gradual or rapid onset, mild to severe throbbing pain, most severe in morning	HYPERTENSION OR HIGH BLOOD PRESSURE HEADACHE	generalized total head pain or encircling "hat-band" pain
Description: throbbing or pounding pain with migraine-like symptoms and muscle spasms in neck	SPINAL TAP HEADACHE	head, neck, and/or shoulder area

UNDERLYING CAUSES AND TRIGGERS	PRIMARY AND SECONDARY TREATMENTS	SELF-CARE TREATMENTS	WHERE IN THE BOOK PAGE #
Causes: inflammation of the temporal arteries (located behind temple) due to an immune-system reaction	see medical doctor		Page 166
Causes: inherited eye disease, digestive/liver dysfunction	see medical doctor; can be supplemented by: ■ acupuncture ■ homeopathy ■ neural therapy ■ nutritional therapy ■ traditional Chinese medicine		Page 167
Causes: injury to head	see medical doctor		Page 167
Causes: unknown	see medical doctor		Page 168
Causes: very high blood pressure (systolic over 200, diastolic over 100)	see medical doctor; can be supplemented by: ■ acupuncture ■ homeopathy ■ neural therapy ■ nutritional therapy ■ traditional Chinese medicine		Page 169
Causes: Lumbar Puncture Diagnostic Test	see medical doctor		Page 169

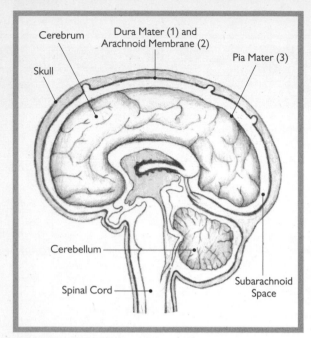

Figure 5.1—The 3 layers of the meninges.

This pain is often described as a tight band around the head that is punctuated with a persistent ache that is concentrated in one distinct spot of the head.

Brain tumor headaches are often aggravated by movements, such as coughing or sudden turns of the head. They can be so devastating that movements as simple as standing up or sitting down become unbearable. Other symptoms may include projectile vomiting, disturbances of vision, smell, or hearing, speech and/or personality changes, problems with balance, gait, or coordination, numbness, fainting, memory loss, disorientation, inexplicable drowsiness, and seizures—all symptoms of impaired brain functioning which may actually precede the headache itself.

MENINGITIS HEADACHE

These headaches are triggered by meningitis, an inflammation of the membranes, or meninges, that surround the brain and spinal cord. Meningitis is brought on by a bacterial or, less commonly, a viral infection which makes its way into the central nervous system through the bloodstream or directly through the ear, nose, or sinuses.

Generally easy to recognize, meningitis-related headaches are intense, generalized headaches of sudden onset, often with fever, intense eye pain, a stiff neck, light sensitivity, vomiting, weakness, mental confusion, and drowsiness. When triggered by a bacterial infection, meningitis is more likely to be fatal than when caused by a viral infection. Antibiotics are administered for bacterial meningitis but are usually ineffective for viral meningitis, which, fortunately, often responds to alternative medical treatment.

ANEURYSM HEADACHE

This type of headache is caused by an aneurysm. A blood vessel or artery in the brain swells and then ruptures or slowly leaks, causing blood to seep into the membranes of the brain. Aneurysm headaches tend to be sudden and severe, with initial symptoms similar to those of migraines or cluster headaches.

A small rupture can cause the aneurysm to leak slowly over a period of minutes to hours, leading to persistent neck pain and stiffness, followed by pain in the back and legs, vomiting, mental confusion, lethargy, paralysis, loss of consciousness, and other signs that warn of an impending stroke. If a blood vessel bursts violently and results in an actual stroke, a person experiences a sudden, unbearable headache, double vision, neck rigidity, followed by a rapid loss of consciousness. Many factors may bring on an aneurysm, including the following:

- high blood pressure
- thickening or hardening of artery walls
- heart disease
- a congenital weakness in blood vessel walls which allows them to become abnormally swollen.
- strenuous physical exertion such as running or sex.

TRIGEMINAL NEURALGIA HEADACHE

These headaches are marked by brief stabbing pains in the facial area, especially the mouth or jaw; although this knifelike pain lasts only a moment to several minutes, it may recur many times throughout the day. Pain is often provoked by cold air, opening the mouth, chewing, or touching the face and jaw.

These headaches are caused by the condition trigeminal neuralgia (also called *tic douloureux*, French for "painful spasm"), a little understood disorder of the trigeminal nerve which supplies feeling to the face, teeth, mouth, and nasal cavity and allows the mouth muscles to chew. Trigeminal neuralgia generally affects late middle-aged or elderly individuals, although it may occur in younger people as a symptom of multiple sclerosis. Some forms of trigeminal neuralgia respond to alternative methods of treatment.

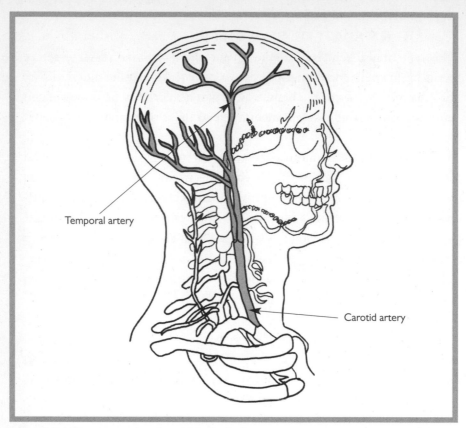

Temporal artery

Carotid artery

Figure 5.2—The temporal and carotid arteries.

OCCIPITAL NEURALGIA HEADACHE

Like trigeminal neuralgia, occipital neuralgia is a nerve disorder which is not well understood, but which is known to produce headaches. The problematic nerve is the occipital nerve, which is responsible for directing sensation to and from the back portion of the scalp. The nerve may have become pinched by tense muscles or scar tissue or inflamed by other conditions.

Although not as intense as those caused by trigeminal neuralgia, occipital neuralgia headaches are also characterized by jabbing or aching, ice pick-type stabs, but in the back of the head. Tenderness in and around the neck and head area is another symptom. These headaches mostly occur among the elderly.

TEMPORAL ARTERITIS HEADACHE

Giving rise to burning, boring, or piercing head pain, temporal arteritis is a rare condition that is marked by the swelling of the temporal artery, the artery located behind the temples, or other scalp arteries. There may even be a visibly red, tender, and swollen artery at the temple where the headache is located. This condition is most common in people over 50, with incidence increasing with age, although in isolated cases it may affect individuals as young as 35.

Localized in the temples or around the ears and the side of the jaw, these headaches are intensified by chewing and increase with severity and duration with time; although they can strike with no other symptoms, these headaches can be accompanied by visual disturbances, weight loss, weakness, low fever, and aches in the body and limbs. Blindness or stroke can result if this type of headache goes untreated.

GLAUCOMA HEADACHE

Often causing referred pain that feels like a headache in its later stages, glaucoma is a disease characterized by intense pressure in the eyes. As glaucoma begins, the sufferer has a milky white film in the eye, and as the disease progresses, it produces severe throbbing pain behind or around the eye and in the forehead. The sufferer will sometimes also have red eyes and see rings around lights. This is a very serious condition; if not promptly treated, it can lead to blindness.

SUBDURAL HEMATOMA HEADACHE

Often caused by a fall or blow to the head, a subdural hematoma is caused when blood accumulates in one part of the head under the skull, very much like a blood blister, a form of hematoma most people have experienced at one time or another. It is known as a subdural hemotoma because the location of the "blister" is beneath the dura mater, 1 of the 3 layers of meninges, the membranes surrounding the brain and spinal cord (see Figure 5.1 on page 164). If the fall or blow to the head is forceful enough, it can tear the veins in the meninges and allow blood to leak out and pool between meningeal layers, thus putting pressure on the brain.

Meninges are the 3 membranous layers that surround the brain and the spinal cord. The 3 layers are the dura mater, the pia mater, and the arachnoid.

Subdural hematoma headaches are accompanied by drowsiness, confusion, mood swings, fatigue, visual disturbances, nausea, weakness or paralysis in isolated areas, or, if left untreated, death. While symptoms can oc-

Organic Conditions Associated with Headaches

HEADACHES—Acoustic neuroma (benign tumor in the cells covering the auditory nerve), anemia, arthritis, carotidynia (inflammation around the carotid artery), cervical spondylosis (arthritis of the vertebral disks in the neck), cholesteatoma (infected cyst in the eardrum or middle ear), common cold, encephalitis (inflammation of the brain), epileptic seizure, fibromyalgia, hydrocephalus (brain swelling caused by over-accumulation of cerebrospinal fluid, the liquid surrounding the brain), hyperpituitarism, hypopituitarism, non-Hodgkin's lymphoma (cancer of the lymph nodes and lymphoid tissue), multiple myeloma (production of malignant plasma cells in the bone marrow), mumps, Paget's disease (a weakening, tightening, and deformity of the bones), palpilledema (swelling of the optic nerves), pheochromocytoma (tumor in central part of the adrenal, the glands above the kidneys), polycythemia vera (an overproduction of red and white blood cells and platelets), pseudotumor cerebri (swelling of the brain), severe kidney failure, sleep apnea (recurrent episodes of breathing cessation during sleep), shingles (nerve condition), stroke, thalamic syndrome (dysfunction of the thalamus brought on by stroke)

HEADACHES WITH FEVER—chronic fatigue syndrome, common cold, genital herpes, heatstroke, flu, HIV, Lyme disease, mastoiditis (inflammation of the mastoid, a bone behind the ear), infectious mononucleosis, peritonsillar abscess (a collection of pus between the tonsils and surrounding tissue due to infection), pharyngitis (inflammation of the pharynx, the part of the throat between the mouth and the esophagus), rabies, rubella (German measles), septic shock (severe drop in blood pressure due to the presence of microorganisms or their toxins in the bloodstream), syphilis, tonsillitis, typhoid fever

HEADACHES WITH FEVER AND NAUSEA—glomerulonephritis (inflammation of the glomeruli, tiny structures that filter blood in the kidneys), Legionnaires' disease, leukemia, malaria, polio, Rocky Mountain spotted fever, systemic lupus erythematosus (inflammation of connective tissues throughout the body), toxic shock syndrome[1]

cur within minutes of injury, they can also build over time, mimicking the symptoms of migraine, until they become increasingly persistent. The elderly are particularly prone to subdural hematomas, since they fall more often and their blood vessels are weak and particularly susceptible to damage. These headaches are treated by surgery.

HEMICRANIA CONTINUA HEADACHE

These headaches are extremely rare, one-sided headaches characterized by dull, throbbing, or pulsating pain interspersed with periods of intense jabs that feel like stabs from an ice pick. Generally, this intense pain persists from 5 minutes to an hour, then subsides and returns again later, as many as 5 times during a 24-hour period. These headaches are also associated with migraine-like symptoms, such as nausea and sensitivity to light. Men and women suffer equally, as do people of all ages. Alcohol or physical exertion can heighten these headaches.

HYPERTENSION OR HIGH BLOOD PRESSURE HEADACHE

This rare type of headache is not related to common high blood pressure but instead is due to a *sudden* rise in blood pressure (such as a reading of 270/130), which may cause swelling and tiny hemorrhages in the brain. The pain feels like a band around the head and is most severe in the morning, slowly improving as the day goes on.

High blood pressure, or hypertension, is a health problem that affects over 15% of the adults in the United States. Although the tendency toward hypertension is inherited, it is often brought about by dietary factors and is worsened by obesity and stress. If not treated, it can lead to hardening of the arteries (arteriosclerosis), and, eventually, heart disease, kidney failure, and aneurysms.

SPINAL TAP HEADACHE

Approximately a third of those who undergo the diagnostic test called the lumbar puncture or spinal tap get these headaches within 48 hours of the procedure (although some get them as long as two weeks afterward). Generally, these headaches are characterized by throbbing, pounding or aching pain in the front or back of the head or in the neck and shoulder area, with a reclining position offering the only relief. They re-

Signs of a Dangerous Headache

If you experience any of the following symptoms, consult a doctor immediately:

- Headaches that appear suddenly, especially if you don't have a history of headaches
- Headaches accompanied by vomiting, nausea, and/or high fever
- Headaches with severe neurological symptoms such as mental confusion, slurred speech, memory loss, sensory disturbance, double vision, loss of motor control, or seizures
- Headaches that do not fit a recognizable pattern of symptoms and pain
- Headaches that prevent you from participating in the activities of daily life
- Headaches that start in early childhood or in old age
- Headaches that grow more severe in intensity, duration, and frequency with time
- Headaches associated with a traumatic head injury
- Headaches that affect your breathing
- Headaches accompanied by clear fluid or blood coming out of the ears or nose
- Headaches accompanied by weakness or numbness on one side

semble migraines, as they are also accompanied by dizziness, nausea, light sensitivity and other visual disturbances; however, again, neck pain and spasm can also occur. Women with a history of headaches, people who are underweight, and young children tend to be more prone to them.

Although no one is certain as to why spinal taps sometimes trigger a headache, researchers suggest that they may be the result of cerebrospinal fluid leaking into the tissues through the puncture wound, causing a further loss in fluids, which brings about a low or negative pressure in the head, producing headaches. This may be why the smaller the needle, the lower the chance of inducing headaches.

Although spinal tap headaches usually go away on their own within a few weeks, persistent attacks are sometimes treated by injecting saline solution near the puncture wound of the initial spinal tap or by injecting the patient's own blood back into the spinal tap area (called an epidermal blood patch).

Diagnosing and Treating Underlying Causes

The treatment for organic headaches is quite different than that used for the other types of headaches explored in this book, because organic headaches result from causes that are normally treated with a combination of conventional and alternative medicine. Conventional medicine can be used to respond to the urgency of the condition through emergency procedures such as surgery or medication, and then, once the crisis is over, alternative medicine can be employed.

Even some of the severe disorders outlined in this chapter can be brought on by the same causes, triggers, and stressors discussed in Chapter 3, "What Causes Your Headache?" and thus can also be improved by most of the alternative therapies in this book. Consulting an alternative physician in addition to a conventional doctor will give your body a chance to recover by helping it to cleanse, repair, and rebuild, thus strengthening your immune system and your body's ability to heal itself.

ALTERNATIVE TREATMENTS

Since organic headaches are rare and best served by combination therapies, it is beyond the scope of this book to cover each one in detail; however, the treatment modalities listed below can help to alleviate symptoms and keep the problem from worsening.

METABOLIC/BIOENERGETIC/ BIOCHEMICAL-BASED THERAPIES

The following therapies, depending upon the symptoms and conditions of the organic problem, may be beneficial as complementary treatments for organic headaches:

See Chapter 17, An A-Z of Alternative Medicine, for more information on each treatment method.

Acupuncture
Ayurvedic Medicine
Detoxification Therapy
Energy Medicine
Environmental Medicine
Herbal Medicine
Homeopathy

Light Therapy
Magnetic Field Therapy
Naturopathy
Nutritional Therapy
Oxygen Therapy
Traditional Chinese Medicine

STRUCTURALLY ORIENTED THERAPIES

Depending upon the nature of the headache condition and underlying cause, the following therapies can also be useful:

Alphabiotics
Bodywork
Biological Dentistry
Chiropractic
Craniosacral Therapy
Neural Therapy
Osteopathy

PSYCHO/EMOTIONAL THERAPIES

Since they are directed toward emotional and psychological wellness, all of these therapies can be useful for those with a life-threatening or other severely disabling disorder:

Aromatherapy
Biofeedback
Flower Essence Therapy
Hypnotherapy
Psychotherapy

SELF-CARE OPTIONS

Again, depending upon the condition, the self-help techniques listed in Chapter 16, "An A-Z of Self-Care Options," can also be helpful for organic headaches.

RECOMMENDED READING

Alternative Medicine: The Definitive Guide. Compiled by the Burton Goldberg Group. Tiburon, CA: Future Medicine Publishing, 1994.

Diamond, Seymour, M.D., and Still, Bill and Cynthia. *The Hormone Headache.* New York: Macmillan, 1995.

Faber, William J., D.O.. *Pain, Pain Go Away.* San Jose, CA: ISHI Press International, 1990.

Herzberg, Eileen. *Migraine: A Comprehensive Guide to Gentle, Safe & Effective Treatment.* Rockport, MA: Element Inc, 1994.

Igram, Cass, M.D. *Who Needs Headaches?* Cedar Rapids, IA: Literary Visions Publishing, 1991.

Lipton, Richard B., M.D., Newman, Lawrence C., M.D., and MacLean, Helene. *Migraine/Beating The Odds: The Doctor's Guide to Reducing Your Risk.* Reading, MA: Addison Wesley Publishing Company, 1992.

National Headache Foundation Fact Sheet. Chicago: National Headache Foundation, October 1994.

Privitera, James R., M.D. "Clots: Life's Biggest Killer." *Health Freedom News* (September 1993), 22-23.

Rapoport, Alan M., M.D. and Sheftell, Fred D., M.D. *Headache Relief.* New York: Simon & Schuster, 1990.

Rapoport, Alan M., M.D. and Sheftell, Fred D., M.D. *Headache Relief for Women.* New York: Little, Brown and Company, 1995.

Robbins, Lawrence, M.D. and Lang, Susan. *Headache Help.* New York: Houghton Mifflin Company, 1995.

Sacks, Oliver, M.D. *Migraine: Understanding a Common Disorder.* Berkeley, CA: University of California Press, 1985.

Stromfeld, Jan and Weil, Anita. *Free Yourself from Headaches: The Natural Drug-Free Program for Prevention and Relief.* Palm Beach Gardens, FL: The Upledger Institute, Frog, Ltd., 1995.

Solomon, Seymour, M.D. and Fraccaro, Steven. *The Headache Book.* Mount Vernon, NY: Consumer Reports Books, 1991.

Chapter 6

Tension Headaches

Tension headaches are associated with cycles of pain because stress of any kind can cause muscle tension, which in turn can cause pain, which can then bring about more stress. Where this stress originates depends entirely on the mind and body of the individual. Nobody has discovered the definitive cause of tension headaches because there isn't one—there are many.

Jackie, a financial broker in her fifties, was a classic type-A personality, the kind of person who made sure that if she did something, she did it well. A superachiever all the way, she had found no challenge too great for her—until she got headaches. Then for the first time in her life, she was losing a battle, and by the time she went to see Judyth Reichenberg-Ullman, N.D., a naturopathic physician in Edmonds, Washington, Jackie was a wreck. She was experiencing daily headaches and was chronically constipated. In her words, "My pain was so bad, I wanted to shoot my head off."

Right away, Dr. Reichenberg-Ullman encouraged Jackie to talk about herself, and as she did, it became clear that Jackie was living a high-energy, fast-paced life that left her stressed out and exhausted. She drank 2 giant cups of coffee and 2 glasses of wine daily. Every day by dinnertime, her muscles would start to ache all over, and then the headache would appear, worsening until she felt as if a band of metal rings was squeezing around her head.

Dr. Reichenberg-Ullman listened to Jackie attentively and looked for insight into her overall condition, not just the state of her body and her head pain. She realized that, besides bringing pain, Jackie's headaches were an expression of imbalanced energy—her mind and body telling her to get out of the race, while her habits kept her running. Keeping this discovery in mind, Dr. Reichenberg-Ullman chose a homeopathic remedy called *Nux vomica* 200C, a high dose of a very diluted form of seeds from a poisonous nut tree. Jackie began taking it daily.

The results were dramatic. Three weeks after starting *Nux vomica*, Jackie's headaches completely disappeared. A month later, she realized that, without really thinking about it, she had begun to eat differently, craving whole grains and vegetables instead of sugar and salt. Her life was simpler and more balanced; she had slowed down, and now, headache free, she was enjoying her life again.

What Is a Tension Headache?

Although Jackie's tension-type headaches were triggered by her stressful life and unbalanced diet, tension headaches can be brought on by many factors. Calling head pain a tension headache is just a simple way of describing a tenseness or a tightness in the head, face, and neck. For one person, this tenseness might occur only in the temples and stay there; for another it may press against the back of the head for a while and then spread across the entire head; and to someone like Jackie, it may get a hold of the head and squeeze it like it plans never to let go.

Even though conventional research says that 90% of all headache sufferers are believed to be afflicted with tension headaches, the tension-type headache is a vastly overused category. Any headache not recognized as a migraine or a cluster is generally tossed into this catch-all type, whether or not it has anything to do with tension.

Even though conventional research says that 90% of all headache sufferers are believed to be afflicted with tension headaches, the tension-type headache is a vastly overused category. Any headache not recognized as a migraine or a cluster is generally tossed into this catch-all type, whether or not it has anything to do with tension. We prefer to substitute the word "stress" for "tension," because stress can mean anything that affects the balance of the body, whether it is repressed emotions, faulty dietary choices, constipation, inadequate sleep, food allergies, hormonal changes, or sensitivities to chemicals or inhalants in your home or workplace.

Symptom Chart—Tension Headaches

SYMPTOMS	HEADACHE TYPE	PAIN LOCATION
Description: gradual onset, mild, steady or dull, aching, sometimes described as viselike squeezing or heavy pressure around head; usually does not throb **Other Symptoms:** knotted, clenched, and uncomfortable feeling in back, shoulders, and neck; stress; anxiety; mood swings; depression **Duration:** can last 1 hour to all day **Frequency:** Episodic—once or twice a week; once a month or less; Chronic—can occur daily or almost daily, more than 15 times per month	MUSCLE CONTRACTION HEADACHE (TENSION HEADACHE)	most often located on both sides of head or as band-like sensation around head or back of neck spreading to whole head sometimes accompanied by aching shoulders

UNDERLYING CAUSES AND TRIGGERS	PRIMARY AND SECONDARY TREATMENTS	SELF-CARE TREATMENTS	WHERE IN THE BOOK PAGE #
Causes: metabolic imbalances, structural disturbances, emotional/psychological factors **Triggers:** dietary and/or environmental sensitivity, hormonal imbalance, autoimmune disturbances, lifestyle factors, structural disturbances, psychological stress	**Primary:** ■ acupuncture ■ detoxification ■ environmental medicine ■ homeopathy ■ naturopathy ■ neural therapy ■ nutritional therapy ■ psychotherapy ■ traditional Chinese medicine **Secondary:** ■ Ayurvedic medicine ■ bodywork ■ chiropractic ■ craniosacral therapy ■ herbal medicine	■ aromatherapy ■ affirmations ■ biofeedback ■ breathing exercises ■ creative visualization ■ exercise ■ flower remedies ■ herbal supplements ■ folk remedies ■ ice and heat ■ journal writing ■ lifestyle changes ■ massage ■ meditation ■ nutritional therapy ■ relaxation techniques ■ support groups	Page 173

The Causes of Tension Headaches

Conventional researchers admit that to them the cause of tension headaches remains unknown. Nobody has discovered the *definitive* cause of tension headaches because there isn't one—there are many.

However, tension headaches are not a hopeless affliction with no end in sight. To an alternative practitioner, tension headaches are just the opposite: They are a chance for people to learn more about themselves, to unravel the dynamics of their own internal and external environments, and to see if they can figure out what their headaches are asking them to change.

Less demanding than migraines, tension headaches are associated with cycles of pain because stress of any kind can cause muscle tension, which in turn can cause pain, which can then bring about more stress, and so on. Stress undoubtedly plays a major role in muscular tension because, as the body tightens and reacts further, more pressure is placed on joints and muscles. As your muscles become chronically overfatigued, they get less and less oxygen and allow chemicals such as histamines to accumulate. This leads to muscle spasms and contractions, which in turn put pressure on nerves—and your headache arrives.

The pain you feel is generally attributed to 2 mechanisms involved in the muscle contraction itself. The first is nerve compression within the muscle, which is typically brought on by factors such as structural misalignment or poor posture. The second is the nerve irritation generated by the buildup of metabolic wastes and is closely related to decreased blood and lymph circulation due to hormonal imbalances, reproductive disorders, emotional stress, or digestive problems.

See Chapter 3, What Causes Your Headache?, for more information on the possible causes of tension headaches.

Today we know that the pain that comes from the tensing and stretching of the scalp and neck is only a component of tension headaches. It may worsen them but is not their primary characteristic. In fact, there is a growing belief among researchers that tension headaches are actually related to migraine, cluster, and other vascular-type headaches, for all of these headaches are marked by alterations of muscle tension, fluctuations of serotonin, the contraction and dilation of blood vessels, and pressure in nerves of the head and neck.

This range of characteristics makes it futile to draw sweeping generalizations about underlying causes or even to attempt to highlight one cause over another. Tension headaches, like all other kinds of headache, are related to stress, but where this stress originates depends entirely on the body and mind of the individual sufferer. One headache may come from a big project that requires long sleepless nights slumped over a computer in an improperly lit room, while another could be the result of a bout of depression or a digestive disturbance caused by a binge of junk food.

Diagnosing and Treating Underlying Causes

Once again, remember, the alternative approach views the body and mind as a functioning whole, each affecting the other. Consider your whole body first:

- **Do you have any digestive disturbances?** These can be noted by red eyes (usually one), mouth sores (canker, not herpes), coated tongue, heartburn, burping, belching, abdominal pain, bloating, flatulence, low back pain, or calloused feet. Remember, most head pain that is linked to digestive disturbances is located in the frontal area of the head.
- **Do you have any pelvic disturbances?** In women, ovarian/uterine; in men, prostate/hemorrhoids; signs include low back pain, neck stiffness, PMS, menstrual cramps, breast tenderness, vaginal discharge; prostate enlargement, lower abdominal pain, and/or rectal pain. Pelvic disturbances usually are manifested as head pain located in the neck and at the back of the head.
- **Do you have both digestive and pelvic disturbances?** People who suffer from

Tension: Stress in Disguise

Stress—be it physical, environmental, emotional, or mental—heavily taxes the body. It hits the internal organs, the liver, thyroid, adrenals, the immune system, the digestive system, and forces the central nervous system (the primary mediator between stress and your body's life force) into overdrive.

When your mind entertains a stressful thought or when you eat a trigger food, the spinal cord and peripheral nerves send distress signals to the internal organs. Your stomach responds by secreting hydrochloric acid, the liver starts synthesizing sugar or cholesterol, the adrenals react by producing more adrenaline and other hormones, the pancreas releases more insulin, the thyroid pumps out hormones that speed up metabolism, and the thymus and its immune system benefits shrink.

Since every one of these responses is connected to your body's ability to manufacture glucose for energy (which is the brain's primary fuel), the reactions described above translate into a sudden internal thud as your blood sugar drops to insufficient levels, your blood clots (during stress, platelets cluster, or aggregate, in preparation for a possible injury and this produces "knots" in your blood), and your blood vessels swell.

179

a combination of these 2 disturbances usually get their headaches at the side or top of the head.

Bearing in mind these physiological disturbances, consult your practitioner and be examined to determine the extent of the condition. Ask your practitioner, for example, to check for the size of the liver, the tension in your stomach, the level of the portal vein blood stagnation, the size of your spleen, and the loudness of the first and second heart sounds. Armed with this information, you and your doctor as a team can plan a treatment strategy.

To discover the cause of stress, different evaluations and treatments are required. The stress of an upcoming presentation that could get you a promotion, for instance, might bring on muscle spasms in your neck, which then could twist your neck joints and give you headaches. A week before the big day, let's say, you go to a chiropractor, and she works on your joints, and your headaches disappear, but the next day they come back. Why? Because unless you do something about the initial stressor, the condition will return again and again; the initiating factor is still part of your life. Ultimately, it is not the chiropractic but the overall changes in the way you live that will determine whether your headaches remain part of your life.

While also treating the obvious cause and pain of your headache, an alternative practitioner will look at it from metabolic, structural, and emotional vantage points, doing whatever is necessary to help you penetrate layer by layer until you reach the cause of your headache—and only then will you be able to bring your body and mind into a state of lasting balance.

ALTERNATIVE TREATMENTS

METABOLIC/BIOENERGETIC/ BIOCHEMICAL-BASED THERAPIES

Tension headaches that are related to nutritional deficiencies, digestive disturbances, allergic reactions and sensitivities, and hormonal imbalances respond well to therapies associated with chemical or metabolic restructuring.

See Chapter 17, An A-Z of Alternative Medicine, for more information on each treatment method.

AYURVEDIC MEDICINE

Cindy, a 38-year-old administrative assistant, lived a stressful life. She had a demanding job that forced her to work long hours and spend many weekends working at her computer, she had 3 stepchildren, and she lived in constant low-grade head pain, which was punctuated by 2 or 3 days of debilitating pain and severe muscle spasm in her neck. When she went to a neurologist for an MRI, her test came back negative, so she was given some muscle relaxants and told that her headaches were due to stress and muscle tension.

Finally at her wit's end, burned out, and groggy from her medication, she went to see Nancy Lonsdorf, M.D., at the Maharishi Ayur-Veda Medical Center in Washington, D.C. Dr. Lonsdorf listened to Cindy's complaints and performed a thorough examination, at which point she determined that Cindy's condition was due to an imbalanced *vata* (1 of 3 metabolic body types), meaning that her constitutional tendencies toward a thin body type and high-energy personality were causing her further anxiety and stress. To bring Cindy's system back into balance, Dr. Lonsdorf prescribed 2 herbal ayurvedic supplements: one to pacify her system, the other to clean out toxins. She gave her sesame oil and instructions on how to massage herself with it every morning. Finally, Dr. Lonsdorf suggested that Cindy resume the meditation practice she had abandoned years earlier.

Within a month, Cindy's energy began to change. Although she still felt stressed, it no longer had the impact it once did, and before long she decided to quit her job and work only part-time. As her feelings of well-being increased, her painful headaches decreased, and only 3 months later, she was 90% headache free.

Ayurveda is the traditional medicine of India, based on many centuries of empirical use. Its name means "end of the Vedas" (which were India's sacred scripts), implying that a holistic medicine may be founded on spiritual principles. Ayurveda describes 3 metabolic, constitutional, and body types (*doshas*), in association with the basic elements of Nature—*vata, pitta,* and *kapha*—and uses them as the basis for prescribing individualized formulas of herbs, diet, massage, and detoxification techniques.

HOMEOPATHY

Ruth, a 34-year-old painter from Ohio, suffered from daily tension headaches which felt like a vise grip exerting a painful pressure around her temples. For 10 years, Ruth would wake up in the morning and start gobbling aspirin like candy. She had been constipated all her life, had terrible menstrual cramps, and drank 4 to 6 cups of black coffee a day. Her husband, a homeopathic M.D., believing that her headaches and other conditions were connected to emotional problems she was having with her family, suggested she see his colleague, Amy Rothenberg, N.D., a naturopath and certified homeopath with a private practice in Enfield, Connecticut.

QUICK DEFINITION

Homeopathy was founded in the early 1800s by German physician Samuel Hahnemann. Today an estimated 500 million people worldwide receive homeopathic treatment; in Britain, homeopathy enjoys royal patronage. Homeopathy is now practiced according to two differing concepts. In classical homeopathy, only one single-component remedy is prescribed at a time in a potency specifically adjusted to the patient; the physician waits to see the results before prescribing anything further. In complex homeopathy, typified by *Hepar compositum*, a prescription involves multiple substances given at the same time, usually in low potencies.

During their first meeting, Dr. Rothenberg asked Ruth to talk about her symptoms, fears, dreams, the foods she liked and the ones she didn't, her family, and the reasons they "drive her crazy." An hour and a half later, Dr. Rothenberg determined that the homeopathic remedy *Staphisagria* (from the seeds of the *staves acre*) was most suited to Ruth's health crisis because it specifically targets head pain and physical and emotional hypersensitivity. But after a one-time 200C dose, Ruth noticed only a subtle overall change, and although it helped her constipation, her headache still persisted.

Then Dr. Rothenberg gave her a one-time 200C dose of *Ignatia* (from the bean of the plant St. Ignatius), a remedy specific to headaches associated with emotions, digestive disorders, coffee sensitivity, and morning headaches. Within weeks, Ruth's headaches began to lift, not suddenly, but gradually becoming a shadow of what had been. Once, a few months later, while she was dealing with a particularly difficult family issue, her headaches suddenly returned. Ruth called Dr. Rothenberg and was again given a 200C dose of *Ignatia*. This time Ruth's headaches went away and never came back.

OTHER METABOLIC/ BIOENERGETIC/ BIOCHEMICAL-BASED THERAPIES

The following therapies, depending upon the symptoms and conditions of your underlying condition, may be beneficial for treating tension headaches:

Primary:
- Acupuncture
- Detoxification Therapy
- Environmental Medicine
- Naturopathy
- Nutritional Therapy
- Oriental Medicine

Secondary:
- Energy Medicine
- Light Therapy
- Magnetic Field Therapy
- Oxygen Therapy

STRUCTURALLY ORIENTED THERAPIES

Tension headaches that are primarily related to poor posture, structural misalignments, and musculoskeletal problems respond especially well to structurally oriented therapies.

BIOLOGICAL DENTISTRY

Alice, 32, had suffered from headaches for 10 years. They had begun as mild tension headaches and had worsened over time, until Alice was experiencing both chronic tension and periodic migraine headaches. Basically, she had a classic case of mixed headache syndrome. When she went for a routine dental exam to Michael Gelb, D.D.S., a dentist with a practice in New York City and White Plains, New York, Dr. Gelb noticed that there was a clicking sound in Alice's jaw and that her face was becoming crooked. He asked if she had any other symptoms, and she told him about her headaches.

Dr. Gelb began to examine Alice's jaw, along with her teeth, and discovered that her chin was slanting to one side. Her symptoms suggested temporomandibular joint syndrome. He measured her and fit her for a mouthpiece in order to raise the side of her mouth that was collapsing. After Alice began wearing the mouthpiece, Dr. Gelb suggested she change the way she sat at her computer and start to exercise more; he also instructed her not to cradle the phone to her chin. At first, her migraine aura switched

HannaSomatics

When he first went to see Eleanor Criswell Hanna, Ed.D., at the Novato Institute for Somatic Research, in Novato, California, Eugene, retired and in his sixties, suffered from chronic pain on the right side of his face, his jaw, his eye, his neck and his shoulder. He had consulted his family physician but been told that nothing was wrong with him.

Upon observation and examination, Dr. Criswell Hanna noticed that Eugene was bending over to the right, meaning that the right side of his body was more contracted than his left. She also noticed that both his head and his body bent forward slightly as he stood and that his pelvis and neck were rotated. Determining that his headaches were due to chronic muscle contraction patterns, she began to guide him in a series of exercises designed to reeducate his brain to muscle communication, assigning home exercises in addition to the ones they did together in her office.

After 4 sessions, Eugene was standing and walking upright, his muscles were no longer chronically contracted, and his headaches were gone—which meant he could once again concentrate on his golf game.

from one eye to the other, and then, in about 6 weeks, with no medication and a couple of adjustments to her mouthpiece, Alice's headaches disappeared, after which time she continued to wear the biplate for another 2 months.

BODYWORK

All styles of bodywork can help to provide relief from the aches and pains of tension headaches. Although it works well for most conditions, bodywork is especially helpful when tension headaches are associated with chronic muscle spasm in the upper back and neck. During an intense muscle spasm, circulation in the muscle is reduced, causing waste products to pool in the area. In a chronic situation, this leads to scarring and calcification, a condition called fibrosis. In cases as severe as this, deep (and, unfortunately, painful) muscle massage is one of the primary ways to break up the calcification and bring blood flow back into the area.

CHIROPRACTIC

Research findings show that spinal manipulation is an effective treatment for tension headaches. In one study, in which doctors compared chiropractic treatments to the use of the antidepressant medication amitriptyline, both groups of headache sufferers improved at a similar rate in all primary outcomes, which included the intensity and frequency of headaches and the patient's over-the-counter (OTC) usage. However, the headache patients who underwent chiropractic care still felt relief 4 weeks after the study had ended, while those who took medication had reverted back to baseline symptoms at the end of 4 weeks.

NEURAL THERAPY

John, retired and in his seventies, had suffered chronic tension headaches for 64 years. He felt depressed, helpless, and, after all his years of pain, he had become a classic case of what physicians refer to as a "passive" patient, depending on others to make him feel better. By the time he sought the treatment of Joseph Schames, M.D., headache specialist and Director of Hollywood Community Hospital in California, John was ready to try a new approach.

Dr. Schames and John became a team: Dr. Schames gave John neural therapy treatments, injecting a ½% solution of the anesthetic procaine into trigger points on his trapezius muscle (from his midback to neck), while John made the commitment to change his diet, stretch and exercise daily, and attend weekly physical therapy sessions.

Within 2 months of beginning their combined effort, John began to go weeks without headaches, and, when he did have one, he reported that the pain was much less intense and usually could be related to a previously identified trigger. To John, having lived with daily headaches all his life, this was a miracle.

OSTEOPATHY

Carl, a farmer who had been a football star in high school, had terrible headaches. His headaches usually matched the description for tension headaches, but every once in a while, he would get a whopper of a migraine. He had been to countless doctors looking for relief before he finally found osteopath Herbert Miller, D.O.

In the intake interview, Carl told Dr. Miller that he had had pelvic and back surgery from a football injury sustained many years earlier. Dr. Miller was not surprised to learn that Carl's headaches started a year or two after surgery. Dr. Miller suspected a correlation between Carl's headaches and the surgery, particularly because Carl had been steadily working long hours as a farmer ever since. When he began to work on the previously injured areas of Carl's body, he found them tender and sore to the touch, sug-

Within 2 months of beginning their combined effort, John began to go weeks without headaches, and, when he did have one, he reported that the pain was much less intense and usually could be related to a previously identified trigger. To John, having lived with daily headaches all his life, this was a miracle.

gesting that these were part of the structural problem underlying Carl's headaches.

Carl began to see Dr. Miller weekly for full-body osteopathic treatments in which Dr. Miller manipulated Carl's muscles from head to toe in an attempt to restore normal functioning. After a few months of treatments, Carl's head pain improved, and within a year and a half of his first visit, not only had Carl given up the stress of farming, but he was relieved of the stress of his chronic tension headaches as well.

OTHER STRUCTURALLY-ORIENTED THERAPIES

Depending upon the underlying cause, the following therapies can also be useful:

- Alphabiotics
- Craniosacral Therapy

PSYCHO/EMOTIONAL THERAPIES

Although all headache sufferers respond well to the therapies listed below, those with tension headaches seem to be particularly responsive to psycho/emotional therapies.

BIOFEEDBACK

Electromyogram (EMG) biofeedback has worked especially well for both the prevention and the relief of tension headache. It is a simple technique that is easy to learn, yet it is extremely powerful because it teaches you how to use your mind to control your body, allowing you to reduce muscle tension in your shoulders, neck, scalp, and elsewhere in your body. By becoming better acquainted with your body, you will also be able to handle sensitive emotions and stressful events more smoothly.

FLOWER ESSENCE THERAPY

Because of their subtle healing properties, flower essences sometimes work when nothing else will. Alana suffered from chronic tension headaches. She had seen her family physician, a naturopath, a chiropractor, and a homeopath; she had undergone CAT scans, elimination diets, and allergy tests. And still her headaches remained a mystery that would not go away. At the end of her tether, she decided to see Patricia Kaminski for flower essence therapy.

Kaminski, a foremost practitioner in the field, asked Alana to go inside her head and give her pain a voice of its own. As her headache spoke, even Alana was surprised, for it began to reflect on her mother and the grief that persisted as a result of her death 2 years earlier. After the headache had its say, Kaminski and Alana talked about the experience. Alana remembered the conflicting feelings she had when her mother died: on the one hand, she was sad to lose her; on the other, she was angry at her. She felt guilty for her anger, so her mind suppressed it, and shortly thereafter her headaches appeared. Suddenly, she saw that unexpressed emotions were poisoning her, and this poison was causing headaches.

Right away, Kaminski knew Alana needed the flower essence *fuchsia*. Fuchsia, a red and purple flower, works to unlock core emotions that have been trapped by suppression and denial and bring about genuine emotional vitality; it is specifically recommended for individuals who, like Alana, mask true feelings with states of hyperemotionality or psychosomatic illness. Kaminski made up an essence remedy combining *Fuchsia* with *Bleeding heart*, a powerful heart cleanser and strengthener, so Alana would be able to cope with her sorrow about her mother's death at the same time. Within the first 24 hours of taking the remedy, Alana felt better, and after several more sessions with Kaminski and 2 months of taking *Fuchsia* with *Bleeding heart*, her headaches disappeared and never came back.

HYPNOTHERAPY

Twelve-year-old Donald suffered from severe tension headaches that seemed to come out of nowhere. His parents took him to see O.T. Bonnett, M.D., a Colorado physician who supplements his regular practice with hypnotherapy. As Donald was holding his head and moaning, Dr. Bonnett suggested they try hypnotherapy to see what was contributing to this otherwise mysterious head pain. Donald agreed, saying that he was willing to do anything if it might help his pain go away.

When Donald was in a trance state, Dr. Bonnett first relieved Donald's current headache through hypnotic suggestion and then asked Donald to remember back to a time before his headaches began. Immediately, Donald began to talk about an event that happened when he was 4 years old and

QUICK DEFINITION

Flower remedies comprise subtle liquid preparations made from the fresh blossoms of flowers, plants, bushes, even trees, to address emotional, psychological, and spiritual issues underlying physical and medical problems. The approach was pioneered by British physician Edward Bach in the 1930s, when he introduced the 38 Bach Flower Remedies, based on English plants and still available today. Since then, an estimated 20 different brands of new flower remedies have appeared, based on plants native to many landscapes, from Australia to India to Alaska, offering about 1500 different blends for a diverse range of psychological conditions.

playing with a group of children, a scene in which a fight erupted and he was hit on the head with a baseball bat. Dr. Bonnett then asked him to recall his next headache, and Donald told of a time when, in the course of a fight with his sister, he had tripped and hit his head. When asked about his third headache, Donald remembered his parents arguing in his room while he was in bed with a bad case of chicken pox which included a high fever and a headache.

Recognizing the connection between Donald's headaches and arguing, Dr. Bonnett asked Donald to "fast forward" and remember what *preceded* his current headache. Donald said he was watching an old cowboy movie on TV and that his headache began the moment the actors started to fight. Once this connection was confirmed, Donald realized that he did not have to experience headaches when he or somebody else was fighting, and through further hypnotic suggestion by Dr. Bonnett, Donald's chronic headaches disappeared.[1]

PSYCHOTHERAPY

In a 1991 study conducted by the Ohio University Department of Psychology, 41 chronic tension headache sufferers were randomly divided into 2 groups, one group receiving psychotherapy (cognitive-behavioral) and the other the antidepressant drug amitriptyline HCL. After 8 weeks, both groups

showed similarly significant improvements, but the group that underwent psychotherapy reported a more positive outlook, citing more control over their perception of pain and less resistance to their daily lives, while the majority of the amitriptyline group reported experiencing mild to substantial side effects.

See Chapter 16, An A-Z of Self-Care Options, for detailed information on each treatment method.

SELF-CARE OPTIONS

No matter what their health condition, everyone can benefit from a little stress management every day, whether it is aromatherapy, exercise, meditation, or another approach. All of the following self-care techniques help you relax, so pick one that you enjoy because if you enjoy it, you will be extra motivated to do it on a regular basis and are twice as likely to benefit.

ACUPRESSURE

The following points may be helpful in relieving tension headaches:

- Governing Vessel 16 (GV 16)
- Gall Bladder 20 (GB 20)
- Bladder 2 (B 2)
- Stomach 36 (St 36)
- Gall Bladder 41 (GB 41)
- Large Intestine 4 (LI 4)
- Liver 3 (Lv 3)

See Chapter 16,
An A-Z of
Self-Care Options,
Acupressure, for more
information on
application.

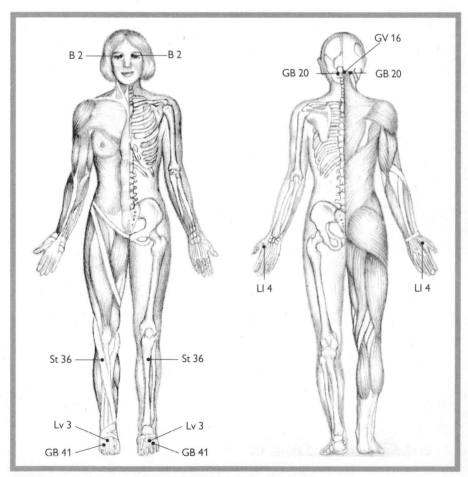

Figure 6.1—Acupressure points helpful for tension headaches.

AFFIRMATIONS/AUTOSUGGESTIONS

Christiane Northrup, M.D., believes that one of the keys to healing tension headaches is to realize that we hold a lot of our tension, especially emotional tension, in our neck. She suggests addressing a source of emotional tension by repeating the following affirmation to yourself: "I release [name of person or situation] to its highest purpose, and I go free." Pay attention to how this declaration feels in your neck, see how it immediately gives you a sense of relaxation. As long as the tension comes back, continue to repeat the affirmation and allow your neck to relax.

AROMATHERAPY

Since aromatherapy has an almost immediate effect on the nervous system, it is an excellent all-around preventative tool for stress management and tension relief. While all essential oils are good for tension headaches, lavender oil and the application methods listed below seem to be the most effective:

INHALATION

Wafting relief: Fill aroma lamp, bowl, or diffuser with water and mix in 4 drops melissa and 2 drops peppermint or Roman chamomile oil.

For aroma to go: Put 2 to 3 drops of melissa, peppermint, and lavender oils on a handkerchief or cloth and inhale throughout the day for prevention.

MASSAGE

Temple rub: Combine lavender (a sedative) and peppermint (a stimulant) oils and rub the mixture on your temples for pain relief.

Sore muscle massage: Mix 10 drops juniper (which adds heat), 8 drops rosemary, 8 drops lavender, and 2 drops of lemon with 2 ounces of vegetable oil and use to massage your neck and shoulders.

BATHS

Aroma soak: For relief of a headache in progress, fill a bath with warm to hot water and add eucalyptus, wintergreen, or peppermint and soak for 20 to 30 minutes.

Muscle relaxant bath: Fill the bath with warm water and add 3 drops chamomile, 3 drops lavender, 2 drops marjoram, 2 drops thyme, 1 drop coriander.

COMPRESSES AND STEAMS

Cold compress relief: Mix 3 drops rose, 1 drop melissa, and 1 drop lavender oils in 2 pints water. Stir thoroughly and place a towel or washcloth in the water. Let it soak 5 minutes, then wring to remove excess water. Lie back and put the compress on the painful area. Rest, change the compress as soon as it reaches room temperature.

Compress for sore muscles: Soak clean cloth in a mixture of 1 drop ginger, 2 drops marjoram, 1 drop peppermint, 1 drop rosemary added to 2 cups hot water; apply to neck and shoulders.

EXERCISE

Exercise is always a good preventative for tension headaches because it mitigates your body's response to stress by producing endorphins, the hormones attributed to the natural euphoria one experiences after exercise. You do not have to become a super-jogger or join in strenuous aerobic activity; a brisk walk with your dog is enough to get the blood moving and put distance between you and whatever is bringing you stress.

FOLK REMEDIES

These home treatments have been used for relief of tension headaches:

- **Hair brushing:** Brushing your hair and scalp with a downward motion every day is a great way to improve blood circulation in the head and keep headaches from occurring. Using a natural bristle brush with rounded tips, begin at your temples and move the brush in tiny circles as you work your way down your scalp, doing the left side, the right side, then return to the middle of your scalp and finish using the same strokes first to the left, then to the right of center.[2]

- **Ginger compress:** Cut and peel one root of fresh ginger, then boil it in 3 cups of water until the water turns cloudy. Soak a washcloth in the mixture, then apply it to the back of your neck. This works well to expand the contracted muscles and relieve dull, steady pain.

■ **Herbal compress:** Boil 3 cups water and pour over 1 tablespoon of lavender and 1 tablespoon of chamomile, letting it steep 20 minutes. Soak a soft cloth in the mixture, then wring it out, and apply to the back of neck or forehead. Cold herbal compresses are also effective.

■ **Try 12 almonds:** Because they contain the natural aspirin salicin, almonds can offer headache relief. This remedy is used in areas of North Africa and Asia where almond trees are common.

■ *Li Shou* **(arm swinging):** This Chinese technique uses motion to relieve headaches by creating a relaxed, meditative state and is taught to school children to relieve stress. Swing your arms back and forth until the blood shifts from your head to your hands, reducing your swollen blood vessels. Next, use your warmed hands to stroke your face, using a circular motion, paying particular attention to the area around your eyes. Repeat the exercise several times.

■ **Wear a headband:** In Korea, people tie a cloth snugly around their heads, just above the eyebrows. This remedy has been somewhat validated by Western science: according to one study, wearing a snug elastic headband helped about a quarter of the participants obtain relief of 50% or more, possibly because the headband restricts blood flow and prevents the dilation of blood vessels.[3]

■ **Wrap rubberbands around your fingers:** Take 10 rubberbands and wrap them around each of your fingers at the first joint, the one closest to your fingernail. Put them on tight, and although they may turn your fingers purplish and hurt a bit, leave them on for no more than 9 minutes to find that your headache has disappeared.

■ **Bite your tongue:** This remedy is not about watching what you say; instead, stick out your tongue about 1/2 inch, then bite on it **gently** for about 9 minutes (not more than 11 minutes), keeping pressure on your tongue the entire time.

HERBAL SUPPLEMENTS

The following herbs can provide relief for all types of tension headaches. Many of the other herbs listed in Chapters 16 and 17 can also be used, depending upon the root cause of your headache.

- **General headache:** angelica, feverfew, meadow sweet, willow bark
- **Musculoskeletal pain and spasms:** cayenne, chamomile, elder, meadow sweet, nettles, qiyelian, turmeric, valerian, vervain, willow bark
- **Stress, anxiety, insomnia, depression, and tension:** cramp bark, feverfew, hawthorn, ginkgo, ginseng, lavender, linden blossom, passion flower, pennyroyal, peppermint, rosehips, skullcap, St. John's wort, valerian, vervain

ICE AND HEAT

Since both cold and heat can relax tense muscles, both can be used effectively for tension headaches. A cold pack on your forehead, eyes, and neck (particularly if you know someone who is willing to give you a neck or shoulder massage at the same time), a hot shower, warm soothing bath with your shoulders and neck submerged, or a foot bath may bring you relief, particularly since these measures comfort and calm the entire body. In some cases, ice packs can be applied to pain sites until the discomfort subsides.

MASSAGE

While all the massage techniques listed in Chapter 16 can be helpful, the following are particularly good for tension headaches:

Carotid Artery Massage
Neck and Shoulder Massage

REFLEXOLOGY

BRAIN—all headaches, circulation, and overall body function
HEAD—all headaches, stress, shoulder and neck tension
JAW—stress, TMJ syndrome
NECK—tension, physical and emotional stress
ARMS AND SHOULDERS—physical and emotional stress and muscle tension

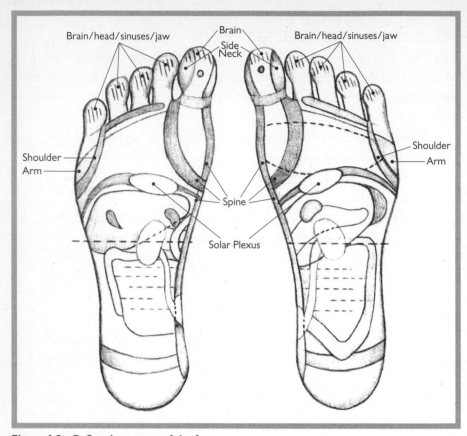

Figure 6.2—Reflexology areas of the feet.

SPINE—all headaches, trauma, stress, tension, digestion

SOLAR PLEXUS—all headaches, stress, anxiety, digestion

RELAXATION EXERCISES

While all of the relaxation exercises listed in Chapters 16 and 17 are beneficial for the relief and prevention of tension headaches, progressive relaxation is especially effective:

1. Lie down on the floor, couch, or bed with your shoes off; you can play soft music or light candles if you want—anything that will help set the stage for relaxation.

2. Spend a few moments watching your breath, paying attention to each inhalation and exhalation, taking at least 5 full-belly breaths.

3. Begin to relax the muscles in your body, group by group, starting

with your feet and working your way up to your neck, face, and head.

As listed in Chapter 16, these self-help techniques also offer excellent relief from tension headaches:

Breathing Exercises
Creative Visualization
Lifestyle Changes
Meditation
Nutritional Therapy/Dietary Changes
Support Groups

RECOMMENDED READING

Alternative Medicine: The Definitive Guide. Compiled by the Burton Goldberg Group. Tiburon, CA: Future Medicine Publishing, 1994.

Benson, Paul, D.O. "Biofeedback and Stress Management." *Osteopathic Annals* 12 (August 1984), 20-26.

Boline, Patrick D. et al. "Manipulation vs. Amitriptyline in Headache." *Journal of Manipulative and Physiological Therapeutics* 18:3 (March/April 1995).

Braly, James, M.D. and Torbet, Laura. Dr. *Braly's Food Allergy and Nutrition Revolution.* New Canaan,CT: Keats Publishing, Inc. 1992.

Clark, Linda, M.A. *A Handbook of Natural Remedies for Common Ailments.* Greenwich, CT: The Devin-Adair Company, 1976.

Dean, Carolyn, M.D. *Dr. Carolyn Dean's Complementary Natural Prescriptions for Common Ailments.* New Canaan, CT: Keats Publishing, Inc., 1994.

Faber, William J., D.O. *Pain, Pain Go Away.* San Jose, CA: ISHI Press International, 1990.

Ford, Norman D. *Eighteen Natural Ways to Beat a Headache.* New Canaan, CT: Keats Publishing, Inc., 1990.

Herzberg, Eileen. *Migraine: A Comprehensive Guide to Gentle, Safe & Effective Treatment.* Rockport, MA: Element Inc., 1994.

Holroyd, Kenneth A. et al. "A Comparison of Pharmacological and Nonpharmacological Therapies for Chronic Tension Headaches." *Journal of Consulting and Clinical Psychology* 59:3 (1991), 387-393.

Igram, Cass, M.D. *Who Needs Headaches?* Cedar Rapids, IA: Literary Visions Publishing, 1991.

Keller, Erich. *The Complete Home Guide to Aromatherapy*. Tiburon, CA: H.J. Kramer, Inc., 1991.

Kunz, Barbara and Kunz, Kevin. *Hand Reflexology Workbook*. Albuquerque, NM: RRP Press, 1994.

Lilienthal, Samuel, M.D. *Homeopathic Therapeutics*. New Delhi: Jain Publishing Co., 1996.

Manahan, William, D., M.D. *Eat for Health*. Tiburon, California: H.J. Kramer, Inc., 1988.

Nambudripad, Devi S., D.C., L.Ac., R.N., Ph.D. *Say Goodbye to Illness*. Buena Park, CA: Delta Publishing, 1993.

National Headache Foundation Fact Sheet, Chicago: National Headache Foundation. October 1994.

Natural Health Secrets from around the World. Boca Raton, FL: Shot Tower Books, 1996.

Northrup, Christiane, M.D. *How to Heal Yourself from Toxic Emotions*. Potomac, MD: Phillips Publishing, Inc., 1995.

Rapoport, Alan M., M.D. and Sheftell, Fred D., M.D. *Headache Relief*. New York: Simon & Schuster, 1990.

Rapoport, Alan M., M.D. and Sheftell, Fred D., M.D. *Headache Relief for Women*. New York: Little, Brown and Company, 1995.

Reed, Daniel. *A Handbook of Chinese Healing Herbs*. Boston, MA: Shambhala Publications, 1995.

Rick, Stephanie. *The Reflexology Workout*. New York: Harmony Books, 1986.

Robbins, Lawrence, M.D. and Land, Susan. *Headache Help*. New York: Houghton Mifflin Company, 1995.

Rothschild, Peter R., M.D., Ph.D. and Fahey, William. *Free Radicals, Stress, and Antioxidant Enzymes: A guide to cellular health*. Honolulu, HI: University Labs Press, 1991.

Simpson, Kristine, et al., eds. *The Experts Speak 1996: The Role of Nutrition in Medicine*. Sacramento: Kirk Hamilton PA-C, 1996, 121-122.

Stromfeld, Jan and Weil, Anita. *Free Yourself from Headaches: The Natural Drug-Free Program for Prevention and Relief*. Palm Beach Gardens, FL: The Upledger Institute, Frog, Ltd., 1995.

Solomon, Seymour, M.D. and Fraccaro, Steven. *The Headache Book*. Mount Vernon, NY: Consumer Reports Books, 1991.

Wilson, Roberta. *Aromatherapy for Vibrant Health & Beauty*. Garden City Park, NY: Avery Publishing Group, 1994.

Chapter 7

Migraine Headaches

"That no one dies of a migraine seems to someone deep in an attack as an ambiguous blessing," says writer Joan Didion. Certainly you can explain the visual disturbances, fatigue, disorientation, nausea, vomiting, even the infamous throb, but unless you have been there, it is nearly impossible to convey the pain and anguish of a migraine. The information in this chapter will change all that.

Florence, 78, suffered from dull, aching, frontal migraines for over 40 years. She had tried nearly every medication, yet she felt no more than partial relief from any of them. Tired of taking so many medications, she came to the Milne Medical Center. She usually got stomach aches a day or 2 before a headache came on; she also admitted to having a strong desire for sweets, especially chocolate.

On physical examination, we noticed that the sclera (the opaque membrane that covers the eyeball and attaches to muscles) in Florence's right eye was red instead of the normal white. She had a yellow, thick, coated area on the back of her tongue, an enlarged liver, tender abdominal areas, and heavy calluses on the bottom of her feet—all signs of a digestive disturbance. We then tested her for allergies using electrodermal screening and discovered she was sensitive to corn, milk, sugar, and chocolate.

After much discussion about allergy and its role in headaches, Florence reluctantly agreed to give up chocolate, sweets, and any other foods containing these ingredients for 1 month to see what happened. One month later, she came back to us *headache free*. Although she was elated, she was also incredulous that not one other doctor in 40 years had even thought to ask about her diet.

QUICK DEFINITION

Electrodermal screening is a form of computerized information gathering, based on physics, not chemistry. A noninvasive electric probe is placed at specific points on the patient's hands, face, or feet, corresponding to acupuncture meridian points, at the beginning or end of energy meridians. Minute electrical discharges from these points are seen as information signals about the condition of the body's organs and systems, useful for a physician in evaluating and developing a treatment plan.

What Is a Migraine Headache?

It is nearly impossible to convey the pain and anguish of a migraine headache to those who have never been in its clutches.

Certainly, you can explain the visual disturbances, fatigue, disorientation, nausea and vomiting, even the infamous throb, but unless you have been there, you lack the frame of reference necessary to appreciate the experience writer Joan Didion captures when she observes, "That no one dies of a migraine seems to someone deep in an attack as an ambiguous blessing."[1]

If you are a migraine sufferer, you are in good company, joining Didion and 8 to 12 million additional Americans who have a "migraine personality." For example, you are probably intelligent, hard-working, and meticulous like migrainers Benjamin Franklin and Charles Darwin. You may be somewhat reclusive and subject to your own whims like migrainers Freud and Caesar. You may gravitate toward leadership like migrainers Abraham Lincoln and Thomas Jefferson. If you have elected to explore this corner of your psyche, you may be capable of feats of imagination like those of Lewis Carroll, George Bernard Shaw, and Edgar Allan Poe. Poe's migraines were so excruciating that he was said to run madly out of the house to bury his head in the snow for relief.

Unfortunately, migraines are on the rise. In the last 10 years, the incidence of migraine among all age groups in America has risen more than 60%. Currently, 1 of every 5 individuals will experience one or more migraines in his or her lifetime. Migraines (literally, pain in one side of the head) are a vascular headache, meaning blood vessels are involved in producing the pain. Although recognizable elements are shared in most migraine-type headaches, each migrainer goes through a different experience before, during, and after a migraine attack, making each case unique. As you read this chapter, keep in mind that we have purposely left room for variance among individuals because migraines are an *overall* symptom that could signify other headaches described in this book.

Regardless of individual cases, migraines are divided into 2 categories:

In the last 10 years, the incidence of migraine among all age groups in America has risen more than 60%. Currently, 1 of every 5 individuals will experience one or more migraines in his or her lifetime. Migraines (literally, pain in one side of the head) are a vascular headache, meaning blood vessels are involved in producing the pain.

Symptom Chart—Migraine Headaches

SYMPTOMS	HEADACHE TYPE	PAIN LOCATION
Warning Signs: no prodromal symptoms, but may have nausea, vomiting, food cravings (especially sweets), depression, exhilaration, hyper- or hypo-activity **Description:** throbbing headache, often synchronized with pulse; steady, but brief jolts of pain, aggravated by activity	COMMON MIGRAINE	generally one-sided, centered above or behind one eye; can begin at the back of head and spread to one entire side of head; sometimes a stiff neck and tender scalp
Prodrome Stage: about 30 minutes before onset, a warning aura consisting of visual disturbances (zigzag lines, blind spots, hallucinations, light flashes); sensory motor disturbances (numbness or tingling in an arm or leg, yawning, smelling strange odors); and/or mental function disturbances (speech impairment, confusion, inarticulation, disorientation) **Other Symptoms:** anxiety, weakness, nervousness, depression; increased urination, urge to move bowels; dizziness, imbalance, lightheadedness, faintness; cold and clammy hands and feet; hot flashes followed by chills; reddened or teary eyes; nausea or vomiting; stomach pain; intolerance for light, noise, and smells; water retention; hyperventilation; nasal congestion **Duration:** from 3 hours to 3 days **Frequency:** rare and occasional to several per week; average is 1 to 3 episodes a month	CLASSIC MIGRAINE	same as common

UNDERLYING CAUSES AND TRIGGERS	PRIMARY AND SECONDARY TREATMENTS	SELF-CARE TREATMENTS	WHERE IN THE BOOK PAGE #
Causes: metabolic imbalances, structural disturbances, emotional /psychological factors **Triggers:** dietary and/or environmental sensitivity, hormonal imbalance, auto-immune disturbances, lifestyle factors, structural disturbances, psychological stress	**Primary:** ■ acupuncture ■ detoxification ■ environmental medicine ■ homeopathy ■ naturopathy ■ neural therapy ■ nutritional therapy ■ psychotherapy ■ traditional Chinese medicine **Secondary:** ■ alphabiotics ■ Ayurvedic medicine ■ bodywork ■ chiropractic ■ craniosacral therapy ■ energy medicine ■ magnetic field therapy ■ osteopathy ■ oxygen therapy ■ psychotherapy	■ aromatherapy ■ affirmations ■ biofeedback ■ breathing exercises ■ creative visualization ■ exercise ■ flower remedies ■ herbal supplements ■ folk remedies ■ ice and heat ■ journal writing ■ lifestyle changes ■ massage ■ meditation ■ nutritional therapy ■ relaxation techniques ■ support groups	Page 197 Page 197

Symptom Chart—Migraine Headaches (continued)

SYMPTOMS	HEADACHE TYPE	PAIN LOCATION
Description: migraine aura without headache, usually occurs in middle age or childhood	**MIGRAINE EQUIVALENT**	one side of the head
Description: paralysis and altered sensation on one side, often accompanied by double vision; most common in children and adolescents	**HEMIPLEGIC AND OPHTHALMOPLEGIC MIGRAINE**	same as common
Description: severe throbbing, sometimes accompanied by lack of coordination; slurred speech; vertigo; double vision; complete or partial blindness in one or both eyes; hearing loss; ringing in ears; depression or confusion; weakness, numbness, or tingling in extremities; vomiting; develops mainly in children and adolescents, especially in young women beginning menstruation	**BASILAR MIGRAINE**	same as common
Description: migraine with blindness or blurring in one eye	**RETINAL MIGRAINE**	same as common but with eye pain
Description: migraine with prolonged aura lasting up to 1 week or symptoms lasting longer or continuously; auras continue past pain phase	**COMPLICATED MIGRAINE**	same as common

UNDERLYING CAUSES AND TRIGGERS	PRIMARY AND SECONDARY TREATMENTS	SELF-CARE TREATMENTS	WHERE IN THE BOOK PAGE #
same as common	same as common	same as common	Page 197
			Page 197
			Page 197
			Page 197
			Page 197

Mixed, Transformed, or "Progressed" Migraine Syndrome

People who begin with occasional attacks of migraine eventually go on to experience milder but more frequent headaches which may even occur daily. Conventional medicine views this phenomenon as a natural progression of the migraine disorder; however, alternative doctors believe that mixed headache syndrome may actually involve rebound headaches that arise due to overmedication.

those with aural, "classic migraine;" and those without aura, "common migraine." While the headache symptoms are generally the same for both, the main difference between the categories is that classic migrainers experience neurological symptoms, an "aura" which warns of the impending attack (called a "prodrome") while common migrainers do not.

Approximately 20% of all migraines are characterized as classic, while 80% are common. It should be noted, however, that both types may produce less obvious warning signs from an hour to a couple of days before the headache occurs, such as depression, irritability, fatigue, moodiness, food cravings (particularly for sweets), frequent yawning, fluid retention, increasing sensitivity to light, and concentration difficulties.

Aura, a term that derives from the Greek word for wind, is like the strong wind that comes before the storm. As a prelude to migraines, it is believed to be related to both electrical and chemical changes in the brain and to a reduction in blood flow to parts of the brain. The aura can consist of visual disturbances, such as flashing lights, zigzag lines, blurring, or bright spots, numbness or tingling on one side of the body, muddled thinking, a sense of unreality, fatigue, anxiety, and/or an overall body weakness. The aura occurs from a half-hour to a few minutes before the onset of the migraine. Some headache experts, such as the late Carl Pfeiffer, M.D., Ph.D., formerly of the Princeton Brain Bio Center (now the Carl C. Pfeiffer Institute), suggested that the first sign of oncoming migraine is the copious production of so-called "water white" urine, which indicates the relaxation of kidney arterioles and indicates the loss of valuable salts such as magnesium, calcium, and potassium.

Both classic and common migraine cause severe pain of a throbbing nature, which often seems to follow the rhythm of the heartbeat and can worsen with activity. This pain is primarily one-sided and usually involves the temple and one eye, although some people may feel pain on both sides; the pain is accompanied by lightheadedness, nausea, vomiting, dizziness, blurred vision, hot and cold flashes, and a marked hypersensitivity to light, noise, and smells. Migraine attacks usually last from 4 hours to 3 days, although in rare cases they can last much longer, in which case the condition becomes known as "status migrainosus" and requires prompt medical attention.

The Causes and Triggers of Migraine Headaches

Although the theories regarding the symptoms and underlying causes of migraines vary considerably, it is widely believed that all migraines ultimately relate to serotonin levels and/or abnormal constriction and swelling of the blood vessels in the head. Getting to the root of a migraine means much more than knowing what makes them hurt so much; it means learning to recognize the complex interplay of conditions and triggers that prompt swelling and pain in the first place.

Like every other type of headache, these causes can be metabolic, structural, or emotional in nature and can arise from an obvious source such as a food allergy just as easily as from a blow to the head or a deeply buried psychological concern. While a more detailed explanation of all of the possible migraine causes and triggers appears in Chapter 3, the following is a brief overview of the causes and theories associated with vascular-type headaches.

GENES

Of all headache types, migraines have the strongest evidence of a genetic correlation. Whether or not they are passed down from family member to family member, migraines can be viewed as a family disorder; when one person in the family has one, all members of the family suffer with them.

See Chapter 3, What Causes Your Headaches?, for more detail on the causes and theories of headaches.

HORMONES

A marked association exists between women's headaches and their menstrual cycles, and in no headache type is this more obvious than in mi-

Visual Disturbances of Migraines

- spots, stars, wavy and straight lines, color splashes, and wave patterns similar to heat waves
- mild loss in vision, with amorphous hallucinations
- flashes of light
- graying or whitening
- shimmering, sparkling, or flickering images
- spots that are often crescent-shaped, generally like zigzags, and often with a shimmering, sparkling, or flickering light at the edges

Children and Migraines

Migraines that strike children almost always take on a different form, which tends to be unique to the physical constitution and personality of the child. For example, a child's migraine pain may be vague rather than localized, or there may be no head pain at all. Instead, the child may just experience the symptoms associated with migraines, such as stomach pains, nausea, dizziness, and confusion. Often these are highly sensitive children who suffer from other conditions, most notably allergies and digestive problems. If left untreated, approximately 50% of children with migraines will simply outgrow the condition. Parents should be aware that children who are prone to motion sickness may also be susceptible to migraines when they reach adulthood.

Diet and Migraine Study

At the Hospital for Sick Children in London, doctors stopped migraine attacks in 82 out of 88 youngsters by putting them on diets free of 55 sensitivity-causing foods. The following foods were most often implicated as a cause of headache:

- cow's milk in 30%
- eggs in 27%
- chocolate in 25%
- oranges in 24%
- wheat in 24%
- cheese in 15%
- tomatoes in 15%

Also on the list were pork, beef, corn, soy, tea, oats, coffee, peanuts, bacon, potatoes, apples, peaches, grapes, chicken, bananas, strawberries, melon, and carrots.

graines. Researchers suggest that 10 to 20% of all women experience some sort of migraine during or around the time of their menstrual period, and that 1 in 7 of all migrainous women experience migraines only around their cycle. This type of migraine is known as menstrual migraine, and it can make women particularly sensitive to other triggers.

ALLERGY/ SENSITIVITY

As with most other health and headache conditions, there is a strong connection between allergies/sensitivities and migraines. Although the percentage is disputed, researchers suggest that between 20 and 90% of all migraines are related to allergy/sensitivity factors.

A groundbreaking study conducted by Joseph Egger of the Hospital for Sick Children in London suggests that the percentage may be even higher. In a carefully controlled study, Egger showed that it was possible to eliminate the incidence of migraine in 93% of the study's 88 migraine sufferers when sensitivity-causing foods were eliminated from their diet. Most of the participants in the study were found to be allergic to more than one type of food, and, as is often the case with food allergies, the foods to which

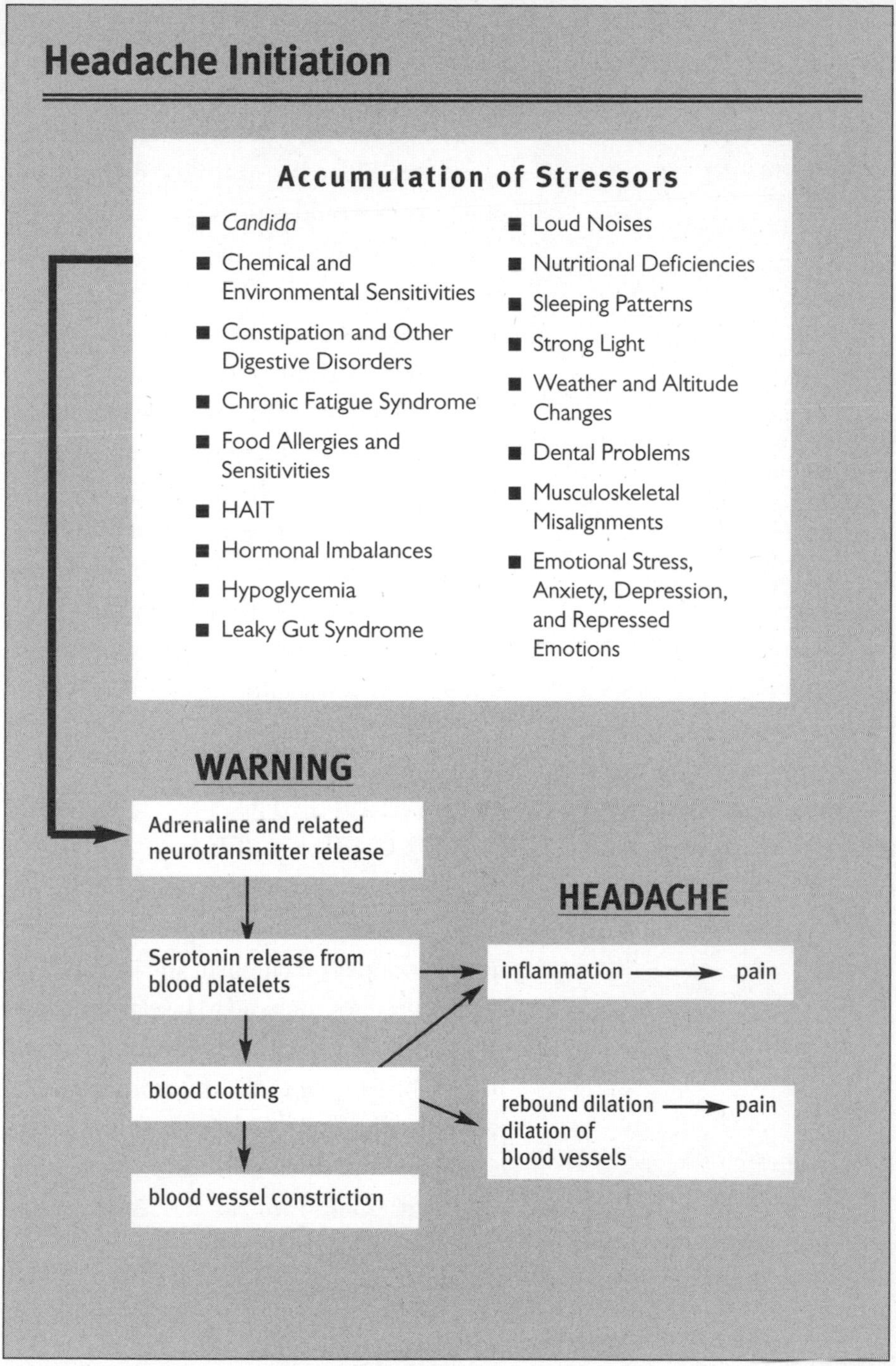

Headache Initiation

Accumulation of Stressors

- *Candida*
- Chemical and Environmental Sensitivities
- Constipation and Other Digestive Disorders
- Chronic Fatigue Syndrome
- Food Allergies and Sensitivities
- HAIT
- Hormonal Imbalances
- Hypoglycemia
- Leaky Gut Syndrome

- Loud Noises
- Nutritional Deficiencies
- Sleeping Patterns
- Strong Light
- Weather and Altitude Changes
- Dental Problems
- Musculoskeletal Misalignments
- Emotional Stress, Anxiety, Depression, and Repressed Emotions

WARNING

Adrenaline and related neurotransmitter release

↓

Serotonin release from blood platelets

↓

blood clotting

↓

blood vessel constriction

HEADACHE

inflammation ⟶ pain

rebound dilation ⟶ pain
dilation of
blood vessels

Figure 7.1—The road to migraine headaches.

A Quick Look at Migraine Triggers

Generally, many of the following triggers work in tandem, so while one event alone will not necessarily bring on a headache, several together probably will.

- alteration of sleep-wake cycle, sleep deprivation, or excess sleep
- changes in time zones
- weather changes
- missing or delaying meal
- sunlight, bright or flickering fluorescent lights, TV and movie viewing
- excessive and/or loud noise
- strong smells
- holidays and travel
- yeast infections
- structural misalignments
- stress, anxiety, anger, depression
- menstruation, oral contraceptives, and hormone replacement drugs
- foods, including cured meats, pork, organ meats, seafood, fatty foods, salt, chocolate, sugar, MSG, NutraSweet, sour cream, aged cheese, yogurt, milk, dairy products, eggs, freshly baked breads, yeast, anything pickled or fermented, alcohol (especially red wine and beer), coffee, tea, cola beverages, wheat, citrus fruits, figs, bananas, red plums, raspberries, corn, avocados, onions, eggplant, potatoes, nuts
- analgesic agents and other drugs
- environmental substances such as smoke, gas fumes, paint fumes

they were allergic were also the foods they craved or ate most frequently. A double-blind placebo test was included as a control, and it was proven that when the offending foods were introduced back into the diet, the migraine pain would return.[2]

BLOOD CLOTTING

Studies have shown that platelet clustering (increased clustering occurs during blood clotting) is altered in migraine patients, which is shown by the decreased sensitivity of platelets to platelet activating factors among migrainers. According to Julian Whitaker, M.D., of Newport Beach, California, migrainers are especially troubled by blood clotting because their platelets release abnormal amounts of serotonin, which then further constricts their arteries.

NUTRITIONAL DEFICIENCIES

Besides the other potential nutritional problems outlined in Chapter 3, people with abnormal copper metabolism and low levels of dietary magnesium tend to be especially given to migraine attacks. Both minerals help to metabolize serotonin and amines that expand blood vessels. One study found a deficiency of ionized magnesium in 40% of patients with migraines. Studies show that not only are brain levels of magnesium reduced during attacks, but that, among migrainers, magnesium levels are low even during headache-free periods.

Sleeping Patterns—Migraines are 3 times

more likely to come on during REM sleep than at any other time of the day or night. Research indicates that 55% of migraine sufferers have also been or are currently sleepwalkers, while 71% suffer from nightmares, and 41% have been known to wet their bed.[3] Furthermore, keep in mind that many sleep disturbances can be traced to food sensitivities that eventually cause digestive and liver disturbances.

Emotional Stress—Some migrainers are thought to exhibit a "migraine personality." Such individuals are often characterized as compulsive workers, perfectionists, those who feel that they have to do everything now and will not rest until their work is done. When they do stop, they let down completely. It is this sudden letting down that is one of the triggers of migraine headaches. When the "go-getter" relaxes, the formerly tightened and restricted head and neck muscles which were squeezing arteries and reducing blood flow suddenly expand and stretch the blood vessel walls, causing an excruciating headache.

Migrainers may also have issues around anger, some being unable to express themselves at all, while others blow up over everything. This suggests that migraines may develop as an energetic response to a sufferer's attempt to control emotional reactions. Repressing intense emotions has a twofold effect on the body: not only can it overstress the system, but the excess hormones secreted during anger (whether or not expressed) may also relate to liver dysfunction as defined by traditional Chinese medicine.

Furthermore, depression is often linked to migraine conditions. In a study of 27- and 28-year-olds conducted in Switzerland, the combination of anxiety disorder and major depression (but not solely one or the other)

The International Headache Society (IHS) Criteria for Migraine Diagnosis

According to IHS researchers, you can determine whether you have a migraine by looking at the following two groups. If you concur with any 2 statements in Group A, plus any 1 in Group B, then, according to the IHS, you have a migraine.

Group A:

- Your pain is located on one side of the head.
- Your pain is throbbing or pulsating.
- Your pain is severe enough to interfere with or keep you from normal activity.
- Your pain is worsened by exertion.

Group B:

- The pain is accompanied by nausea or vomiting.
- The pain is accompanied by sensitivity to light and noise.

SOURCE: Dr. Jerome Walker, M.D., Michael Norman, M.D., and Sharon Parisi, Ph.D., "Controlling Headache: Question and Answers." DeKalb Medical Center, Headache Treatment Center, in Decatur, Georgia.

proved to be closely associated with migraine, suggesting that anxiety, depression, and migraine may deserve to be classified as a distinct syndrome of its own. We believe, however, that the true underlying factors were not considered in this study.

Kathleen Merikangas, Ph.D., coauthor of a study at the Yale University School of Medicine concludes:

"Headache and depression tend to be almost identical; they are both a physiological response to stress, like a steam valve with different thresholds. In general, migrainers have hypersensitive nervous systems that make them more highly in tune to both their inner and outer environments. And, while this can express itself as a food or chemical allergy in one person, it can just as easily get translated into depression or a shy personality in another. We are finding that more and more migrainers have a propensity for both."[4]

Migrainers may also have issues around anger, some being unable to express themselves at all, while others blow up over everything. This suggests that migraines may develop as an energetic response to sufferer's attempt to control emotional reactions.

This implies that headaches and depression themselves are results of the hypersensitive nervous system; but we contend that the truth of the matter is that the underlying causes express themselves as headache and depression.

Diagnosing and Treating Underlying Causes

As with other headaches, prevention is the cure for migraines. Yet, since migraines can be the symptom of a vast number of conditions, locating their source and preventing them from happening is not always easy. Fortunately, you and your alternative practitioner have a powerful array of diagnostic tools, such as a headache questionnaire, physical exam, hormone analysis, allergy testing, hypoglycemia testing, elimination diet, structural manipulation, and/or nutritional analysis.

Once the cause has been identified, regardless of what your practitioner is capable of doing, healing your headaches becomes *your* job. You may have to change your lifestyle, eat better, sleep more regularly, avoid your triggers, exercise, release emotional baggage, and think positive thoughts. It takes more effort to heal a migraine than it does to stuff it deeper inside with a prescription drug. But once you have come out the other side, your migraines are gone and your life is your own again; then you will be glad you took the time to do the job the way it needs to be done.

ALTERNATIVE TREATMENTS

METABOLIC/ BIOENERGETIC/ BIOCHEMICAL-BASED THERAPIES

Due to their vascular nature, migraines tend to respond best to metabolic/bioenergetic/biochemical-based therapies, especially when combined with structural and psycho/emotional therapies and self-care. The following case studies give an idea of the variety, versatility, and vitality of therapies available from alternative physicians.

The Chinese Medical View of Migraines

In the vocabulary of Chinese medicine, migraines are a symptom of a deep energetic imbalance in the blood system. Generally, this imbalance is linked to either the liver and the gallbladder or the kidney and the bladder. Classically, the migraine expression (as well as that of the sensitivity headache) tends to be along a "yang" meridian, even though its root is in the "yin" organ. Yang means active, warm energy while yin mean passive, cool energy. Since the gallbladder's yin partner is the liver, it is really the liver that is the source of the headache. Most commonly, there is a blood deficiency in the liver, so it cannot perform its role of lubricating and spreading energy through the body. Instead, the energy creates friction and gets caught, creating pain.

See Chapter 17, An A-Z of Alternative Medicine, for more information on each treatment method.

ACUPUNCTURE

According to Joseph Carter, L.Ac., C.M.T., of Berkeley, California, migraine headaches are linked closely to liver functioning and digestion. Dr. Carter's patient Sally came to him with debilitating migraines that came up from her neck and along one side of her head, lodging behind her eye.

As he took her history, Dr. Carter discovered that Sally's headaches tended to come on just before the onset of menstruation and that over the last 3 years, since she began experiencing headaches, her periods had become progressively heavier, accompanied by more severe head pain. For the previous year, Sally had been unable to go to work during her periods, having to lie in a dark room for 2 to 3 days and wait until the headache went away. Sally was also overweight and had long-term problems with her digestion.

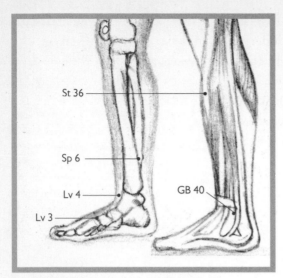

Figure 7.2—Acupuncture/acupressure points.

Dr. Carter knew immediately that the cause of Sally's headaches was her liver, so, after her first acupuncture treatment, he showed her 3 balancing points on the feet, 2 corresponding to the liver and 1 to the gallbladder. Whether or not Sally was experiencing a headache, Dr. Carter instructed her to hold (as often as possible throughout the day) specific points such as Stomach 36 (St 36), Spleen 6 (Sp 6), to build up her blood, Liver 3 (Lv 3), Liver 4 (Lv 4), and Gallbladder 40 (GB 40) to regulate her liver. Each point is actually a pair of points, one on each leg.

QUICK DEFINITION

Eight Treasures
includes rehmannia root, angelica, *dong quai*, condonopsis root, poria fungus, peony root, atractylodes rhizome, ligusticum rhizome, and licorice root.

In addition, he gave her 2 blends of Chinese herbs to build up her blood: 3 tablets, 3 times a day of *Eight Treasures* from the end of her period to the middle of her cycle and 3 tablets, 3 times a day of *Xiao Yao Tong* from ovulation to the start of her period. *Xiao Yao Tong* contains bupleurum root, paeonia root, angelica dong quai, poria fungus, tractylodes rhizome, ginger, licorice root, and mentha leaf. Dr. Carter also gave Sally acupuncture treatments every other week, prescribed a multimineral supplement, and had her drink lots of water and begin a regular exercise routine. By the time her second menstruation came, Sally reported that her feet had become very hot while he had been stimulating the points, and then her headaches disappeared.

"The fact that her feet were warm meant that blood was staying there, or that her energy had begun traveling more efficiently along the gallbladder meridian, which runs from the head to the feet," explains Dr. Carter. Eventually, after a few more cycles, Sally's headaches stopped altogether.

With all the toxins in our food, water, and air, it is no wonder the liver, the organ responsible for filtering toxins, is having a difficult time these days. Furthermore, since Chinese medicine considers the liver to be the primary emotional organ, it is the first place in the body to feel the effects of stress and worry. This also explains why women tend to get more liver-related headaches than men. As they bleed every month, their blood is more prone to deficiencies.

A good example of this phenomenon can be seen by looking at the case of Samantha, a part-time clerk for a stock brokerage firm who had been experiencing severe migraines with every menstrual cycle since her early teens and now was suffering from daily tension headaches as well. She had tried drugs, and she had eliminated coffee, chocolate, and cheese, but still her headaches worsened. Then, at the urging of a friend, she came to the Milne Medical Center.

During the initial evaluation, we immediately noticed that, in addition to the hormonal connection, Samantha's headaches revolved around outbursts of anger. Her pulse confirmed the liver connection and we began treating her for an "overactive liver and heart fire" condition, inserting needles into the points that would sedate the liver and heart meridians. We also put her on a strict diet, which we supplemented with herbs for hormonal imbalances, including wild yam, *vitex*, *bupleurum* root, peony, *dong quai*, and blue cohosh. After 6 acupuncture treatments conducted over a 6-week period, her liver improved and her headaches cleared up completely.

AYURVEDIC MEDICINE

When Donna, 29, first visited Vivek Shanbhag, M.D., Chairman of the Ayurvedic Medicine Department at Bastyr University in Seattle, she had been experiencing migraines twice a week for 7 years. They usually came early in the morning and frequently were preceded by visual disturbances which quickly disappeared and were replaced by nausea and hyperacidity. Her right knee and ankle hurt as well.

After taking a detailed history and physical exam, Dr.

Vitamin B2 Is Better Than Aspirin for Migraines

High doses of vitamin B2 (riboflavin) can be an effective, low-cost substitute treatment for aspirin in the treatment of migraine headaches, and without any side effects, according to Belgian researchers reporting in the medical journal *Cephalagia* in 1994. In the study, 49 patients with migraine received 400 mg of vitamin B2 daily before breakfast for 3 months; 25 of these patients also received 75 mg of aspirin every day. Both groups experienced a 68% improvement in symptoms, indicating that vitamin B2 performed as well as aspirin.

QUICK DEFINITION

Acupuncture meridians are specific pathways in the human body for the flow of life force or subtle energy, known as *Qi* (pronounced *CHEE*). In most cases, these energy pathways run up and down on both sides of the body, and correspond to individual organs or organ systems, designated as Lung, Small Intestine, etc. There are 12 principal meridians and 8 secondary ("extraordinary") channels. Numerous points of heightened energy, or *Qi*, exist along the meridians and are called acupoints. Along the 14 principal channels, there are 361, but there are an estimated 1000 such acupoints on the body's surface, each of which is potentially a place for acupuncture treatment.

Triphala and *Suta Shekar* are available through Ayurvedic Naturopathic and Nutrition Clinic, 23700 Edmonds Way, Edmonds, WA 98029. tel: 206-783-2873

QUICK DEFINITION

Ayurveda is the traditional medicine of India, based on many centuries of empirical use. Its name means "end of the Vedas" (which were India's sacred scripts), implying that a holistic medicine may be founded on spiritual principles. Ayurveda describes 3 metabolic, constitutional, and body types (*doshas*), in association with the basic elements of Nature—*vata, pitta,* and *kapha*—and uses them as the basis for prescribing individualized formulas of herbs, diet, massage, and detoxification techniques.

Shanbhag determined that Donna's constitution was predominately *pitta* in body type (marked by her medium build, warm ruddy skin, intense personality, and need to eat and sleep regularly), with a secondary *kapha* body type component (determined by her slow digestion and oily hair). He diagnosed her problems to be related to an "aggravated *pitta*," due much to her high-stress job, irregular diet (which included 5 to 6 cups of coffee a day and 2 to 3 glasses of wine a week), and lack of time for her family.

To start with, Dr. Shanbhag gave her a special diet to follow, including instructions to eliminate tomatoes and garlic and cut down on coffee and red meat. He then started her on 2 ayurvedic formulas of mixed herbs, specifically *Triphala* for detoxification and *Suta Shekar* for overall repair. He also taught her techniques and exercises to do at home on her own, which included inserting drops of essential oil in her nostrils, simple stretching postures, and a breathing technique. Within 3 visits, Donna's headaches were 75% better, and eventually they faded away completely.

ENVIRONMENTAL MEDICINE

When 39-year-old Cheryl first went to see Ellen W. Cutler, D.C., at the Tamalpais Pain Clinic in Corte Madera, California, she had experienced a severe migraine during the 3 weeks before menstruation ever since her periods started at age 11. Doctors had put her on birth control pills to regulate her periods and had her taking the conventional drug Imitrex, which, although it worked for her migraines, often left her completely exhausted and incapable of functioning. Her color was poor and her life force was drawn, almost as if she had given up altogether.

To evaluate the cause of Cheryl's problem, Dr. Cutler performed 4 diagnostic examinations: an abdominal palpation, a 24-hour urine analysis, a

test for enzyme deficiencies and digestive and assimilation imbalances, and muscle testing for allergies/sensitivities. Cheryl's
enzyme test showed that she was sugar-intolerant and that she
was not deriving full benefit from the foods she was eating, so
Dr. Cutler supplemented her diet with enzymes to help her digest sugar and to assimilate her food.

Furthermore, Cheryl's allergy tests revealed that she was
allergic to eggs, vitamin C, sugar, minerals, salt, vinegar, certain fruits and berries, alcohol, radiation, and her own progesterone, thyroid, and adrenaline. Dr. Cutler used chiropractic, acupuncture, and NAET to desensitize Cheryl to all of
these substances. Finally, Dr. Cutler supplemented
Cheryl with a natural basic vitamin, natural progesterone cream, vitamin C, and evening primrose oil.
Within a short period of time and without the use of
Imitrex, Cheryl's premenstrual migraines disappeared.

NAET stands for
Nambudripad Allergy
Elimination Technique.
It was developed by
Devi S. Nambudripad,
D.C., L.Ac., R.N.,
Ph.D., and involves the
use of acupuncture
meridians to desensitize
the nervous system so
that it no longer reacts
to foods or substances
as allergens. For more
information on NAET,
see Chapter 10,
Allergy/Sensitivity
Headaches.

HERBAL MEDICINE

When 14-year-old Sandy called the office of Deborah
Frances, N.D., she complained of acute migraines.
Interviewing Sandy over the telephone, Dr. Frances
recognized that Sandy's headaches fit the description
of a classic migraine, including a sudden onset of visual symptoms, such as "weird lights flashing in her
eyes," followed by terrible head pain.

Since Sandy's headaches were of recent origin,
Dr. Frances recommended that Sandy take 30 drops
of liquid feverfew every 15 minutes for a total of 4
doses and then call back if she was not feeling better. When Dr. Frances
saw Sandy a few days later, Sandy reported that her headache disappeared
after just 2 doses.[5]

In Robert's words, "I had thousands of dollars worth of tests, CAT scans, MRIs, all kinds of things, but they didn't cure anything. Then in a simple nutritional supplement, I was handed the key to my headaches."

HOMEOPATHY

Melinda, a 32-year-old sales manager for a computer software manufacturer in Boston, had incapacitating migraines that, besides their pain, also
made her feel as if she were suddenly going crazy. She could not think; if

driving, she had to pull off the road. Generally, she would have an entire day in which she felt as if someone were trying to split her head in two with an ax, during which time she would be constipated and could not urinate. Sometimes she would vomit clear bile-like liquid. The worst of it was the depression and suicidal thoughts that would overcome her during her headaches. With every headache, Melinda had visions of guns blowing her head off, or of driving her car off the road; it was all she could do to stop herself from acting on her thoughts.

On her first visit to Paul Herscu, N.D., a naturopath specializing in homeopathic medicine, in Enfield, Connecticut, Melinda spent over an hour talking about her symptoms. Dr. Herscu gave her 1 dose of *Natrum muraticum* 200C, a homeopathic headache remedy (from table salt) that was most closely aligned with Melinda's reported symptoms.

About 6 weeks into her treatment, when she was not improving as much as he had expected, Dr. Herscu decided that he needed to treat Melinda's most severe complaint—her depression and thoughts of suicide. This time he prescribed 1 dose of *Helleborus niger* 200C, a homeopathic headache remedy (from Blackhellebore or Christmas rose) that is also effective for treating depression, and her condition began to improve. At first, it was like an on/off switch, where she would get headaches with the depression one time and depression without headaches the next, but eventually, after a total of 6 months' treatment, her headaches went away.

NUTRITIONAL THERAPY

Essential Fatty Acid (EFA) Supplements—Robert, 52, a real estate broker, got his first migraine when he was 35. He practically lived on Excedrin, Bufferin, and Alka Seltzer, until about 4 years ago, when his migraines increased to 1 or more a week, with tension headaches almost daily. In his desperate search for relief, Robert went from doctor to doctor and tried many different drugs. However, since he objected to feeling like a "walking zombie," he kept looking for a doctor who could help him. He eventually found Kelly Sutton, M.D., a family physician who complements her practice with homeopathy and herbs.

After taking a thorough history and conducting a physical examination, Dr. Sutton took him off the beta blockers and started him on fish oil pills 3 times daily along with 10 mg of the

Some of the 41 Headache Drugs Doctors Prescribed for Mary over a 2-Year Period

Prednisone	Ansaid	ne w/APAP
Ogen	Lidex CR	Metoclopramide
Provera	Amicillin	Propox NAP
Synthroid	Terpin Hydrate/Codeine	Verelan
Prozac	Seldane	Vicodin ES
Mevacor	Diazepam	Monopril
Kronofed A	Methocarbamol	Hemorrhoidal HC Supp.
Hismanal	Codeine	Carafate
Pen VK	Amoxil	Midrin
Robaxisal	Butalbital/	Imipramine
Triam/HTZ	APAP/CAF	Desipramine
Tagamet	Hydrocodo	6 Phenazo
Zantac	Voltaren	pyridine pyridium
Micro-K	Lorazepam	Septra
SMZ Trimethoprim	Phenergan Supp.	

antidepressant amiltryptaline from a previous doctor's prescription. When Robert's headaches disappeared 3 months later, Dr. Sutton told him that it was time to take him off the antidepressant. She switched his daily supplements from fish to flaxseed oil, another EFA, and Robert slowly tapered off his dosage of amiltryptaline.

At first, Robert's headaches came back once or twice a month, but they were less severe and shorter in duration. Finally, Robert's headaches disappeared entirely. In Robert's words, "I had thousands of dollars worth of tests, CAT scans, MRIs, all kinds of things, but they didn't cure anything. Then with a simple nutritional supplement, I was handed the key to ending my headaches."

Enzyme Therapy—Mary, 73 was suffering from chronic, debilitating migraines when she went to see Dennis Crawford, D.C., a practitioner who combines chiropractic with nutritional therapy. Mary had seen 13 doctors, had been prescribed 41 drugs, including hormones, antibiotics, tranquilizers, and painkillers, and had already spent over $30,000 on medical tests. At the time, she was taking 13 different drugs

QUICK DEFINITION

Fats and oils are made of building blocks called **fatty acids.** Of these long-chain molecules (comprising atoms of carbon, hydrogen, and oxygen) the "fatty" end does not dissolve in water, while the "acid" end does. Fats are also called triglycerides as they consist of 3 (tri) fatty acid molecules joined to one molecule of glycerol, a kind of sugar. Unsaturated fats required in the diet are called **essential fatty acids,** and include linoleic acid (which is an omega-6 oil), found in corn and beans, and alpha linolenic acid (which is an omega-3 oil), found in fish, flaxseeds, and walnuts.

QUICK DEFINITION

Enzymes are fundamental to all living processes in the body, necessary for every chemical reaction and the normal activity of our organs, tissues, fluids, and cells. There are hundreds of thousands of these Nature's "workers". Enzymes are specialized living proteins and enable your body to digest and assimilate food. There are special enzymes for digesting proteins, carbohydrates, fats, and plant fibers. Specifically, protease digests proteins; amylase digests carbohydrates; lipase digests fats; cellulase digests fiber; and disaccharidases digest sugars.

every day, which "only took the edge off" her pain. Her face was "puffed up like a basketball," her mind was cloudy, she had difficulty talking, she vomited frequently, and her head hurt so badly that she had to sleep sitting up.

Dr. Crawford's diagnosis revealed that Mary was deficient in 2 essential enzymes, namely cellulase (digests plant fibers) and protease (digests proteins). Cellulase deficiency is associated with facial nerve pain while a shortage of protease is related to temporomandibular joint problems. The lack of these enzymes helped create the conditions leading to her chronic headaches. In addition, Dr. Crawford noted that Mary panted, or hyperventilated, from anxiety as she lay on his examination table. To help relieve this, Dr. Crawford gave Mary a blend of hawthorn berries, Collinsonia root, motherwort, rosemary leaf, and willow bark with selected enzymes.

Dr. Crawford also gave Mary chiropractic adjustments and a series of enzyme formulas to redress the lack of cellulase and protease. The cellulase enzyme formula also contained citrus bioflavonoids, carrot, fenugreek, garlic, rose hips, grape seed extract, and pau d'arco, while the protease blend featured calcium lactate and kelp.

Immediately following this, Mary's facial and headache pain disappeared, her appearance improved, and her vitality was much better. Soon after, she reduced, then eliminated, all her drugs, including prednisone. Mary commented, "I feel better and have more freedom now than in the past 18 months."

TRADITIONAL CHINESE MEDICINE

Billy, 7, had been experiencing terrible migraine headaches for 3 years. He had gone from doctor to doctor, undergone countless neurological exams, even went to the Mayo Clinic, but still nobody could help him. One after another, doctors told him that he would have to learn to live with his problem, which meant he was facing the rest of his childhood going to school only half the time and missing out on countless outings and adventures with his friends.

Determined to find a solution, Billy's parents took him to see David Krofcheck, O.M.D., D.Ac., C.A. of the Health and Energy Professional Corporation in Kalamazoo, Michigan. During the initial evaluation, Dr. Krofcheck did muscle testing in which he had Billy hold a bottle of *Candida* yeast mold extract as Dr. Krofcheck tested Billy's muscles for signs of weakness. Billy's muscles showed that he had a sensitivity to *Candida*, indicating that he had a yeast infection. He had been given antibiotics when he was younger for recurring ear infections, thus setting the stage for a bacterial overgrowth.

Dr. Krofcheck gave Billy one acupuncture treatment, in which he focused on the meridian systems most involved with the weakened large intestine and spleen, and prescribed a diet of less-complex carbohydrates and more raw foods, as well as herbs, including rosemary, thyme, pau d'arco, and caprylic acid. Two weeks later, Billy's "incurable" headaches disappeared.

OTHER METABOLIC/BIOENERGETIC/ BIOCHEMICAL-BASED THERAPIES

The following therapies, depending upon the symptoms and underlying causes or conditions, may also be beneficial for treating migraine headaches:

- Detoxification Therapy
- Energy Medicine
- Light Therapy
- Magnetic Field Therapy
- Naturopathy
- Neural Therapy
- Oxygen Therapy

STRUCTURALLY ORIENTED THERAPIES

Many forms of physical medicine can be useful in the treatment of migraine, especially when used in conjunction with metabolic therapies, psycho/emotional therapies, and healthy lifestyle changes. While these structurally oriented therapies sometimes work on their own, they are often more effective in shortening the frequency, duration, and severity of the attack than they are at actually curing the disorder.

ALPHABIOTICS

Tanya, an architect living in Phoenix, suffered from debilitating migraines for 4 years. Her migraines started after her car was rear-ended while she was driving in rush hour traffic. The force of the blow left her with a severe case of whiplash, and a few months later her headaches began. Her headaches progressively worsened with each episode, until the smell of food made her vomit and bright lights and noise caused her to writhe in pain. She tried painkilling drugs, but nothing worked for her; her only option during her 3 days of pain was to lock herself in a darkened room.

For more information about alphabiotics, see Chapter 17, An A-Z of Alternative Medicine.

At the urging of her sister, Tanya finally agreed to go see William LaVelle, M.D., L.Ac., for an alphabiotic alignment. The Alphabiotic Alignment Process is a painless structural aligning method designed to reset the central nervous system and coordinate the activities of both brain hemispheres. At first, Tanya was confused, as Dr. LaVelle did not seem interested in hearing the details of her headache. Instead, he instructed Tanya to lie on the table, and then went, in his words, "to the root of the problem—the brain stem." Miraculously, from her first alignment, Tanya's migraines disappeared.

BIOLOGICAL DENTISTRY

Catherine, a 40-year-old Californian, suffered from migraines accompanied by severe facial pain for about a year before she saw Dwight Jennings, D.D.S., a dentist specializing in orthopedic dental medicine. While examining her, Dr. Jennings observed that Catherine's back teeth were too short for her jaw, forcing her skull and jaw to compensate—a problem he believed was the underlying cause of her migraines.

Using computerized equipment, Dr. Jennings measured the shape and movement patterns of Catherine's mouth and jaw and then custom-made 2 dental appliances for her, one for day and another one for night. The appliances built up Catherine's back teeth and allowed her jaw to be supported in a more forward position. Immediately after she began wearing her appliances, Catherine's headaches disappeared, and a few years later, after her jaw joint had been retrained to a healthy position, she stopped wearing the appliances and remained headache free.

CHIROPRACTIC

Tamera's migraines were devastating. They came on with no warning, caused immense pain, were accompanied by projectile vomiting, and created visual disturbances that became so severe that black was all she could see. She had taken painkilling drugs, had the inside of her sinuses scraped, had given up caffeine, but all that helped was, again, crawling into a dark room and sleeping. If she was lucky, her migraine would be gone when she woke up again.

Then she went to Jay Holder, D.C., Ph.D., for chiropractic treatments; after her first few adjustments, her attacks became less frequent. Then one day she relapsed and experienced another full-blown migraine. She was in excruciating pain and could not drive, so, rather than waste time and money going to the hospital for another pharmaceutical injection, she came by ambulance to Dr. Holder.

As soon as Tamera was on the table, Dr. Holder discovered that partial dislocations, or subluxations, of her coccyx and sphenoid bones were causing her problem. Subluxations create nerve interference in the spine. As he adjusted her, Tamera's headache went away on the spot. From that point on, Tamera's headaches were never as severe, and over time they gradually faded away.

PSYCHO/EMOTIONAL THERAPIES

Christiane Northrup, M.D., likens migraines to mini-explosions inside the head, associated with 2 emotional factors: the inability to express anger and the drive to be perfect and achieve in the world. She believes that her own migraines, which began when she was 12 years old, were the result of her emotions. She notes:

"I was virtually the poster child of migraine headache sufferers. I was an overachiever who wasn't satisfied with anything less than straight A's. Though my father tried to persuade me to relax and smell the roses, I was very driven and hard on myself. I now realize that I resented some of my mother's driven qualities but felt helpless to create something new."[6]

BIOFEEDBACK

Since the hands and feet of many migrainers feel cold when at the height of their headache attacks, thermal biofeedback, a biofeedback technique in which the imagination is used to warm the hands and draw blood away from the head, can be helpful for migraines.

SELF-CARE OPTIONS
AFFIRMATIONS/ AUTOSUGGESTIONS

See Chapter 16, An A-Z of Self-Care Options, for more information on self-treatment methods.

In *You Can Heal Yourself*, Louise Hay points out that migraines seem to follow an emotional pattern that seeks to deflate the overachieving, perfectionist tendencies of hardworking people. Migraines are your body's way of saying "I dislike being driven" or, "You are resisting the flow of life," says Hay. When you wake up in the morning, don't jump out of bed; instead, lie there, in warmth and comfort, and repeat one or more of the affirmations listed in Chapter 16 or make something up on your own. Here are a few samples: *I feel healthy, relaxed, and free of pain.* Or: *I approve of myself and I am safe to be who I am.* The basic idea you want to establish and affirm is that life is easy and that it is okay to relax because everything will work out as it is supposed to.

AROMATHERAPY

The following aromatherapy techniques can be useful for migraine headaches:

INHALATION

Wafting relief: Fill aroma lamp, bowl, or diffuser with water and mix in 4 drops melissa and 2 drops peppermint or Roman chamomile oil.

For aroma to go: Put 2 to 3 drops of melissa, peppermint, and lavender oils on a handkerchief or cloth and inhale throughout the day for prevention.

MASSAGE

Temple rub: Combine lavender (a sedative) and peppermint (a stimulant) oil and rub the mixture on your temples for pain relief.

Good oils for vascular-type headaches: anise, basil, chamomile, coriander, eucalyptus, lavender, lemon, marjoram, melissa, onion, peppermint, rosemary.

BATHS

Aroma soak: For relief of a headache in progress, fill a bath with warm to hot water and add eucalyptus, wintergreen, or peppermint and soak for 20 to 30 minutes.

COMPRESSES AND STEAMS

Icy migraine compress: 2 drops peppermint, 1 drop ginger, and 1 drop marjoram oils added to 1 quart ice water; soak a clean cloth and apply to head, forehead, or neck at first inkling of approaching migraine; if desired, apply an icepack over the compress to keep it from heating up. Avoid contact with your eyes.

Lavender and peppermint compress for vascular headache: At first sign of headache, make 2 compresses, a lavender and peppermint compress for the forehead, and a hot marjoram (a vasodilator, stretches blood vessels) for the back of the neck; this combination provides a combination of relaxing, stimulating, and vasodilating effects.

Aromatherapy steam: Boil 2 pints of water and pour into a large bowl; add 1 drop melissa, 2 drops peppermint, and 2 drops lavender oil. Put your head over the bowl and cover your head and the bowl with a large towel. Inhale deeply through your nose for about 10 minutes.

FOLK REMEDIES

The following techniques have been used for migraine headache relief:

Vinegar compresses: Soak a washcloth with vinegar and place it in the refrigerator until it is sufficiently chilled. Then apply the compress to your forehead, temples, and neck. You can also inhale vinegar for even faster relief. Boil equal parts vinegar and water, pour mixture into a bowl, and place a towel over the bowl and your head as you inhale the rising steam.

Warm salt pack: To make a salt pack, roast 1 cup salt in a dry frying pan until salt is warm to the touch, being careful that it does not overheat. Pour salt into a thin dish towel, then fold it so you can apply it to your head; rub the painful areas rather than keeping the pack in one place.

Herbal foot bath: This is an excellent way to draw blood and congestion away from your head. Place 1 tablespoon of powdered mustard or ginger in a deep basin big enough for both feet. Fill the basin with water as hot as you can bear, then sit in a comfortable chair and slowly immerse your feet in the water. Drape a thick towel over the basin to keep the heat in, and place a cool or cold towel on your neck or forehead. Close your eyes and relax, breathing deeply for about 15 minutes.

Icy foot bath: Fill a basin with ice water (refrigerated water with ice) and soak your feet. Believe it or not, your feet will actually start to feet warm after a few minutes. When you are finished, dry off, get under the covers of your bed, and relax.

Cold hip-sitz bath: Fill a tub with 2 inches of warm water. Sit in the tub, and then turn on the cold water and let it run till it covers your hips. Dry off with a coarse towel and cover up. A muscle massage is especially beneficial after this treatment.

Alternating hot and cold showers: To improve blood circulation, try alternating hot and cold showers once a day for 2 or 3 months; this remedy works to abort vascular-type headaches because the heat further dilates the blood vessels (which may temporarily cause pain) while the cold makes blood vessels contract.

Cold water and hot water wrist baths: If you feel a headache coming on fill a sink with cold water and then hot water on your wrists, alternating back and forth until you feel the headache pass.

Drink a headache tonic: Fill a large pot with water and mix in small pieces of fresh ginger root, coriander seeds, diced garlic, and a little honey to taste. Boil off half the liquid and drink what is left periodically throughout the day.

Apple cider vinegar and honey tonic: To offset the causes of a digestive headache, particularly one related to excess acid production, D.C. Jarvis, M.D., in *Vermont Folk Medicine*, suggests taking apple cider vinegar in water and/or 2 teaspoons honey every day to help regulate the body's pH balance. Dr. Jarvis has observed that, when taken as a rescue remedy, this mixture will stop any headache, including a migraine, within a half-hour. If you do not like the taste, you can place equal parts apple cider vinegar and water in a steamer, place your face over it with your head covered with a towel, and inhale 75 breaths.

Try 12 almonds: Because they contain the natural aspirin salicin, almonds can offer headache relief. This remedy is used in areas of North Africa and Asia where almond trees are common.

A spoonful of honey: A tablespoon of raw honey at first inkling of an impending headache can abort a vascular headache; take a spoonful, wait a half-hour, and if it has not worked, take another tablespoon with 3 glasses of water.

Wear a headband: In Korea, people tie a cloth snugly around their heads, just above the eyebrows. This remedy has been somewhat validated by Western science: according to one study, wearing snug elastic headband helped about a quarter of the participants obtain relief of 50% or more, possibly because the headband restricts blood flow and prevents the dilation of blood vessels.

The paper bag trick: Because your exhaled breath is composed largely of carbon dioxide (CO_2) and carbon dioxide is known to dilate the cerebral arteries, some say breathing into a bag and rebreathing your expired air at the earliest sign of a vascular headache can abort the approaching attack. This works especially well when classic migraine sufferers do it the minute they see a warning aura. Try breathing into the bag for 15 to 20 minutes and then lying down for 20 minutes. If the headache has not gone away, repeat the breathing cycle one more time.

Blinking red light: While too high-tech to be a folk remedy, this may be the home cure of the future. Developed by John Anderson, M.D., of Great Britain, this treatment involves a pair of goggles that blink red light at different speeds before your eyes. In one study, 72% of those who used the treatment reported that their migraines stopped within an hour of beginning the treatment. Those who reported the most success credited some of it to their ability to adjust the speed and brightness of the light to a level they found soothing. (Similar light goggles can be purchased through Sharper Image or Tools for Exploration, listed in Appendix A.)

HERBAL SUPPLEMENTS

The following herbs can be considered effective in preventing and relieving headaches and their associated systemic conditions:

Allergy/sensitivity or digestive disorders: black horehound, cayenne, chamomile, fenugreek, feverfew, ginger, nettle, passion flower, peppermint, rosemary, safflower, slippery elm, St. John's wort, wood betony.

Constipation/detox: aloe, burdock, dandelion, goldenseal (root), milk thistle, nettle, Oregon grape root, senna, vervain, wood betony.

Hormonal/reproductive problems: black cohosh, blackhaw, cayenne, chamomile, chasteberry, cramp bark, dong quai, lavender, Jamaican dogwood, passion flower, skullcap, St. John's wort, wild yam.

Stress, anxiety, insomnia, depression, and tension: cramp bark, feverfew, hawthorn, *Ginkgo*, ginseng, lavender, linden blossom, passion flower, pennyroyal, peppermint, rosehips, skullcap, St. John's wort, valerian, vervain.

Vascular imbalances: balm, basil, black willow, cayenne, elder flower, feverfew, garlic, ginger, *Ginkgo*, goldenrod, Jamaican dogwood, lavender, marjoram, peppermint, rosemary, rue, thyme, sage, willow bark, wood betony, wormwood.

Also, depending on the related symptoms and causes of your migraines, such as if they occur in conjunction with your menstrual cycle or are linked to your digestion, one of the following herbal teas can be beneficial:

Hormonal headache relief tea: Combine 3 parts lemon balm, 3 parts chamomile, 1 part skull cap, and 1 part passionflower to make a total of 2 to 4 tablespoons. Place herbs in a glass tea jar and pour 1 quart boiling water over them, letting it steep 20 minutes. Strain and drink ¼ cup every 30 minutes until headache is gone.

Migraine tea: Use equal parts black horehound, meadowsweet, and chamomile; make an infused tea, and drink to relieve vascular headaches accompanied by vomiting.

Tea for digestive problems: Combine ½ teaspoon each of chamomile leaves, catnip flowers, fennel seed, and peppermint leaves. Pour 1 quart boiling water over the herbs, and let it steep 10 minutes.

Antinausea headache tea: Simmer 1 teaspoon fresh ginger in a pot of water for 7 minutes; let it steep another 10 minutes.

LIFESTYLE CHANGES

In addition to the self-care regimens outlined in Chapter 16, such as establishing regular sleeping habits, eating a healthy diet, and maintaining good posture, the following simple changes in your lifestyle and behavior can help you avoid getting "let-down" or weekend migraines:

- Wind down slowly rather than suddenly, from a tense deadline or project, relaxing a little at a time to give blood vessels a chance to relax slowly and thereby better handle increases in blood flow.
- Try to intersperse work with rest and rest with play, keeping a balance among the 3 so you do not get tense or overworked.
- If neither of these do the trick, try to maintain your Monday-through-Friday schedule on weekends, such as getting up and eating meals at the same time or drinking your cup of coffee at the same time as you do during the week.

The following self-help techniques can also be helpful for migraine headaches:

- Breathing Exercises
- Creative Visualization
- Exercise
- Ice and Heat
- Massage
- Meditation
- Nutritional Therapy/Dietary Changes
- Relaxation Exercises
- Support Groups

RECOMMENDED READING

Alternative Medicine: The Definitive Guide. Compiled by the Burton Goldberg Group.

Tiburon, CA: Future Medicine Publishing, 1994.

The American Council on Headache Education, with Lynee M. Constantine and Suzanne Scott. *Migraine: The Complete Guide*. New York: Dell Publishing, 1994.

Braly, James, M.D.. and Torbet, Laura. *Dr. Braly's Food Allergy and Nutrition Revolution. New Canaan*, CT: Keats Publishing, Inc., 1992.

Carper, Jean. *Food: Your Miracle Medicine*. New York: Harper Collins, 1993.

Clark, Linda, M.A. *A Handbook of Natural Remedies for Common Ailments*. Greenwich, CT: The Devin-Adair Company, 1976.

Diamond, Seymour, M.D. and Still, Bill and Cynthia. *The Hormone Headache*. New York: Macmillan, 1995.

Faber, William J. , D.O. *Pain, Pain Go Away*, San Jose, CA: ISHI Press International, 1990.

Ford, Norman D. *Eighteen Natural Ways to Beat a Headache*. New Canaan, CT: Keats Publishing, Inc., 1990.

Hanington, E. "The Platelet and Migraine." *Headache*, 1986.

Herzberg, Eileen. *Migraine: A Comprehensive Guide to Gentle, Safe & Effective Treatment*, Rockport, MA: Element Inc., 1994.

Hills, Hilda Cherry. *Good Food to Fight Migraine*. New Canaan, CT: Keats Publishing, Inc., 1979.

Igram, Cass, M.D. *Who Needs Headaches?* Cedar Rapids, IA: Literary Visions Publishing, 1991.

Jensen, Bernard, D.C., Ph.D. *Tissue Cleansing through Bowel Management*, 10th ed. Escondido, CA: Bernard Jensen Publishing, 1981.

Jouanny, Jacques, M.D. et al. *Homeopathic Therapeutics: Possibilities in Chronic Pathology*. France: Editions Boiron, 1994.

Joutel, A., Bousser, M.G., Olson, T.S., et al. "A Gene for Familial Hemiplegic Migraine Maps to Chromosome 19," *Nat Genet 5* (1993), 40-45.

Keller, Erich. *The Complete Home Guide to Aromatherapy*. Tiburon, CA: H.J. Kramer, Inc., 1991.

Kunz, Kevin and Kunz, Barbara. *Hand Reflexology Workbook*. Albuquerque, NM: RRP Press, 1994.

Leach, Robert A., A.A., D.C., F.I.C.C. *Chiropractic Theories, Principles and Clinical Applications*. Baltimore, MD: Williams & Wilkins, 1994.

Lilienthal, Samuel, M.D. *Homeopathic Therapeutics*. New Delhi: Jain Publishing Co., 1996.

Lipton, Richard B., M.D., Newman, Lawrence C., M.D., and MacLean, Helene. *Migraine/Beating the Odds: The Doctor's Guide to Reducing Your Risk*. Reading, MA: Addison-Wesley Publishing Company, 1992.

Lipton, Richard B., M.D. and Stewart, Walter F., MPH., Ph.D. "Migraine in the United

States: A Review of Epidemiology and Health Care Use." *Neurology* 43, suppl. 3 (1993) S6-S10.

Manahan, William, D., M.D. *Eat for Health.* Tiburon, CA: H.J. Kramer, Inc., 1988.

Nambudripad, Devi S., D.C., L.Ac., R.N., Ph.D. *Say Goodbye to Illness.* Buena Park, CA: Delta Publishing, 1993.

National Headache Foundation Fact Sheet. Chicago: National Headache Foundation, October 1994.

Natural Health Secrets from Around the World. Boca Raton, FL: Shot Tower Books, 1996.

Pritivera, James R., M.D. "Clots: Life's Biggest Killer." *Health Freedom News* (September 1993): 22-23.

Rapoport, Alan M., M.D. and Sheftell, Fred D., M.D. *Headache Relief.* New York: Simon & Schuster, 1990.

Rapoport, Alan M., M.D. and Sheftell, Fred D., M.D. *Headache Relief for Women.* New York: Little, Brown and Company, 1995.

Robbins, Lawrence, M.D. and Lang, Susan. *Headache Help.* New York: Houghton Mifflin Company, 1995.

Rothschild, Peter R., M.D., Ph.D. and Fahey, William. *Free Radicals, Stress, and Antioxidant Enzymes: A guide to cellular health.* Honolulu, HI: University Labs Press, 1991.

Sacks, Oliver, M.D. *Migraine: Understanding a Common Disorder.* Berkeley, CA: University of California Press, 1985.

Shealy, C. Norman, M.D., Ph.D. and Myss, Caroline M., M.A. *The Creation of Health: Merging Traditional Medicine with Intuitive Diagnosis.* Walpole, NH: Stillpoint Publishing, 1988.

Simpson, Kristine, et al., eds. *The Experts Speak 1996: The Role of Nutrition in Medicine.* Sacramento: Kirk Hamilton PA-C, 1996, 121-122.

Stang, P.E. and Osterhaus, J.T. "Impact of migraine in the United States: data from the National Health Interview Survey." *Headache* 33 (1993), 29-35.

Stromfeld, Jan and Weil, Anita. *Free Yourself from Headaches: The Natural Drug-Free Program for Prevention and Relief.* Palm Beach Gardens, FL: The Upledger Institute, Frog, Ltd., 1995.

Solomon, Seymour, M.D. and Fraccaro, Steven. *The Headache Book.* Mount Vernon, NY: Consumer Reports Books, 1991.

Wilson, Roberta. *Aromatherapy for Vibrant Health & Beauty.* Garden City Park, NY: Avery Publishing Group, 1994.

A good mechanic wouldn't dream of touching your car until he figured out why you brought it to him in the first place. Nor should you expect to get help from a system of medicine that starts tinkering around with your head without listening to how your body runs. If you have already heard, "There's nothing more we can do for you," don't despair. You have the opportunity to work with an alternative medical practitioner and find real healing.

Chapter 8

Cluster Headaches

Their devastating pain and puzzling array of symptoms make cluster headaches among the most challenging headaches to eliminate. The pain, coming in frequent stabbing bursts caused by the abnormal contraction and expansion of blood vessels, often impels cluster headache sufferers to do almost anything to distract their attention from the pain.

Once named "Horton's neuralgia" or "Harris' neuralgia," after 2 of the physicians who first studied and described the syndrome, and still known in Britain as "episodic migrainous neuralgia," cluster headaches are among the worst kinds of pain known to humanity—worse than the pain of childbirth or accidental amputation, according to its sufferers. Although cluster headaches appear to be the result of the same vascular syndrome as migraines, the pain of clusters is so severe that migraines feel mild by comparison.

Although migraines are made worse with movement, clusters seem to be intensified when the sufferer lies down; since pain comes in frequent bursts and it causes intense agitation, it is difficult to rest even in quiet periods. Cluster headaches often begin with a sense of fullness in one ear, progressing to a stab of unilateral pain near the eye, forehead, or cheek, then, within minutes, become a full-blown cluster.

> *I used to bang my head against the wall just to alter the feeling in my head.*
>
> —Erica, a former cluster victim

Cluster head pain is so devastating that sufferers, although embarrassed to admit it, are often driven to inflict pain on other areas of their bodies, twisting a steel blade between their teeth, cutting or bruising an arm or leg, or applying boiling water to the forehead. However bizarre this might sound, studies of cluster sufferers have shown this behavior to be far from crazy but, instead, a common coping mechanism among those who will do anything to distract their attention from the pain in their heads.

Cluster sufferers tend more than other headache sufferers to fit a certain profile. The typical cluster victim is a 20- to 50-year-old male. (Clusters strike 1 in 250 men and only 1 in 1,000 women.) He is taller than average. If Caucasian, he tends to have hazel eyes, and a red, rugged complexion that is distinguished by thick skin with deep, coarse lines around forehead, mouth, and chin (qualities attributed by Chinese medical diagnosis to a constitution marked by poor digestion). He is often described as a hard-striving, dynamic, highly active, type-A personality, who rarely expresses his emotions, drinks heavily, and smokes between 2 and 3 packs of cigarettes a day. Some research suggests that female cluster sufferers tend to be more masculine in appearance and have atypical clinical profiles.[1]

Despite these distinguishing characteristics, cluster headaches are regularly mistaken for other types. For example, they may be misdiagnosed as TMJ headaches because of the way the pain radiates around the jaw, or an organic headache because of the sheer intensity of pain the sufferer feels; they may also be thought to be allergy or sinus headaches because of the related symptoms of stuffed or runny nose and teary, reddened eyes. Many cluster sufferers endure unnecessary diagnostic tests and treatments, including needless nasal surgery, before finding a practitioner who is able to recognize their symptoms and help to relieve them.

Cluster Subcategories

There are 3 main variations of cluster headaches:

EPISODIC CLUSTER
The most common type of cluster headache (affecting 80 to 90% of cluster sufferers), these generally come in 4-to 9-week periods, with at least 2 attacks per week, and are followed by a remission from headache symptoms that lasts from 5 to 12 months or more.

CHRONIC CLUSTER
Affecting 10% of cluster sufferers, these differ from episodic only in that the remission period tends to be shorter or nonexistent, with many sufferers experiencing daily or near-daily attacks throughout 6-to 12-month periods or longer.

ATYPICAL CLUSTER
(also known as cluster variant or chronic paroxysmal hemicrania)
As its name suggests, this headache is like a cluster, but it affects more women than men and the head pain comes in shorter but more frequent attacks, with as many as a dozen attacks, each lasting 10 to 30 minutes; in some cases, the pain can jump from one side of the head to the other.

Symptom Chart—Cluster Headaches

SYMPTOMS	HEADACHE TYPE	PAIN LOCATION
Description: rapid onset, burning, boring, sharp or throbbing; can be knifelike; excruciating and among the worst pain known; affects men more frequently **Other Symptoms:** sweating on forehead, abdomen, and trunk; red and teary eyes; stuffy nose and drainage of clear fluid from one nostril; drooping eyelid; flushed face; exhaustion after pain subsides **Duration:** usually 15 minutes to 3 hours; tends to occur in early morning, often awakens patient from sleep **Frequency:** Episodic: 1 to 6 times per day for several weeks or months; can go into remission for months or years, but cluster cycle generally comes every 10 months Chronic: daily or almost daily without relief for 6 months or more	**CLUSTER HEADACHE**	on one side of the head, felt most intensely behind or around one eye; moderate pain can occur in forehead, temple, cheek, nose, and ear areas and at side of head right above neck; mild discomfort may occur above lip and/or in chin and jaw areas
Description: symptoms similar to above; chronic; mostly strikes in women **Other Symptoms:** same as typical cluster **Duration:** briefer than typical cluster headaches, lasting from a few minutes to no more than an hour **Frequency:** equal frequency during the day and night, can occur as few as 4 and as many as 40 times a day	**CHRONIC PAROXYSMAL HEMICRANIA HEADACHE** (also called **Atypical Cluster or Cluster Variant Headache**)	pain can occur in places other than behind eye and can shift locations

UNDERLYING CAUSES AND TRIGGERS	PRIMARY AND SECONDARY TREATMENTS	SELF-CARE TREATMENTS	WHERE IN THE BOOK PAGE #
Causes: metabolic imbalances, structural disturbances, emotional/psychological factors **Triggers:** dietary and/or environmental sensitivity, hormonal imbalance, autoimmune disturbances, lifestyle factors, structural disturbances, psychological stress	**Primary:** ■ acupuncture ■ detoxification ■ environmental medicine ■ homeopathy ■ naturopathy ■ neural therapy ■ nutritional therapy ■ psychotherapy ■ traditional Chinese medicine **Secondary:** ■ alphabiotics ■ Ayurvedic medicine ■ bodywork ■ chiropractic ■ craniosacral therapy ■ energy medicine ■ magnetic field therapy ■ osteopathy ■ oxygen therapy ■ psychotherapy	■ aromatherapy ■ affirmations ■ biofeedback ■ breathing exercises ■ creative visualization ■ exercise ■ flower remedies ■ herbal supplements ■ folk remedies ■ ice and heat ■ journal writing ■ lifestyle changes ■ massage ■ meditation ■ nutritional therapy ■ relaxation techniques ■ support groups	Page 231

Page 231

Do You Have Cluster Headaches?

If you answer yes to 4 or more of these questions, consider yourself among those who suffer from cluster headaches:

Do your headaches generally come for 1 to 3 months at a time, then go away for months or years, sometimes coming back at a certain time of the year?

When in the headache cycle, do you have between 1 and 6 or more attacks per day?

Do your attacks occur at night or during some other predictable time (such as after work)?

Is your pain excruciating and located on one side of your head?

Do these attacks last somewhere between 10 minutes and 2 hours?

Is one side of your nose stopped up or running during an attack?

Does your face, forehead, and trunk sweat during an attack?

Does the eye on your painful side get red and teary? Does the eyelid droop?

Are you restless and constantly moving during an attack?

Are headache cycles marked by depression and insomnia?

Do you sometimes get the urge to hurt yourself during an attack?

The Causes and Triggers of Cluster Headaches

Their devastating pain and puzzling array of symptoms make cluster headaches among the most challenging headaches to eliminate. Most theories seem to have been offered in a vain attempt to make sense of the disorder, even though researchers have little idea why the same apparent conditions result in a cluster in one person and a migraine in another.

The following are the causes most commonly linked to cluster headaches:

VASCULAR IRREGULARITIES

Most researchers agree that cluster headaches are directly related to the abnormal contraction and expansion of blood vessels, but, as is the case with all so-called vascular-type headaches, this understanding offers few clues to the actual cause, as a wide range of factors, from allergies and digestion to physical structure and emotions, can bring about the vascular changes that often result in headaches.

MALFUNCTIONING HYPOTHALAMUS

Perhaps the most intriguing of the cluster theories put forth today is the idea that a disturbance in the hypothalamus gland contributes to the periodic or cyclic nature of the cluster syndrome. As the seat of the body's biological clock, the hypothalamus is responsible for normal body rhythms, such as appetite, sleep, and hormone (including serotonin) secretion; those rhythms being faulty seems to trigger a chain of reactions that ultimately results in a headache. The relationship between bodily rhythm and clusters is substantiated by the regularity of the cluster cycle in some sufferers;

some can accurately predict the exact time and day of the next occurrence.

A 10-year study of 400 sufferers over the course of 900 cycles has provided further proof of a faulty time-keeper by showing that cluster cycles worsen as the days become shorter or longer, peaking in January and July, the times of year when this change is most pronounced.

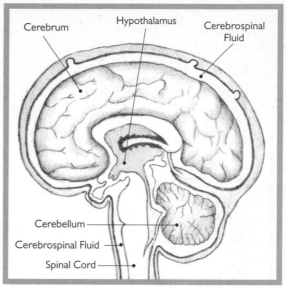

Figure 8.1—Brain and spinal cord.

HORMONE IMBALANCES

Since the majority of cluster sufferers are male, scientists are searching for a link between cluster and male sex hormones, hoping to establish a connection similar to the link between migraine headaches and estrogen fluctuations in women. Although inconclusive, there is some evidence among cluster sufferers of abnormalities in male hormone secretion, since testosterone is found to be lower during an active cluster cycle than when clusters are in remission.

DIGESTIVE DISORDERS

Digestion is a major factor of overall health, and whenever this essential process is malfunctioning, the overall condition of the body, particularly its ability to sustain itself by absorbing nutrients, is at stake. A number of conditions may coexist with and in fact create greater risk than more obvious causes of cluster headaches, including peptic ulcers, leaky gut syndrome, constipation, toxicity, low blood sugar (hypoglycemia),

A 10-year study of 400 sufferers over the course of 900 cycles has provided further proof of a faulty timekeeper by showing that cluster cycles worsen as the days become shorter or longer, peaking in January and July, the times of year when this change is most pronounced.

Candida, stress, and food and environmental allergies/sensitivities.

HISTAMINE FLUCTUATIONS

Another possible cause of clusters deals with the production of histamine, the hormone that is released in abnormal amounts when the skin or membranes of the body are exposed to an allergen. Research has shown excess levels of histamine in the tissues of those suffering from cluster attacks.

Since the majority of cluster sufferers are male, scientists are searching for a link between cluster and male sex hormones, hoping to establish a connection similar to the link between migraine headaches and estrogen fluctuations in women.

NERVE DYSFUNCTION

It is quite possible that clusters are related to swelling and inflammation in the nerves behind the eye, which exerts pressure on the large vein, called the cavernous sinus vein, that carries blood from the eyes to the head.

OXYGEN DEPRIVATION

It is suggested that low blood levels of oxygen contribute to a cluster attack. This theory derives from the facts that oxygen is often useful in treating clusters and that the brain gets 65 to 90% less oxygen during Rapid Eye Movement (REM) sleep, the time when clusters are known to appear.

Clusters are triggered by many of the same substances and events that incite just about every other headache, especially migraines and other vascular headaches. These include the range of metabolic triggers (blood clotting, chronic fatigue syndrome, food, chemical and environmental allergies/sensitivities, nutritional deficiencies, sleep disturbance, weather, and altitude changes); structural triggers (dental problems and musculoskeletal misalignments); and emotional/psychological triggers (stress, anxiety, and repressed emotions).

The cause-and-effect relationship between clusters and the myriad of triggers is unclear, however, due to the limited research that has been done on the mechanism of cluster headaches. Even so, a few correlations seem to be apparent, particularly the fact that these triggers are mainly active during a cluster cycle and not at other times. For example, a person may be able to drink as much as he wants until a cluster period begins, at which point a sip could be enough to bring on another attack.

The following triggers are most closely linked to the occurrence of cluster headaches:

ALCOHOL

Drinking alcohol during an episode of cluster headaches can immediately bring on an attack; furthermore, since 91% of cluster sufferers say they drink regularly, two-thirds classifying themselves as heavy drinkers, it is quite possible that a presently unknown link exists between clusters and the consumption of alcohol.

DRUGS

Cluster sufferers, desperate to try anything that might reduce their pain, often take an ill-advised assortment of drugs. This eventually adds to the overall syndrome, fostering other problems, such as liver toxicity and digestive disturbances and quite possibly triggering rebound or other headache types.

See Chapter 3, What Causes Your Headache?, for more details on the causes and triggers of headaches.

SMOKING

Some relationship exists between clusters and cigarette smoking, for studies that have examined the habits of cluster sufferers have shown 94% to be heavy smokers; although smoking is believed to worsen attacks, studies have not proved that the incidence of clusters decreases after the sufferer stops smoking.

ALTERNATIVE TREATMENTS

METABOLIC/BIOENERGETIC/BIOCHEMICAL-BASED THERAPIES

ACUPUNCTURE

Barbara, a 64-year-old, part-time accountant from Michigan, had suffered from cluster headaches for 4 years, chronic headaches for 20. Each episode lasting from 5 to 6 weeks, Barbara's clusters had taken over her life:

"It felt like something was chewing on the bones of one side of my face and head, as if someone were trying to separate my right side from my left. My right eye would swell shut, my jaw would lock in place, my nose would run on the right and I would drool— and usually this went on for about 3 hours. By the time they stopped, I would be completely exhausted, but then they would start all over again."

The first doctor who treated Barbara diagnosed her condition as a sinus infection and put her on antibiotics; when that did not work he put her on painkillers; later he sent her to a dentist who pulled teeth and did root canals. When all this failed to work, Barbara went to an ear, nose, and throat doctor who suggested surgery, which, based on past experience, Barbara opted not to have.

Finally, she ended up seeing a neurologist at a headache clinic. After a barrage of expensive tests, he diagnosed her condition as cluster headaches and told her that although there was no cure for cluster headaches, medication could help—medication with which the pharmacist warned her to be careful because too much could cause her blood vessels to collapse.

This medication cut the duration of pain to about a third of what it had been, but Barbara still had clusters, and the reduction was short-lived. When clusters returned full-force, the neurologist gave her lithium, which also worked only for a short while. Then, while Barbara was in the middle of yet another full-fledged episode, a coworker left the telephone number of David Krofcheck, O.M.D., D.Ac., C.A., on her desk, and Barbara tried acupuncture.

Barbara reported:

"On the first visit, he took all my pulses, looked into my mind with his questions, put needles all over me, covered me up, turned off the lights, and I went to sleep—something which is unheard of in a cluster. The relief lasted until the next day. I called him up and went in for another treatment, and this one lasted until 3 nights later. I went back the next day, and, after our session, I asked him when I should I come back; he said not until you have another one. This was in early 1990, and I haven't had another cluster since. To me, it feels like a miracle."

DETOXIFICATION THERAPY

Jackson, a carpenter in his early fifties, suffered from a typical case of cluster headaches. On his first visit to the Milne Medical Center, he described his cluster episode the night before. That day he had awakened from an afternoon nap with a sharp, excruciating pain above his right eye, his eyes and nose were watering, and he knew he was in for it because he had slept through the early warning signs and his regular medications were not going to help. Eventually the pain and pressure became so unbearable that he had his wife drive him to the hospital for a pain shot. He came to us hoping that we might be able to offer him something other than prescriptions.

Upon examination and allergy testing, it became obvious that Jackson was suffering from internal toxicity and digestive problems which were triggered and worsened by his frequent ingestion of corn. He ate popcorn almost every day. We immediately put him on an elimination diet and started an internal detoxification program that consisted of daily coffee enemas and an herbal bowel cleanser that consisted of Epsom salts in warm water. We also had him add wheat grass and vitamin supplements to his daily diet. Although this caused significant diarrhea, Jackson said it was the first thing that relieved the feeling of pressure in his head. We then gave Jackson acupressure to help open up his energy stagnation and taught him some acupressure techniques to do at home.

Jackson followed our instructions as if his life depended on it, and, although it took a complete change of his diet and lifestyle—which meant much hard work and dedication—his clusters eventually went into remission. Now, 3 years later, Jackson feels 20 years younger and happier and healthier than ever.

ENVIRONMENTAL MEDICINE

Devi S. Nambudripad, D.C., L.Ac., R.N., Ph.D., of Buena Park, California, reports a 90 to 95% success rate with cluster-type headaches. In one case, a newly married woman named Jane moved into a condominium with her husband and immediately began to experience cluster headaches. For a year and a half, she tried various treatments, but nothing worked until she consulted Dr. Nambudripad and tried the Nambudripad Allergy Elimination Technique (NAET), an allergy-testing and desensitization tech-

For more information about NAET, see Chapter 10, Allergy/Sensitivity Headaches.

nique that uses muscle testing and acupuncture stimulation to teach the nervous system not to react to specific substances.

After a thorough interview and examination, Dr. Nambudripad tested Jane for various substances and discovered she was allergic to oak, and, not surprisingly, Jane's condominium had oak cabinets. Dr. Nambudripad desensitized Jane to oak and then gave her a series of acupuncture, acupressure, and chiropractic treatments. Today, Jane's cluster headaches are gone.

OXYGEN THERAPY

People who snore and wake up suddenly with a cluster headache may do so because they have low levels of oxygen in their blood. This is why breathing pure oxygen through an oxygen mask for a few minutes can often stop an oncoming attack. Some sufferers rent a tank, keep it at work or at home, and use it for 15 minutes at the first sign of an impending cluster. Studies have shown this method to be an effective way to abort a cluster in progress as much as 80% of the time.

CAUTION

If you have respiratory problems, do not use pure oxygen without first consulting a qualified practitioner.

Renting an oxygen tank and mask is relatively easy and inexpensive. You can find one by either contacting a nearby hospital or buying one through your local medical supply store. To use the oxygen tank, remain seated with your body bent slightly forward. Place the mask on your face and inhale 100% oxygen at 7 to 10 liters per minute for 15 to 20 minutes. You can use oxygen longer if needed; however, do not use it for more than 1 hour a day.

OTHER METABOLIC/BIOENERGETIC/ BIOCHEMICAL-BASED THERAPIES

Depending upon underlying symptoms and conditions, the following therapies may be beneficial for treating cluster headaches:

- Acupuncture and Traditional Chinese Medicine
- Ayurvedic Medicine
- Energy Medicine
- Homeopathy
- Light Therapy
- Magnetic Field Therapy
- Naturopathy
- Nutritional Therapy

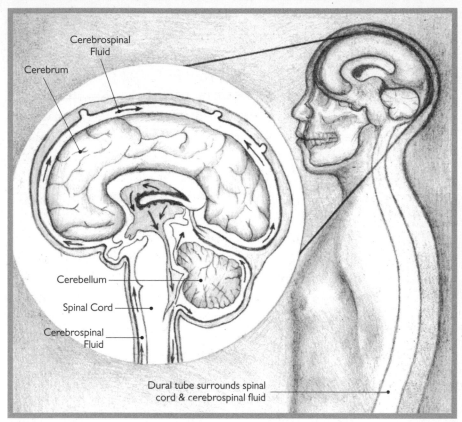

Fig 8.2—The craniosacral system.

Labels within figure:
Cerebrospinal Fluid
Cerebrum
Cerebellum
Spinal Cord
Cerebrospinal Fluid
Dural tube surrounds spinal cord & cerebrospinal fluid

STRUCTURALLY ORIENTED THERAPIES
CRANIOSACRAL THERAPY

Bob, a successful sports agent in his mid-thirties, had suffered from clusters for over 5 years. He tried prescription drugs, but felt that they either made him tired or dopey, and neither state was conducive to the level of performance expected of him in his job. Finally, after much searching, he came upon Benjamin Shield, Ph.D., of Santa Monica, California, a clinician who uses Rolfing, craniosacral therapy, herbs, and acupressure to treat a wide range of conditions associated with structural imbalances, including headaches.

Right away, Dr. Shield could see that Bob's clusters were related to an extremely tight bone where the cranial base meets the first vertebra (called the atlas), which was squeezing blood and energy pathways like fingers pressing on a hose. Without ample blood flow, vital nutrients, oxygen, and energy could not reach his brain, thus causing blood vessels to dilate and produce headaches. In addition, by perennially bracing himself for the next headache, Bob had developed poor posture.

First, Dr. Shield eased the musculoskeletal system and soft tissues with a session of deep, full-body Rolfing; then he used the light pressure of craniosacral therapy to adjust the bones of the skull and normalize the swollen areas in the skull. Over the course of 15 weekly sessions, Bob's cluster cycles tapered off and stopped completely. Now he is headache free.

OSTEOPATHY

Herbert Miller, D.O., an osteopathic physician from Indiana, uses a combination of osteopathy, nutritional therapy, and exercise to treat cluster headaches. One patient, a farmer in his mid-forties, had been suffering from clusters for more than 10 years. He had traveled to many different doctors and had been put on all the usual headache medications, but his clusters persisted.

Dr. Miller realized that the man's headaches were being caused by repeated traumas to his musculoskeletal structure incurred as he bounced across the fields in his tractor. After 6 months of weekly sessions in which Dr. Miller performed full body osteopathic massage, and 20 minutes daily of simple stretching exercises on the part of the patient, the cluster cycle was broken. Now, Dr. Miller sees him 4 times a year to keep his body in shape because the man still drives a tractor.

OTHER STRUCTURALLY ORIENTED THERAPIES

Depending upon the underlying cause, the following therapies can also be useful:

Alphabiotics

Biological Dentistry

Bodywork

Chiropractic
Neural Therapy

PSYCHO/EMOTIONAL THERAPIES
FLOWER ESSENCE THERAPY
The following flower essences may help to relieve the emotional and physiological causes and effects of cluster headaches:

ALLERGY/SENSITIVITY
- **Dill**—for those who are overwhelmed, hypersensitive, or over-stimulated; known to enhance digestive function
- **St. John's Wort**—used for headache accompanied by light sensitivity or vulnerability to environmental stress, including allergies
- **Yarrow**—strengthens the sensitivity that occurs when body tries to deal with input overload, either through the environment or through digestion

TRAUMA
- **Arnica**—for severe trauma in which it feels like you have left your body; restores conscious embodiment
- **Five Flower Remedy** (also called Rescue Remedy)—for panic, disorientation, or loss of consciousness; used to restore calm and stability in emergencies or during intense stress; contains cherry plum, clematis, impatiens, rock rose, star of Bethlehem
- **Self Heal** (the flower *Prunella vulgaris*)—used to restore the physical body after a blow or injury, especially when damage seems overwhelming; restores a vital sense of self

STRESS AND TENSION
- **Dandelion**—for stress and tension held in the muscles of the body; brings about dynamic, effortless energy
- **Impatiens**—for people who are constantly rushing, impatient, intolerant, tense; creates acceptance and patience
- **Iris**—for tension, especially in the neck region; and inability to feel inner freedom

- **Mimulus**—for those who are frequently in fear of their next headache attack
- **Five Flower Remedy**—helps in coping with stress in general

GENERAL HEADACHE
- **Lavender**—good overall headache remedy; used to dispel nervousness and overstimulation, which deplete the physical body
- **Five Flower Remedy**—good overall stress remedy

See Chapter 16, An A-Z of Self-Care Options, for more information on self-treatment methods.

OTHER PSYCHO/EMOTIONAL THERAPIES

The following therapies can also be beneficial for cluster headaches:

Biofeedback

Hypnotherapy

Psychotherapy

SELF-CARE OPTIONS
SELF-ACUPRESSURE

The following points (see Figure 8.3) can be helpful to relieve the pain of cluster headaches as well as improve your overall system and help eliminate cluster cycles altogether:

- Governing Vessel 20 (GV 20)
- Governing Vessel 16 (GV 16)
- Gall Bladder 20 (GB 20)
- Bladder 2 (Bl 2)
- *Yin Tang* point (GV 24.5)
- Stomach 3
- Stomach 36
- Liver 3 (Lv 3)
- G-Jo #13 (LI 4)

AROMATHERAPY

The following aromatherapy blends are suggested as a supplemental therapy for cluster prevention and relief:

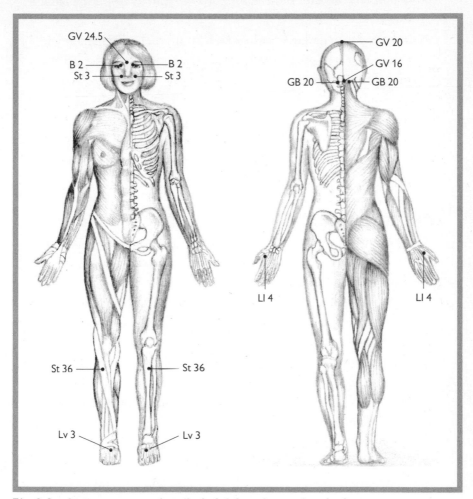

Fig 8.3—Acupressure points helpful for cluster headaches.

INHALATION

Wafting relief: Fill aroma lamp, bowl, or diffuser with water and mix in 4 drops melissa and 2 drops peppermint or Roman chamomile oil.

For aroma to go: Put 2 to 3 drops of melissa, peppermint, and lavender oils on a handkerchief or cloth and inhale throughout the day for prevention.

MASSAGE

Temple rub: Combine lavender (a sedative) and peppermint (a stimulant) oils and rub the mixture on your temples for pain relief.

Good oils for vascular-type headaches: Anise, basil, chamomile, coriander, eucalyptus, lavender, lemon, marjoram, melissa, onion, peppermint, rosemary

BATHS

Aroma soak: For relief of a headache in progress, fill a bath with warm to hot water and add eucalyptus, wintergreen, or peppermint and soak for 20 to 30 minutes.

COMPRESSES AND STEAMS

Cold compress relief: Mix 3 drops rose, 1 drop melissa, and 1 drop lavender oils in 2 pints water. Stir thoroughly and place a towel or washcloth in the water. Let it soak for 5 minutes, then wring to remove excess water. Lie back and put the compress on the painful area. Rest; change the compress as soon as it reaches room temperature.

Lavender and peppermint compress for vascular headache: At the first sign of headache, make 2 compresses, a lavender and peppermint compress for the forehead, and a hot marjoram (a vasodilator, stretches blood vessels) for the back of the neck; this combination provides a combination of relaxing, stimulating, and vasodilating effects.

Aromatherapy steam: Boil 2 pints of water and pour into a large bowl, add 1 drop melissa, 2 drops peppermint, and 2 drops lavender oils. Put your head over the bowl and cover your head and the bowl with a large towel. Inhale deeply through your nose for about 10 minutes.

BREATHING EXERCISES

The self-care version of oxygen therapy, breathing exercises can be useful for the cluster sufferer since they increase the oxygen supply in the body and can thereby help to prevent cluster headaches.

Three-Part Breath—This technique is designed to draw air deep into the diaphragm so it can oxygenate the entire system. Basically, it is done by dividing a deep inhalation into 3 parts, with the first part lifting the belly, the second filling the lungs, and the third extending into the upper chest. Hold for 3 seconds and release in one long exhalation. Do not strain or force your breathing. Repeat 5 times.

Wu **Breathing Exercise**—*Wu* is a Chinese breathing technique known to relieve headaches. Lie down in a relaxed position with your head on a low pillow and your arms reaching down your sides, your feet a little more than hip-width apart. Place the tip of your tongue on the roof of your mouth, just past where the front teeth meet the gums, and breath naturally but deeply through your nose. Imagine the breath coming through your nose and the top of your head down to the center of your belly. Continue this for about 20 to 30 minutes, concentrating on the breath coming in through your head. Practice in the morning and at night.

Pulse Breathing—This technique involves diaphragm breathing and a pulsed, hard exhalation—much like a karate expert yells as he hits the brick. To start, take a deep breath and exhale, then inhale and exhale forcefully (called a pulse breath). Then take 2 deep breathing cycles and a pulse; 3 breathing cycles and a pulse; 4 breathing cycles and a pulse; 5 breathing cycles and a pulse. Perform this exercises twice daily and any time you are under stress.

> *Cayenne is the number one herb for treating clusters. In one study, 11 out of 16 cluster patients who used cayenne experienced a complete disappearance of their attacks, while 2 others reported 50% reduction.*

FOLK REMEDIES

The following folk remedies may also be helpful as supplementary treatments for cluster headaches:

Herbal compress: Boil 3 cups water and pour over 1 tablespoon lavender and 1 tablespoon chamomile, letting it steep for 20 minutes. Soak a soft cloth in the mixture, then wring it out and apply on the back of neck or forehead. Cold herbal compresses are also effective.

Herbal foot bath: This is an excellent way to draw blood and congestion away from your head. Place one tablespoon powdered mustard or ginger in a deep basin big enough for both feet. Fill the basin with water as hot as you can bear, then sit in a comfortable chair, and slowly immerse your feet in the water. Drape a thick towel over the basin to keep the heat in, and place a cool or cold towel on your neck or forehead. Close your eyes and relax, breathing deeply for about 15 minutes.

Alternating hot and cold showers: To improve blood circulation, try alternating hot and cold showers once a day for 2 or 3 months; this remedy works to abort vascular-type headaches because the heat further dilates the blood vessels (which may temporarily cause pain), while the cold makes blood vessels contract.

Cold water and hot water wrist baths: If you feel a headache coming on and you are away from familiar territory, look for a sink and run cold water and then hot water on your wrists, alternating back and forth until you feel the headache pass.

Drink a headache tonic: Fill a large pot with water and mix in small pieces of fresh ginger root, coriander seeds, diced garlic, and a little honey to taste. Boil off half the liquid and periodically drink what is left throughout the day.

Apple cider vinegar and honey tonic: To offset the causes of a digestive headache, particularly one related to excess acid production, D.C. Jarvis, M.D., in *Vermont Folk Medicine*, suggests taking apple cider vinegar in water and/or 2 teaspoons honey every day to help regulate the body's pH balance. Dr. Jarvis has observed that when taken as a rescue remedy this mixture will stop any headache, including a migraine, within a half-hour. If you do not like the taste, you can place equal parts of apple cider vinegar and water in a steamer, place your face over it with your head covered with a towel, and inhale 75 breaths.

A spoonful of honey: A tablespoon of raw honey at first inkling of an impending headache can abort a vascular headache; take a spoonful, wait a half-hour, and if it has not worked take another tablespoon with 3 glasses of water.

Li Shou (arm swinging): This Chinese technique uses motion to relieve headaches by creating a relaxed, meditative state and is taught to school children to relieve stress. Swing your arms back and forth until the blood shifts from your head to your hands, reducing your swollen blood vessels. Next, use your warmed hands to stroke your face, using a circular motion, paying particular attention to the area around your eyes. Repeat the exercise several times.

Wrap rubberbands around your fingers: Take 10 rubberbands and wrap them around each of your fingers at the first joint, the one closest to your fingernail. Put them on tight, and although they may turn your fingers purplish and hurt a bit, leave them on for no more than 9 minutes to find that your headache has disappeared.

Bite your tongue: This remedy is not about watching what you say; instead stick out your tongue about $1/2$ inch, then bite on it *gently* for about 9 minutes (not more than 11 minutes), keeping pressure on your tongue the entire time.

The paper bag trick: Because your exhaled breath is composed largely of carbon dioxide (CO_2) and carbon dioxide is known to dilate the cerebral arteries, some say breathing into a bag and rebreathing your expired air at the earliest sign of a vascular headache can abort the approaching attack. This works especially well when classic migraine sufferers do it the minute they see a warning aura. Try breathing into the bag for 15 to 20 minutes and then lying down for 20 minutes. If the headache has not gone away, repeat the breathing cycle one more time.

HERBAL SUPPLEMENTS

Cayenne is the number one herb for treating clusters. Although numerous studies of the impact of herbs on clusters have been undertaken, the most impressive was conducted in Italy. In this study, 11 out of 16 cluster patients who used cayenne experienced a complete disappearance of their attacks, while 2 others reported 50% reduction.[2]

One way to administer cayenne is to rub a cayenne preparation inside and outside the nostril on the affected side. Another way is to add powdered capsicum (the active ingredient of cayenne pepper) to a mild skin cream and rub it on your temples or in your nostrils. Although sneezing is a known side effect of cayenne, this usually does not last long and eventually, after cayenne is used for a while, subsides altogether.

Depending upon the severity of the headache, additional herbal supplements can be used as an adjunct to other therapies, since herbs can relieve symptoms and help to strengthen the body. Although still other herbs may be used to treat and relieve associated symptoms and underlying or preexisting conditions, the following herbs can be effective in cases of cluster headaches:

Allergy/sensitivity or digestive disorders—black horehound, cayenne, chamomile, fenugreek, feverfew, ginger, nettle, passion flower, peppermint, rosemary, safflower, slippery elm, St. John's wort, wood betony

Brain function—ginseng, *Ginkgo*, rosemary

Circulation—cayenne, feverfew, hawthorn, garlic, rosemary

Constipation/detox—aloe, burdock, dandelion, goldenseal (root), milk thistle, nettle, Oregon grape root, senna, vervain, wood betony

General headache—angelica, feverfew, meadowsweet, willow bark

Head trauma and swelling— coriander, skullcap, St. John's wort

Hormonal/reproductive problems—black cohosh, blackhaw, cayenne, chamomile, chasteberry, cramp bark, *dong quai*, lavender, Jamaican dogwood, passion flower, skullcap, St. John's wort, wild yam

Immune system— echinacea, garlic, ginger, *Ginkgo*, ginseng, golden seal, nettle, rosehips

Musculoskeletal pain and spasms—cayenne, chamomile, elder, meadowsweet, nettles, *qiyelian*, turmeric, valerian, vervain, willow bark

Sinus congestion—lavender, rosemary, peppermint, eucalyptus

Stress, anxiety, insomnia, depression, and tension— cramp bark, feverfew, hawthorn, ginkgo, ginseng, lavender, linden blossom, passion flower, pennyroyal, peppermint, rosehips, skullcap, St. John's wort, valerian, vervain

Vascular imbalances—balm, basil, black willow, cayenne, elder flower, feverfew, garlic, ginger, *Ginkgo*, goldenrod, Jamaican dogwood, lavender, marjoram, peppermint, rosemary, rue, thyme, sage, willow bark, wood betony, wormwood

REFLEXOLOGY

Applying light pressure on the following reflexology areas can help to relieve the pain of cluster headaches as well as improve your overall constitution, and thus eliminate cluster cycles altogther.

- **Brain**—all headaches, circulation, and overall body function
- **Head**—all headaches, stress, shoulder and neck tension
- **Pituitary**—hormonal imbalance, allergy/sensitivity, digestive, migraine, cluster
- **Sinuses**—sinus, allergy
- **Neck**—tension, physical and emotional stress
- **Spine**—all headaches, trauma, stress, tension, digestion
- **Solar Plexus**—all headaches, stress, anxiety, digestion

See Chapter 16, An A-Z of Self-Care Options, Reflexology, for information on application.

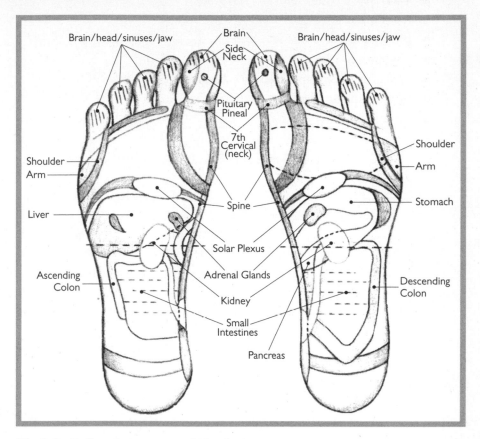

Fig 8.4—Reflexology areas of the feet.

- **Adrenal Gland**—hypertension, hormonal imbalance, digestion, toxicity
- **Stomach**—digestion, sensitivity/allergy, migraine
- **Pancreas**—hypoglycemia, digestion
- **Intestines**—digestion, sensitivity/allergy, migraine
- **Kidney**—vascular, allergy/sensitivity, toxicity, migraine
- **Liver**—digestion, circulation, toxicity

OTHER SELF-CARE OPTIONS

The following self-help techniques can also be helpful for cluster headaches:

- Affirmations/Autosuggestions
- Creative Visualization

- Exercise
- Ice and Heat
- Lifestyle Changes
- Meditation
- Nutritional Therapy/Dietary Changes
- Relaxation Exercises
- Support Groups

RECOMMENDED READING

Alternative Medicine: The Definitive Guide. Compiled by the Burton Goldberg Group. Tiburon, CA: Future Medicine Publishing, 1994.

The American Council on Headache Education, with Lynee M. Constantine and Suzanne Scott. *Migraine: The Complete Guide.* New York: Dell Publishing, 1994.

Benson, Paul, D.O. "Biofeedback and Stress Management." *Osteopathic Annals* 12 (August 1984), 20-26.

Blau, J.N. "Behaviour During a Cluster Headache." *The Lancet* 342 (September 18, 1993), 723-725.

Braly, James, M.D. and Torbet, Laura. *Dr. Braly's Food Allergy and Nutrition Revolution.* New Canaan, CT: Keats Publishing, Inc., 1992.

Clark, Linda, M.A. *A Handbook of Natural Remedies for Common Ailments.* Greenwich, CT: The Devin-Adair Company, 1976.

Diamond, Seymour, M.D. and Still, Bill and Cynthia. *The Hormone Headache.* New York: Macmillan, 1995.

Faber, William J., D.O. *Pain, Pain Go Away.* San Jose, CA: ISHI Press International, 1990.

Ford, Norman D. *Eighteen Natural Ways to Beat a Headache.* New Canaan, CT: Keats Publishing, Inc. 1990.

Herzberg, Eileen. *Migraine: A Comprehensive Guide to Gentle, Safe & Effective Treatment.* Rockport, MA: Element Inc., 1994.

Igram, Cass, M.D. *Who Needs Headaches?* Cedar Rapids, IA: Literary Visions Publishing, 1991.

Jensen, Bernard, D.C., Ph.D. *Tissue Cleansing through Bowel Management*, 10th ed. Escondido, CA: Bernard Jensen Publishing, 1981.

Jouanny, Jacques, M.D. et al. *Homeopathic Therapeutics: Possibilities in Chronic Pathology.* France: Editions Boiron, 1994.

Keller, Erich. *The Complete Home Guide to Aromatherapy.* Tiburon, CA: H.J. Kramer, Inc., 1991.

Kunz, Kevin and Kunz, Barbara. *Hand Reflexology Workbook*. Albuquerque, NM: RRP Press, 1994.

Lilienthal, Samuel, M.D. *Homeopathic Therapeutics*. New Delhi: Jain Publishing Co., 1996.

Lipton, Richard B., M.D., Newman, Lawrence C., M.D., and MacLean, Helene. *Migraine/Beating the Odds: The Doctor's Guide to Reducing Your Risk*. Reading, MA: Addison-Wesley Publishing Company, 1992.

National Headache Foundation Fact Sheet. Chicago: National Headache Foundation, October 1994.

Natural Health Secrets from around the World. Boca Raton, FL: Shot Tower Books, 1996.

Rapoport, Alan M., M.D. and Sheftell, Fred D., M.D. *Headache Relief*. New York: Simon & Schuster, 1990.

Rapoport, Alan M., M.D. and Sheftell, Fred D., M.D. *Headache Relief for Women*. New York: Little, Brown and Company, 1995.

Rick, Stephanie. *The Reflexology Workout*. New York: Harmony Books, 1986.

Robbins, Lawrence, M.D. and Land, Susan. *Headache Help*. New York: Houghton Mifflin Company, 1995.

Simpson, Kristine, et al., eds. *The Experts Speak 1996: The Role of Nutrition in Medicine*. Sacramento: Kirk Hamilton PA-C, 1996, 121-122.

Stang, P.E. and Osterhaus, J.T. "Impact of Migraine in the United States: Data from the National Health Interview Survey." *Headache* 33 (1993), 29-35.

Stromfeld, Jan and Weil, Anita. *Free Yourself from Headaches: The Natural Drug-Free Program for Prevention and Relief*. Palm Beach Gardens, FL: The Upledger Institute, Frog, Ltd., 1995.

Solomon, Seymour, M.D. and Fraccaro, Steven. *The Headache Book*. Mount Vernon, NY: Consumer Reports Books, 1991.

Wilson, Roberta. *Aromatherapy for Vibrant Health & Beauty*. Garden City Park, NY: Avery Publishing Group, 1994.

Alternative medical practitioners will treat your headache as part of the whole complex system which is your body. They tend to look for imbalances in that system which may be producing the headache. By addressing the imbalance, rather than treating the symptom, they can help you eliminate your headaches.

Chapter 9

Trauma Headaches

Affecting 1.5 million Americans a year, trauma headaches are those that occur after an injury to the head, neck, or spine, striking anywhere from 24 hours to months, even years, after the accident. A seemingly minor bump on the head can bring on chronic headaches, even when evidence of injury does not show up in neurological exams.

Ten-year-old Timmy came to the Milne Medical Center complaining of chronic headaches that had begun after he had fallen from his treehouse and suffered a concussion. Although his skull X rays and MRI scan had turned out negative, 3 months later he was still experiencing almost daily neck and total head pain, which was not helped by aspirin or Tylenol, and kept Timmy from his favorite activity, playing soccer after school.

After evaluation, we decided to use a combination of acupuncture and homeopathy to help resolve the bruising and energy stagnation that had resulted from Timmy's fall. We treated him with acupuncture stimulation at tender trigger points around his neck and head and gave him *Arnica* and *Natrum sulfuricum*. Over the course of 2 weeks, which included 3 acupuncture treatments and 3 doses daily of these homeopathic remedies, Timmy's symptoms gradually went away and his headaches disappeared.

What Is a Trauma Headache?

Affecting over 1.5 million Americans a year, trauma headaches are headaches that occur after an injury to the head, face, neck, or spine. Often characterized as a symptom of posttrauma or postconcussion syndrome, these headaches can be confounding as there is often no rhyme or reason to their symptoms. Sometimes they strike within 24 to 48 hours of the initial trauma, while in other cases it takes months, sometimes even years, for them to appear.

Making matters worse, the severity of the initial injury and the severity of the pain are often disproportionate; a seemingly minor bump on the head can bring on a devastating bout of chronic headaches, while a fractured or lacerated skull may produce only localized pain.

Another confusing aspect of trauma headaches is that they can produce symptoms and pain that mimic migraine or tension headaches, sometimes both. Trauma headache pain can involve muscular contraction as well as the neurological or metabolic symptoms that are associated with vascular or systemic disturbances. Trauma headaches can be localized or generalized, throbbing or dull, with or without an aching neck, shoulder, and/or back.

Sometimes pain is accompanied by dizziness or spinning sensations (called vertigo), mood changes, insomnia and/or fatigue, irritability, a reduced attention span, depression, blurred vision, ringing in the ears, sensitivity to noise or bright lights, nausea, intolerance for alcohol or medication, and a diminished desire for sex. Frequently, these symptoms are worsened by exertion and, in about 10% of cases, are also accompanied by fainting spells.

In a majority of cases, trauma headaches will build in intensity and then taper off within a few weeks. About a third of all trauma headache sufferers, however, have headaches that last more than 2 months after the injury. For these individuals, once the headache develops, it usually occurs daily and is fairly resistant to treatment.

CAUTION

Subdural Hematoma: A headache following a head injury must be closely watched, since it could be the sign of a more serious condition. Headaches that appear within 24 hours and worsen over time, then gradually decrease, may only be an expression of postconcussion syndrome, but those that do not gradually disappear, especially when accompanied by drowsiness, may be signs of a broken blood vessel bleeding into the lining of the brain. This ruptured blood vessel is called a subdural hematoma, a very serious condition that requires immediate medical attention.

Causes and Triggers of Trauma Headaches

The types of head injuries generally associated with trauma headaches are known as closed-head injuries, meaning that the skull escaped fracture or penetration during the injury. Closed-head injuries produce excessive pain because, unlike fractures in which the blow is mainly absorbed by the bone, the brain must take most of the force.

This vibration may bruise the brain and interfere with the activity of the neurotransmitters and/or the nerve connections, leading to the associated symptoms of reduced mental abilities, erratic personality changes, and heightened perception of pain. In addition, whiplash-type injuries can also damage the inner ear, producing sensations such as vertigo and ear ringing. Essentially, then, a trauma can have lasting effects, on both a structural and

Symptom Chart—Trauma Headaches

SYMPTOMS	HEADACHE TYPE	PAIN LOCATION
Description: dull, aching, stabbing and sharp or excruciating pain at site of injury **Other Symptoms:** can mimic migraine or tension headache symptoms, including runny or stuffy nose, sneezing, postnasal drip, diarrhea and/or fever; sweating on forehead above drooping eye and on abdomen and trunk; redness and tearing eye; visual and/or other sensory disturbances; limited attention span, insomnia, anxiety, weakness, irritability, shakiness, blacking out, intolerance for light and noise, nausea, vomiting. **Duration:** 20 minutes to all day **Frequency:** in clusters or continuous; daily or rarely	**TRAUMA HEADACHE**	where the head injury occurred or can mimic location of tension or migraine headache
Description: persistent headache that worsens with time; sleepiness, confusion, disturbances of vision; nausea or vomiting; weakness or numbness in one part of body	**SUBDURAL HEMATOMA HEADACHE**	

UNDERLYING CAUSES AND TRIGGERS	PRIMARY AND SECONDARY TREATMENTS	SELF-CARE TREATMENTS	WHERE IN THE BOOK PAGE #
Causes: blow to head or fall; can be worsened by metabolic imbalances, structural disturbances, emotional/psychological factors	**Primary:** ■ acupuncture ■ bodywork ■ chiropractic ■ craniosacral therapy ■ homeopathy ■ neural therapy ■ osteopathy ■ traditional Chinese medicine **Secondary:** ■ alphabiotics ■ Ayurvedic medicine ■ detoxification ■ energy medicine ■ environmental medicine ■ herbal medicine ■ magnetic field therapy ■ naturopathic medicine ■ oxygen therapy	■ aromatherapy ■ affirmations ■ biofeedback ■ breathing exercises ■ creative visualization ■ exercise ■ flower remedies ■ folk remedies ■ herbal supplements ■ ice and heat ■ journal writing ■ lifestyle changes ■ massage ■ meditation ■ nutritional therapy ■ relaxation techniques ■ support groups	Page 257
	see medical doctor		Page 257

Traumas Most Often Associated with Headache

HEAD IS INJURED BY A FALL OR BLOW TO THE HEAD:

These are the most common types of head injuries.

FORGOTTEN TRAUMA: These can be the result of something that happened when you were young—trauma ranging from bumping heads with a playmate to the press of forceps or complications at birth. When you think of the number of times a toddler falls, it is easy to imagine how a physical trauma can develop much later into a structural problem that can result in chronic headaches.

WHIPLASH (sometimes called an "acceleration-deceleration" injury): Even without an actual blow, the force of being bounced or jerked around can exert undue pressure against the muscles, ligaments, or tendons of the head, neck, and spine, setting the stage for muscle contractions and spasms similar to those of tension headaches. In addition, such a trauma can damage nerves and bruise blood vessels in the brain.

See Chapter 3, What Causes Your Headache?, for more detail on what triggers headaches.

a functional or metabolic level.

One theory as to why the head pain of a trauma is delayed or hard to predict is that the mechanism that heightens the headache actually occurs after the trauma. For example, a blow to the head results in damaged tissues, nerves, and membranes that then become engorged with fluid. Such swelling can further disrupt the blood-brain barrier and allow otherwise excluded particles and substances, including toxins, into the brain and spinal cord, adding additional damage to an already impaired brain.

Another theory suggests that the delayed onset of trauma headaches is attributable either to the buildup of scar tissue in the scalp or to the gradual worsening of the misalignments caused by the fall or injury.

The brain contains billions of nerve cells, each responsible for making at least a thousand or more connections with other nerve cells, and even a minor injury can affect this complex web of connections. This injury often serves to worsen an already damaged system, putting further strain on an already overburdened mechanism. Existing conditions can often intensify the symptoms of a trauma and make it difficult, if not impossible, for the body to sustain enough energy to heal through its own accord.

These conditions include metabolic/biochemical imbalances such as problems with blood clotting, candidiasis, chronic fatigue syndrome, chemical and environmental sensitivities, constipation and other digestive disturbances, food allergies and sensitivities, hypoglycemia, leaky gut syndrome, nutritional deficiencies, and changes in sleeping patterns, weather, and altitude; structural imbalances such as dental problems, musculoskeletal misalignments, and poor posture; and emotional/psychological factors such as stress, anxiety, and repressed emotions.

Diagnosing and Treating Underlying Causes

Depending upon the degree of the trauma, trauma headaches generally (1) heal on their own, (2) stabilize at a certain point of distortion or dysfunction, or (3) worsen and affect other bodily systems to create imbalances or magnify already existing conditions.

Unless there are signs of serious damage, trauma headaches do not show up during neurological examinations, a fact which can be particularly troublesome if the headache is related to a long forgotten trauma. Further compounding an already difficult prognosis, physical pain causes psychological distress, putting further physiological demands on the brain and body.

Nonetheless, alternative practitioners are detectives who are accustomed to such complexity and trained not only to ask probing questions that may uncover past injuries but also to use their eyes, ears, and hands to see what even you may not consciously remember or correlate to your headache. It is the practitioner's job, for instance, to notice that a distant injury can sometimes cause one shoulder to sit lower than the other or make the head and neck rigid and restrict their range of motion, no matter how subtly. The practitioner looks for food allergies, hormonal imbalances, stress patterns, and every other factor and condition that may be contributing to the head pain. When these factors are completely understood, the practitioner begins to treat the headache.

It is the practitioner's job to work with you to determine the therapies that will effectively heal your headaches. Every head injury is different, so treatments must be individualized to fit the particular headache pattern. The basic therapy categories—metabolic, structural, and psychological/emotional—must be evaluated and addressed, either by the practitioner or through your own initiative. The therapies listed below are used most frequently to treat trauma headaches.

ALTERNATIVE TREATMENTS

METABOLIC/BIOENERGETIC/ BIOCHEMICAL-BASED THERAPIES

HOMEOPATHY

See Chapter 17, An A-Z of Alternative Medicine, for more information on possible treatment methods.

Like herbal medicine, homeopathy is often used to relieve pain and stimulate the body's innate healing capacity. In cases of trauma, homeopathy is especially useful when combined with structural therapies. A perfect example of the good pairing of therapeutic modalities is the case of Jake, a 10-year-old boy who accidentally fell and hit his head on the sidewalk while he was rollerblading through his city neighborhood.

Because Jake had neglected to wear his helmet, the fall caused him to lose consciousness for 2 to 3 minutes. His parents rushed him to the emergency room where, after a series of tests, it was determined that the damage to his head was not serious. He was diagnosed as having a concussion and told he would feel better in a few days.

His headaches did not go away with his concussion, however. Instead they got progressively worse until Jake began to suffer from daily headaches which began at the back of his head and worked their way up to create a hot feeling at the top of his head. Aspirin and Tylenol proved ineffective. So, recognizing the probability that a conventional doctor would put Jake on more serious drugs, his parents took him to the Milne Medical Center.

Upon evaluation, we determined that Jake would respond best to a combination of approaches: homeopathy, a blended remedy of *Arnica montana* 3X and *Natrum sulphuricum* 3X (from Sodium Sulfate), to help him overcome the emotional and physical shock of his trauma; and craniosacral therapy, in which gentle rhythmic adustments were used to move Jake's cranial bones and stimulate the flow of energy to the brain. Jake noticed an improvement right away. After 3 cranial treatments and a month of 3 doses daily of homeopathy, Jake's headaches were gone, and he was once again rollerblading—with a helmet.

The following homeopathic remedies are a sampling of those that can be useful for trauma headaches. Keep in mind, however, that homeopathic remedies work best when prescribed by a qualified practitioner; when self-administered, these remedies should be taken only in doses of 6X or lower.

For Structural Misalignments and Trauma—*Actae Racemosa, Arnica montana* (bruise-like ache, worsened by movement, associated with physical exhaustion or trauma); *Byronia, Calcarea carbonica* (physical overexertion); *Colocynthis, Ranunculus bulbosus* (head pain associated with postural problems, pains in the back and side); *Rhus toxicodendron* (physical overexertion); *Silicea* (pain in the nape of the neck associated with nervous exhaustion).

For Headaches without Symptoms Characteristic of a Particular Remedy—*Aconitum nappellus* (taken at the onset of any acute headache); *Apis mellifica* (migraines accompanied by swelling); *Secale cornutum* (migraines); *Serotoninum* (congestive headaches, particularly with unstable blood pressure).

OTHER METABOLIC/BIOENERGETIC/ BIOCHEMICAL-BASED THERAPIES

All of the following therapies are also useful for the treatment of trauma headaches:

- Acupuncture
- Ayurvedic Medicine
- Detoxification Therapy
- Energy Medicine
- Environmental Medicine
- Light Therapy
- Magnetic Field Therapy
- Naturopathic Medicine
- Nutritional Therapy
- Oxygen Therapy
- Traditional Chinese Medicine

STRUCTURALLY ORIENTED THERAPIES

BODYWORK

Although all types of bodywork can be effective for headaches, this chapter highlights 2 techniques, myotherapy and Rolfing. Remember, however, that deep massage is also often good for traumas that occurred long ago, since it helps to break up calcified or scarred areas of the muscles.

Myotherapy—Fifteen-year-old Craig had been experiencing what doctors believed to be migraines since the age of 6. He saw stars, vomited, and missed 1 out of 4 school days because of his headaches. Doctors had put him through every test and the gamut of medications, yet nothing relieved his pain. Then his mother took him to see myotherapy founder, Bonnie Prudden, C.B.M.P. As she examined him, Prudden asked if Craig had ever hit or harmed his head in any way before the headaches began. Craig's mother remembered a time when, at the age of 4, Craig had knocked heads with another little boy and got a terrible lump on his forehead; she realized at the same time that Craig's forehead still swelled when his headaches struck.

Prudden recognized this as the clue she was looking for and determined that the site of Craig's injury contained very active trigger points. Through 3 sessions of myotherapy by Prudden, plus daily self-myotherapy techniques performed at home to work his jaw, neck, and face, Craig's "migraines" went away, and Craig was finally pain free and able to enjoy a normal life. [1]

Myotherapy is a technique of pain relief developed by physical fitness and exercise therapy expert Bonnie Prudden. The myotherapist applies deep manual pressure, usually with fingertips, on the skin for 5-7 seconds, to precise sites of muscular pain, called "trigger points." Prudden found that this technique can relieve pain for about 90% of all muscle-related pain conditions, making it unnecessary to use painkilling injections.

Rolfing, also known as Structural Integration, is a vigorous form of therapeutic, stress-releasing bodywork developed by Ida Rolf, Ph.D. (1896-1979). It uses a series of hand-delivered physical manipulations and adjustments of the myofascial tissue to help reorient the body to gravity. Dr. Rolf taught that human function is improved when the body segments (head, torso, pelvis, legs, feet) are properly aligned. Rolfers apply pressure through the fingers, knuckles, and elbows to loosen up the rigidified fascial tissue, which is the thin, elastic, semifluid membrane that envelops every muscle, bone, blood vessel, nerve, and organ.

Rolfing—Kathy, a woman in her early forties, had been in a devastating car accident in which a driver had run a red light and slammed into her in an intersection. The accident had damaged Kathy's rib cage and shoulder, and 4 months later, the trauma had worked its way down her spine and up her neck and finally resulted in head pain that was accompanied by jaw pain, visual disturbances, mental confusion, and fatigue.

When she went to see Jan Henry Sultan, L.M.T., a Rolfing practitioner and licensed massage therapist in New Mexico, Kathy's body had become so misaligned that her head was tilting to compensate, her face was crooked, and her entire body was in pain. Kathy wanted to have another baby but was afraid that her body could not successfully carry a pregnancy.

After a series of treatments, in which Sultan massaged the trunk of Kathy's body to reorganize the relationship between the rib cage and the spine, especially from the rib cage to the shoulder since these were the areas of direct impact, Kathy's headaches disappeared, and her body straightened up to the point where she was able to have another baby.

CHIROPRACTIC

Ellen Cutler, D.C., who uses a combination of chiropractic, the Nambudripad

Allergy Elimination Technique (NAET), and nutritional therapy in her Corte Madera, California, practice, treated a 13-year-old girl who had been diagnosed with chronic migraines. Whenever the young girl encountered a stressful situation, she would be struck with excruciating migraines accompanied by vomiting and almost total disability.

The girl had been getting nowhere with conventional treatments. Upon examination, Dr. Cutler immediately discovered that the girl's tailbone was misaligned in relation to her head and spine. Dr. Cutler performed the needed adjustments; when the treatment was finished, the girl, without warning or prompting, reexperienced an intense emotion which was connected to a forgotten trauma that had occurred when she was 3 years old. As the trauma was released, so were the girl's headaches.[2]

CRANIOSACRAL THERAPY

Three years after her car accident, Page, a 27-year-old mother of 2, was still suffering from chronic head, neck, and back pain. She had seen conventional doctors, and they had put her through CAT scans, MRIs and X rays, had given her medications, and finally, when nothing seemed to work, had told her that she was going to have to learn to live with her pain. Desperate, she went to see Don Ash, R.P.T., a registered physical therapist with a private practice in New Hampshire.

In their first session, while Dr. Ash was working on Page's skull, using a very light touch in conjunction with a gentle rocking technique, Page suddenly rolled into a fetal position and began crying. She complained of aching wrists, ankles, and shoulders and said she saw the color red. Recognizing her behavior as a sign of deep emotional release which often occurs during craniosacral therapy, Dr. Ash asked Page to stay with the feelings and sensations as they came up.

Page complied, and 10 to 15 minutes later, she recalled the complete details of her car accident—even though she had previously been unable to recover this memory due to blacking out during the accident. Through her body, Page was able to remember going 60 miles per hour and seeing a red car coming toward her; she described how, when she hit the car, her ankles curled underneath the seat, her wrists locked against the

Craniosacral therapy refers to correcting imbalances in the relationship among breathing, the sacrum, and bones of the skull (cranium) especially the occiput. The sacrum (or hip bone) acts as a pump to propel cerebrospinal fluid up the spine to the brain; the cranial bones contract and pump it back down. Health depends on a smoothly functioning sacro-occipital pump; craniosacral work, as delivered by a chiropractor, restores the sacrum to full motion and balance with respect to the cranial bones.

steering wheel, and her neck snapped.

Dr. Ash explains:

"Such emotional release is the by-product of craniosacral therapy. Page had what is termed a somato-emotional release. As she relived the car accident, the collective energy of this trauma was released from her body—both the physical and the emotional parts of it. The net result was that she was able to let go of her headaches. However, it took 3 craniosacral therapy sessions and 2 moist head massages, as well as some gentle head, neck, and back stretching at home, for her headaches to disappear entirely."

NEURAL THERAPY

Neural therapy can be an effective treatment for those suffering from trauma headaches, particularly if the pain has persisted for more than a couple of months. This is because neural therapy fosters the growth of new tissues and cells at the trauma site, which in turn speeds up the process of recovery.

An excellent example of this therapy is the case of Beth, a 42-year-old legal secretary who had suffered a concussion and laceration after her car was hit head-on by another car. Since the accident, Beth had experienced almost daily headaches that were marked by sharp, shooting pain around the area of the scar on her head. Her scar was tender to the touch, and Beth did not like brushing her hair. She went to multiple specialists, including neurologists and neurosurgeons, who could offer only drug therapy.

Forgoing this traditional route, Beth opted instead to visit the Milne Medical Center. Upon examination of her head, we discovered that Beth had a 5-inch jagged scar near the top of her head, which was tender to palpation. We treated her with neural therapy consisting of injections of a 1% solution of the anesthetic lidocaine and vitamin B12 in and around the scar. This one treatment provided Beth with immediate pain relief from both her headache and the pain around her scar.

OSTEOPATHY

David, a 25-year-old actor living in Hollywood, California, injured his head while doing stunt work on location for a film in North Carolina. He had taken a fall in which he blacked out, but it was not until 3 months later that he felt pain in his head, which he described to feel as if someone were trying to push a nail into the back of his head. At first he did not tell anyone about his accelerating head pain, but then after passing out in front of a friend, he went to a doctor.

The doctor put him through an avalanche of tests, including CAT scans and MRIs, and told him he was suffering from a complicated, post-traumatic migraine that was caused by a blow to the head—nothing David did not already know. David was then sent from neurosurgeons to interns to psychologists, 18 in all, none of whom took him seriously when he told them that he felt that there was something structurally wrong with his head. He asked for a cranial specialist and was told that there was no such doctor, and instead was prescribed pills that he did not want to take.

Giving up on conventional medicine, David visited a naturopath, and after a month of homeopathy in conjunction with herbs, the naturopath determined that David's problem was structural and strongly recommended that David see an osteopath. Relieved to finally get the information he had been seeking, David visited Stefan Hagopian, D.O., an osteopathic physician practicing in Los Angeles, California.

By simply palpating David's skull, Dr. Hagopian confirmed that David's head was so compressed that it was affecting the energy flow to the rest of his body. Dr. Hagopian then began to perform adjustments, and as he did, David felt his energy open up and felt relief for the first time in a year. Today, after seeing Dr. Hagopian on and off for about 2 years, David says that, despite sometimes feeling pain, his headaches are 90% better than they were and he is living a normal life again.

PSYCHO/EMOTIONAL THERAPIES
BIOFEEDBACK
Biofeedback is an effective way to get you in touch with the underlying mechanisms and holding patterns associated with your physical pain so that you can learn to release it. Since trauma headaches often express themselves as either tension or migraine headaches, either thermal or muscle response techniques can be learned, depending on the headache symptoms.

FLOWER ESSENCE THERAPY
Since flower essences get to the core of the emotional conditions that lie beneath a headache rather than to the headache itself, these essences can be

By simply palpating David's skull, Dr. Hagopian confirmed that David's head was so compressed that it was affecting the energy flow to the rest of his body. Dr. Hagopian then began to perform adjustments, and as he did, David felt his energy open up and felt relief from his headache for the first time in a year.

used as an adjunct to other therapies, particularly when the trauma headache is being aggravated by stressful or unexpressed emotions. The following essences are most closely related to the emotional symptoms that are associated with traumas or injuries.

Trauma—Arnica, Five Flower Remedy, Queen Anne's Lace, Rescue Remedy, St. John's Wort, Self Heal

Stress and Tension—Dandelion, Fuschia, Impatiens, Rescue Remedy

General headache—Lavender, Rescue Remedy

HYPNOTHERAPY

Hypnotherapy can be a useful tool for uncovering forgotten or repressed traumas that may be connected to the headache syndrome. In one study, David Cheek, former president of the American Society of Clinical Hypnosis, reports that when hypnosis was used to age-regress patients back to the time of their birth, they made head and shoulder movements that exactly matched those made by fetuses during childbirth, movements that are not commonly known nor part of everyday movement patterns. He goes on to suggest that the very fact that this phenomenon exists suggests a correlation between types of birth experiences and health problems in later life.

Among other cases, Cheek cites the example of a physician with chronic, severe headaches who, under hypnosis, experienced memories of a painful birth marked by a difficult delivery. In Cheek's opinion, the patient's gesturing looked as if it were in response to forceps being applied to his head in a manner common to "high forceps delivery," a fact of the actual delivery later confirmed by the patient's mother.

Once this memory was uncovered, it became clear that the patient's headaches, which came on only when he was under extreme stress, were a conditioned response to pressure, which, because of his birth experience, meant pain. Cheek used a series of hypnotic suggestions to change the patient's response by recreating the event without pain and trauma, and the headaches disappeared.[3]

PSYCHOTHERAPY

Psychological counseling can help your headache in a number of ways. First, if the trauma you experienced was especially devastating or terrifying, counseling provides a way to talk about the event, helping you understand and work through the feelings and emotions surrounding it. In addition, counseling can help to relieve any stress or emotional tension that is worsening the pain you already feel. Finally, for some, psychological testing offers a way to determine the degree to which the headache has caused damage to mental functioning—for example, the degree of memory impairment or difficulty concentrating.

SELF-CARE OPTIONS

Besides the self-care options outlined in Chapter 16, it is important to take the standard precautions to prevent head injury, such as driving carefully, wearing a seat belt while driving or a helmet while bike riding, and so on. Furthermore, to avoid rebound headaches in addition to trauma headaches, stay away from potentially habit-forming painkillers and other medications. The best way to take care of yourself after a trauma injury is to eat a healthy diet and try some or all of the techniques listed below.

Under hypnosis, a physician with chronic severe headaches experienced memories of a painful birth marked by a difficult forceps delivery. Once this memory was uncovered, it became clear that the patient's headaches were a conditioned response to pressure, which because of his birth experience, meant pain.

See Chapter 16, An A-Z of Self-Care Options, for more information on self-treatment methods.

ACUPRESSURE

G-Jo #13: *G-Jo*, which translates as "first-aid," is a type of acupressure that can be used under nearly every painful circumstance. Although there are more than 20 different *G-Jo* acupressure points, *G-Jo* #13 (also called *Hoku*, "Joining the Valley," or Large Intestine 4) is probably the best general acupoint for just about any headache (although not for pregnant women).

Using the thumb and index finger of your left hand, press the area located in the fleshy web between your thumb and index finger on the backside of your right hand. Experiment with it until you find the tender spot,

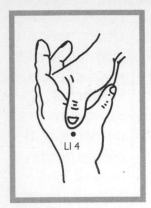

Figure 9.1—G-Jo acupressure point.

and, once there, hold it firmly down toward the bone, pressing as deeply as is comfortable. Do this for 20 seconds to a minute and then reverse hands. As you do this, you should feel some warmth or a slight flush of perspiration across your forehead, neck, or shoulders. Most people find that they feel immediately relaxed, and others say *G-Jo* "erases" their headache.

AROMATHERAPY

The following aromatherapy techniques have been used to treat those suffering from trauma headaches:

MASSAGE

Temple rub: Combine lavender (a sedative) and peppermint (a stimulant) oils and rub the mixture on your temples for pain relief.

Sore muscle massage: Mix 10 drops juniper (which adds heat), 8 drops rosemary, 8 drops lavender, and 2 drops of lemon with 2 ounces vegetable oil and use to massage your neck and shoulders.

BATHS

Muscle relaxant bath: Fill the bath with warm water and add 3 drops chamomile, 3 drops lavender, 2 drops marjoram, 2 drops thyme, 1 drop coriander.

COMPRESSES AND STEAMS

Cold compress relief: Mix 3 drops rose, 1 drop melissa, and 1 drop lavender oils in 2 pints water. Stir thoroughly and place a towel or washcloth in the water. Let it soak for 5 minutes, then wring to remove excess water. Lie back and put the compress on the painful area. Rest; change the compress as soon as it reaches room temperature.

Compress for sore muscles: Soak clean cloth in a mixture of 1 drop ginger, 2 drops marjoram, 1 drop peppermint, and 1 drop rosemary oils added to hot water; apply to neck and shoulders.

EXERCISE

Cranial stretch—These simple exercises should be done at least twice a week and used whenever relief is needed. Perform them while sitting comfortably with your back straight. Hold each posture for 15 to 30 seconds, breathing comfortably and gently throughout.

Hair Grasp #1: Start at the forehead along the hairline on the right side of the head; make a fist and grab your hair, squeezing your fingers until you feel mild discomfort and hold. Continue this exercise all the way around your hairline to the back of your head, then return to the forehead, and start again, this time 2 inches from your hairline. When you have finished, use your left hand and do the same steps on the left side.

Hair Grasp #2: Using your right hand over your right ear and your left hand over your left ear, take both hands and grasp your hair, keeping the right elbow low and the left elbow high. Then slowly lower your left elbow and raise your right elbow until you feel mild discomfort, hold, and wait for release. Do this several times and then repeat the above steps using the reverse motion, starting with your left elbow low and your right elbow high.

Hair Grasp #3: Keeping your elbows high, grasp the hair above your forehead with your left hand, and grasp the hair at the base of the neck with the right hand; slowly bring the elbows down until you feel mild discomfort, then hold, and wait for release. Do this several times and then do the same steps on the other side, with your left hand in back and your right hand in front.

Osteopathic Exercises—These exercises can help you to improve mobility and lessen the stiffness and pain that often accompany a traumatic injury. Move only as far as is comfortable. Do not strain to do these exercises, and be sure to breathe comfortably throughout:

- Sit with your elbows resting on a table and your head resting in your open hands. As you hold this position, breathe in and tilt your head sideways against your right hand, exerting pressure with your head with about a fourth of your muscle strength. Hold your breath as you exert this pressure for about 5 to 7 seconds, then relax the pressure and your breath simultaneously. Repeat this 2 times, and then tilt to the left and perform the same movement 3 times.

- Place your hands together over your forehead and let your head rest in your hands with your neck flexed. Take a deep breath and push your hands against your forehead and your forehead against your hands, hold the contraction for 7 seconds, then release slowly as you breath out. Repeat 2 times.

- Flex your neck, gently tuck your chin to your chest, and place both hands against the back of your head. Breath in and push your head backward against the weight of your hands, hold for 5 to 7 seconds, and release as you breathe out. Repeat times.

- Carefully tilt your head backward and look up at the ceiling. Place your hands on your forehead, and using only about 10% of your strength (any more could cause discomfort), slowly attempt to push your head back into its upright position. Repeat 2 times.

- Sit upright and pull your chin toward the back of your neck as if you were trying to make a double chin. Breathe in and place a hand on your chin as resistance while trying to return chin to its normal position. Hold the contraction for 5 to 7 seconds. Release as you breathe out. Repeat twice.

- Place your left hand on your left check and use it as resistance as you breathe in and try to turn your head to the left. Hold the contraction for 5 to 7 seconds. Repeat the exercise on the right side.

HERBAL SUPPLEMENTS

Depending upon the severity of the headache, herbal medicine is used either alone or as an adjunct to other therapies, since it can relieve symptoms and help to strengthen the body. Although other herbs are also used to deal with associated symptoms and underlying or preexisting conditions, the following herbs can be effective in cases of trauma headaches:

Brain function—*Ginkgo*, rosemary
Circulation— feverfew, garlic, rosemary
General headache—angelica, feverfew, meadowsweet, willow bark

Head trauma and swelling—coriander, skullcap, St. Johns wort

Musculoskeletal pain and spasms—cayenne, chamomile, elder, meadowsweet, nettles, *qiyelian*, turmeric, valerian, vervain, willow bark

OTHER SELF-CARE OPTIONS

The following techniques can also be helpful:

- Affirmations/Autosuggestions
- Breathing Exercises
- Creative Visualization
- Folk Remedies
- Ice and Heat
- Lifestyle Changes
- Meditation
- Nutritional Therapy/Dietary Changes
- Relaxation Exercises

RECOMMENDED READING

Alternative Medicine: The Definitive Guide. Compiled by the Burton Goldberg Group. Tiburon, CA: Future Medicine Publishing, 1994.

Blaylock, Russell L., M.D. *Excitotoxins: The Taste That Kills.* Santa Fe, NM: Health Press, 1994.

Clark, Linda, M.A. *A Handbook of Natural Remedies for Common Ailments.* Greenwich, CT: The Devin-Adair Company, 1976.

Faber, William J., D.O. *Pain, Pain Go Away,* San Jose, CA: ISHI Press International, 1990.

Ford, Norman D. *Eighteen Natural Ways to Beat a Headache.* New Canaan, CT: Keats Publishing, Inc., 1990.

Goleman, Daniel. "Severe Trauma May Damage the Brain as Well as the Psyche." *New York Times* (Aug 1, 1995).

Igram, Cass, M.D. *Who Needs Headaches?* Cedar Rapids, IA: Literary Visions Publishing, 1991.

Erich, Keller. *The Complete Home Guide to Aromatherapy.* Tiburon, CA: H.J. Kramer, Inc., 1991.

Lilienthal, Samuel, M.D. *Homeopathic Therapeutics.* New Delhi: Jain Publishing Co., 1996.

"Maladjustment May Be Result of Birth Events." *Brain Mind Bulletin* 1:7 (February 16, 1976), 1-2.

Manahan, William, D., M.D. *Eat for Health*. Tiburon, CA: H.J. Kramer, Inc., 1988.

National Headache Foundation Fact Sheet. Chicago: National Headache Foundation, October 1994.

Natural Health Secrets from around the World. Boca Raton, FL: Shot Tower Books,1996.

Prudden, Bonnie. *Pain Erasure: The Bonnie Prudden Way*. New York: Ballantine Books, 1980.

Rapoport, Alan M., M.D. and Sheftell, Fred D., M.D. *Headache Relief*. New York: Simon & Schuster, 1990.

Rapoport, Alan M., M.D. and Sheftell, Fred D., M.D. *Headache Relief for Women*. New York: Little, Brown and Company, 1995.

Robbins, Lawrence, M.D. and Lang, Susan, *Headache Help*. New York: Houghton Mifflin Company, 1995.

Simpson, Kristine, et al., eds. *The Experts Speak 1996: The Role of Nutrition in Medicine*. Sacramento: Kirk Hamilton PA-C, 1996, 121-122.

Solomon, Seymour, M.D. and Fraccaro, Steven, *The Headache Book*. Mount Vernon, NY: Consumer Reports Books, 1991.

Speed, William G., M.D., "Headache Following Injury." *ACHE Newsletter* (September 1993).

Stromfeld, Jan and Weil, Anita. *Free Yourself from Headaches: The Natural Drug-free Program for Prevention and Relief*. Palm Beach Gardens, FL: The Upledger Institute, Frog, Ltd., 1995.

Walker, Morton, M.D. *DMSO Nature's Healer*. Garden City Park, NY: Avery Publishing Group, Inc., 1993.

Ward, Thomas N., M.D. and Johnson, Lawrence R. "Post-traumatic Headache." American Council for Headache Education, ACHE's Electronic Network Support Committee, Sept 15, 1995.

Wilson, Roberta, *Aromatherapy for Vibrant Health & Beauty*. Garden City Park, NY: Avery Publishing Group, 1994.

Chapter 10

Allergy/
Sensitivity
Headaches
Food/Chemical/Environmental

A surprising number of people are unaware of the role allergies and sensitivities to foods, chemicals, and other substances play in causing headaches. Some practitioners estimate that reactions of this type are responsible for 70% or more of all headaches.

Tiffany, a 25-year-old retail sales clerk in a major department store, had suffered for 3 years from "migraine" headaches which came on at the end of her work week. Doctors had been giving her increasing doses of pain medication, which her system did not tolerate well and which caused an acidic stomach, mouth sores, and tender, acne-like lesions on her face and chest. During her initial evaluation at the Milne Medical Center, Tiffany reported that she was frustrated by her need for more potent medications and by her increasing battles with depression.

As we delved deeper into her history, she revealed that she tended to sneeze whenever she walked through the perfume department of her store. She was also very sensitive to tobacco smoke, which would cause her eyes to water and her nose to run. Electrodermal screening confirmed that she was especially sensitive to chemicals found in perfume, including hydrocarbon and phenolic compounds, as well as formaldehyde and tobacco smoke.

We determined that her best treatment strategy was first to limit her exposure to these environmental compounds as much as possible. Then we further reduced her sensitivity by using allergy neutralization therapy in which she took diluted forms of these allergens under her tongue each day before going to work and again if she was exposed. Furthermore, we recommended that Tiffany stop eating refined carbohydrates and increase her intake of raw fruits and vegetables.

Finally, in order to speed up her detoxification process, we had her take nutritional supplements for detoxification, including the amino acids N-acetyl-L-15, L-glutathione, L-glutamine, L-methionine, vitamins C, E, B-complex, folic acid, biotin, and quercetin, and the minerals magnesium, zinc, copper, molybdenum, and manganese. Due to her almost daily exposure to allergens, Tiffany's response was slower than it might have been; however, 2 months after she began therapy, she was promoted to an administrative job that allowed her to eliminate her exposure—and her headaches.

What Is an Allergy/Sensitivity Headache?

Imagine being so sensitive that you would get a headache from anything you did not buy from a special catalog; you could not have a pet or houseplants, wear perfume, eat in restaurants, or go outside during the spring. You could not even see your friends and family unless they promised to use special soaps and shampoos and have their cotton-only clothes specially laundered. For such individuals, every new substance or chemical brings a new threat of headache.

Whether or not this describes your current situation, the prohibitions sketched above suggest a frustrating life with few spontaneous pleasures. Although such extreme cases are rare, they warn of the problems confronting 21st-century humans. We are living in an environment that has changed considerably over the past decades. We are eating laboratory-manufactured foods, pesticide-laced produce, meats filled with hormones and antibiotics; we are breathing in formaldehyde in our office buildings; our streets are steeped in the invisible effects of carbon monoxide; and we are filling our bloodstreams with pharmacological agents, such as birth control pills, antibiotics, and headache medicines. Our bodies, unable to keep up with such reckless changes, are starting to break down.

Allergy/sensitivity headaches are a prime example of this process in motion. Alternative physicians, especially clinical ecologists, know this and

QUICK DEFINITION

Electrodermal screening is a form of computerized information gathering, based on physics, not chemistry. A noninvasive electric probe is placed at specific points on the patient's hands, face, or feet, corresponding to acupuncutre meridian points, at the beginning or end of energy meridians. Minute electrical discharges from these points are seen as information signals about the condition of the body's organs and systems, useful for a physician in evaluation and development of a treatment plan.

Amino acids are the basic building blocks of the 40,000 different proteins in the body, including enzymes, hormones, and the key brain chemical messenger molecules called neurotransmitters. About 20 amino acids cannot be made by the body and must be obtained through the diet; others are produced in the body but not always in sufficient amounts. The body's "amino acid pool" consists of: alanine, arginine, asparagine, aspartic acid, carnitine, citrulline, cysteine, cystine, GABA, glutamic acid, glutamine, glutathione peroxidase, glycine, histidine, isoleucine, leucine, lysine, methionine, ornithine, phenylalanine, proline, serine, taurine, threonine, trytophan, tyrosine, and valine.

Symptom Chart—Allergy/Sensitivity Headaches

SYMPTOMS	HEADACHE TYPE	PAIN LOCATION
Description: dull, aching, or throbbing, generalized pain, felt either continuously or in brief jolts; worsened by activity **Other Symptoms:** sneezing or nasal congestion, watery eyes; anxiety, weakness, nervousness, depression; increased urination, urge to move bowels; dizziness, weakness, lightheadedness, faintness; cold and clammy hands and feet; hot flashes followed by chills; nausea or vomiting; stomach pain; diarrhea; intolerance for light and noise; alcoholic hangover **Duration:** 1 hour to all day or longer **Frequency:** rarely to daily and usually about 4 to 12 hours after contact with or ingestion of offending substance	**ALLERGY/ SENSITIVITY HEADACHE** (Food/Chemical/ Environmental)	anywhere on or all over head, although sometimes located in forehead, back of head and/or neck; above or behind one eye

UNDERLYING CAUSES AND TRIGGERS	PRIMARY AND SECONDARY TREATMENTS	SELF-CARE TREATMENTS	WHERE IN THE BOOK PAGE #
Causes: metabolic imbalances, structural disturbances, emotional/psychological factors **Triggers:** dietary and/or environmental sensitivity, hormonal imbalance, autoimmune disturbances, lifestyle factors, structural disturbances, psychological stress	**Primary:** ■ acupuncture ■ detoxification ■ environmental medicine ■ homeopathy ■ naturopathy ■ nutritional therapy **Secondary:** ■ Ayurvedic medicine ■ bodywork ■ chiropractic ■ craniosacral therapy ■ energy medicine ■ herbal medicine ■ magnetic field therapy ■ osteopathy ■ oxygen therapy ■ traditional Chinese medicine	■ affirmations ■ aromatherapy ■ biofeedback ■ breathing exercises ■ creative visualization ■ exercise ■ flower remedies ■ folk remedies ■ herbal supplements ■ ice and heat ■ journal writing ■ lifestyle changes ■ massage ■ meditation ■ nutritional therapy ■ relaxation techniques ■ support groups	Page 277

A surprising number of people are not aware of the role allergies/ sensitivities play in causing head- aches. Some prac- titioners estimate that allergies/ sensitivities are responsible for 70% or more of all headache cases.

are doing everything within their power to educate people and end needless suffering. Nonetheless a surprising number of people are not aware of the role allergies/sensitivities play in causing headaches, de- spite the fact that some practitioners estimate that allergies/sensitivities are responsible for 70% or more of all headache cases. It is understandable that the connection between allergies/sensitivities and headaches often goes unnoticed, because allergy/sen- sitivity headaches can resemble tension, migraine, cluster, trauma, or sinus headaches, and are easily mislabeled as one of these more familiar types.

Allergy/sensitivity headaches may also be missed because they are rarely caused by a single allergy or sensitivity but are the result of a combination of factors. Over prolonged exposure, these overwhelm the brain's regulatory mechanisms as if too much input were short-circuiting the ability to respond. For example, if you are a woman and have your period and it is Thursday night and you are stressed over a Friday deadline, a glass of red wine may be the last straw that acti- vates an allergy/sensitivity headache.

COMMON SIGNS OF AN ALLERGIC/ SENSITIVITY REACTION TO FOOD

If the following symptoms accompany your headache, it is possible that your headache stems from a food allergy or sensitivity:

Mental or physical fatigue—Feeling tired, particularly after eat- ing or upon waking in the morning, can mean the body is working over- time in its efforts to ward off antigens.

Water retention—Holding onto water is one of the ways the body dilutes the power of the tissue-bound allergens so, when under attack, your body will not release fluids. Other clues include unexplained weight gain, bloating after meals, and excessive thirst.

Dark circles, puffiness, or wrinkles under the eyes—Called "al- lergic shiners," these are all signs of a food allergy.

Excessive mucus—Coughing up phlegm after meals (especially af- ter dairy or bread products), a chronically congested nose, postnasal drip, and mucus in the stools suggest that there is a digestive problem.

Type I vs. Type II & III Allergic Reactions

Even today the thinking of most conventional allergists is outdated, for the traditional view all but ignores Type II and III immunological reactions and concerns itself mainly with Type I reactions. Associated with inhalant and airborne allergens such as pollen, Type I allergies are those in which symptoms appear within an hour or so of contact and affect only limited areas of the body such as the skin (hives), airways (wheezing), or digestion (upset stomach).

Generally, Type I allergies are associated with the antibody called immunoglobulin E (IgE), the antibodies most commonly detected by skin testing and the IgE RAST blood test. Because these symptoms are readily visible, these allergies are classified as "active allergies."

Type II and III reactions, on the other hand, are classified as "hidden allergies" because they deal with hard-to-recognize sensitivities to foods, odors, natural gas, chemicals and symptoms that usually do not show up until an hour to as long as 3 to 7 days after contact. These reactions involve the antibody immunoglobulin G (IgG), and they can affect any system, organ, or tissue in the body. Type II reactions involve antibodies localized to a particular tissue or cell type, while damage caused by Type III reactions affects those organs where the antigen-antibody complexes are deposited. Besides headaches, Type II and III reactions involve other symptoms often associated with headaches, including numbness, mood and behavior changes, fatigue, visual disturbances, burning or flushing of the skin, and muscle and joint aches.

Both IgE and IgG antibodies are formed during the course of the reactions and both antibodies seem to be involved in the problems associated with delayed allergic symptoms. However, most food allergies are primarily the result of Type II and III reactions, which is why they are harder to detect.

Digestive disturbances—Integral to food allergies, digestive disturbances include bloating, cramping, gas, burping, coated tongue, bad breath, vomiting, nausea, constipation alternating with diarrhea, blood or mucus in the stools, and anal itching.

Emotional symptoms—Inability to focus and concentrate, unexplained irritability and depression, anxiety, crying jags, hyperactivity, and bulimia can stem from and worsen the effects of food allergies.

Recurrent infections—particularly in children, chronic upper respiratory problems, such as sore throats, colds, and ear infections, flourish when the immune system is overworked.

Chronic pain—Besides headaches, examples of chronic pain include arthritis, muscle cramps and aches, and PMS.

SUBCATEGORIES OF ALLERGY/ SENSITIVITY HEADACHES

Although all of the following headache types fit under the catch-all classification of allergy/sensitivity, they tend to be so common that they often get a secondary category of their own.

HYPOGLYCEMIC, LOW BLOOD SUGAR, OR HUNGER HEADACHE—Low blood sugar, or hypoglycemia, is a common, often missed cause of headache. Shaky hands, sharp words, and the sinking feeling you get when your lunch is long gone and dinner is not on the table are all signs that your headache is probably due to a drop in your blood sugar. These generalized, sometimes throbbing headaches often occur an hour or 2 after eating too much sugar, coffee, and/or processed junk foods, although they can also be due to skipped meals or irregular mealtimes.

NUTRITIONAL DEFICIENCY HEADACHES—These headaches are attributed to vitamin/mineral deficiencies that come about because of a poor diet or a malfunctioning digestive system. Often they are marked by low iron or B-complex deficiencies, pH imbalances (especially overacidity), or poor protein assimilation; however, nutritional excesses, such as too much copper, can also causes headaches.

CONSTIPATION HEADACHES— These headaches are linked to stagnant or irregular bowel movements which allow toxins in the stool to be absorbed back into the bloodstream. These headaches are characterized by a low-grade head pain, sometimes accompanied by discomfort in the abdomen, lightheadedness, fatigue, and general malaise.

HANGOVER HEADACHES—These are the nightmares with which people awaken after a night (or afternoon) of overindulgence, especially when alcohol products are mixed. These headaches appear to be the result of metabolic disturbances in the brain (a side effect caused by lowered blood sugar and excessive blood vessel dilation) and the dehydration which occurs as the body works to rid itself of the excess alcohol. Coming on any time from several hours after drinking to the next day, hangover headaches are characterized by throbbing, severe, often migraine-like pain and are frequently accompanied by nausea, light sensitivity, malaise, and overall skin pallor.

ICE CREAM HEADACHES— These icy headaches sneak up on you when you eat or drink cold things and can feel like someone shot an arrow through your forehead. Quick bites of ice cream, smoothies, milk shakes, and iced drinks hit the roof of your mouth and overstimulate the nerve endings in the mouth and palate, sending a shock wave from the mouth's surface to the cranial nerve in the head. Generally, the pain of an ice cream headache is brief and intense and is sometimes located at temples or behind the ears as well as in the forehead. It arises and fades away within a few minutes.

MSG HEADACHES—These headaches come about as a result of eating foods flavored with monosodium glutamate (MSG), an additive often found in Chinese foods, potato chips, processed foods, and seasoning salts. Symptoms of an MSG headache include migraine-like throbbing pain in the temples and forehead, pressure and tightness in the face, burning sensations in the trunk, neck and shoulders, pressing chest pain, dizziness, perspiration, and abdominal cramps. Although a definitive link between MSG and headaches has yet to be pinned down, research suggests that certain people poorly metabolize this flavor-enhancer, so that it builds up in the bloodstream until it causes a chemical overreaction.

HOT DOG HEADACHES—These headaches are triggered by sodium nitrate or sodium nitrite, a headache-provoking ingredient used to preserve cured meats such as hot dogs, bologna, sausage, bacon, salami, pepperoni, and ham. These headaches usually come on about 30 minutes after eating and last for several hours. Often they are accompanied by facial flushing.

CARBON MONOXIDE HEADACHES— These headaches are caused by exposure to carbon monoxide, the silent killer which prevents the normal delivery of oxygen to the brain tissues. Normally, this happens when exposure is 10% or more. Since carbon monoxide is colorless, odorless, and tasteless, it is important to be aware of it in poorly ventilated rooms, in cars, and around faulty furnaces, air conditioning systems, and gas stoves.

Janet's Hypoglycemic Headache

" I used to drink a pot of coffee for breakfast, a frozen yogurt and muffin for lunch, then drink more coffee, and wonder why I'd get a headache every afternoon around 3 or 4 o'clock. I thought all I had to do at this point was eat a candy bar and my headache would go away. When it came back, it made the afternoon headache look like a trip to an amusement park," says Janet, a 50-year-old accountant in Los Angeles.

Janet has since learned to control her headaches by eating more frequent meals, eliminating coffee ("the hardest thing I've ever done—but worth it"), and cutting back on sweets and refined carbohydrates.

The symptoms of these headaches often mimic typical flu, cold, or hangover complaints, include throbbing, generalized head pain, dizziness, weakness, body aches and pains, and nausea. If more than one member of your household is experiencing similar headaches and signs, you should test for carbon monoxide poisoning by ordering a special blood workup called a carboxyhemoglobulin level. (Routine blood tests don't detect carbon monoxide.)

Causes of Sensitivity Headaches

As we have previously mentioned, allergy/sensitivity reactions are often linked to an immune system that has become overburdened with toxins. How do these toxins get in the system in the first place? One way unwanted substances enter is through the nose, another through the skin, but the most frequent is through the mouth. When it takes in such substances, the body reacts as if it were being invaded by an enemy, known scientifically as an antigen, and sets off a chain of events in a concerned effort to destroy it.

This process works without fail when the body is healthy or only comes upon such unwanted visitors occasionally; however, when it becomes run down by other conditions or exposure to unwanted substances becomes chronic, these reactions become commonplace. At this point, the body becomes further imbalanced and can no longer remove the food antigens through its normal process.

As the second line of defense, the natural tendency of the digestive tract is to step in and do everything possible to fend off these unwanted substances. Thus, the white blood cells stationed along the small intestine wage a digestive war, creating antibodies in droves and sending them out to neutralize food antigens, until there is so much commotion that the body no longer knows the difference between wanted and unwanted substances.

This is the stage at which the digestive system begins to leak (leaky gut syndrome) and release toxins into the liver. If this goes unchecked, the liver also becomes so overburdened that antigens begin pouring into the blood-stream, where they then travel anywhere the blood flows, moving on to other organs and organ systems. Once there, they invade tissues and disrupt the system, causing a wide variety of abnormal reactions.

A QUICK LOOK AT FACTORS CONTRIBUTING TO ALLERGY/SENSITIVITY HEADACHES

Allergy/sensitivity headaches are especially associated with antigen-antibody reactions which affect the temporal arteries in the skull, expanding blood vessels, thinning vessel walls, and leaking fluid into surrounding tissues. The pain occurs as the brain begins to swell, pressing against the inflexible skull and stretching sensitive tissues. Yet constant exposure to a food or environmental substance is not the only factor that brings about an allergy/sensitivity headache. Other factors that can contribute to an allergy/sensitivity reaction include:

- hormonal imbalances
- physical trauma
- malnourishment or nutritional deficiencies
- enzyme deficiencies
- leaky gut and other digestive disturbances, (associated with food intolerances, chemicals, overeating, and food addictions)
- constipation
- pollution
- circulation problems
- compromised immune system.

Initially, these allergy/sensitivity reactions appear isolated or seemingly unrelated to any observable fact. But with continued exposure over the course of months or years of subtle reactions, the damage reaches a threshold and suddenly explodes into massive symptoms, such as constant debilitating headaches, fatigue, depression, and chronic digestive disorders.

Just how and when an allergic reaction will manifest is most likely determined more by constitution and genetics than anything else. Everyone has strong and weak points, so while oranges may give you a headache, someone else may get mouth sores from them. Researchers have discov-

Researchers have discovered that in cases where both parents have allergies, over 70% of their children also have allergies, while the number drops to less than 10% for children of allergy-free parents.

See Chapter 3, What Causes Your Headache?, for more detail on the causes and triggers of headaches.

ered that in cases where both parents have allergies, over 70% of their children also have allergies, while the number drops to less than 10% for children of allergy-free parents. Thus the real trick to unraveling allergy/sensitivity headaches—and the source of dedicated detective work—is identifying your trigger foods and substances and eliminating your exposure to them.

There is no limit to the number of substances that can cause a reaction; nearly every substance around us, from newspaper print to sunlight, can trigger and probably has triggered, an allergy/sensitivity headache. On average, those with allergy/sensitivity headaches tend to react to 1 to 20 substances, although there are especially sensitive people, called "universal reactors," who are so sensitive that their body produces antibodies to just about every substance with which they come in contact. There is no such thing as a predetermined, definable allergic response; people are individuals, and the same substance can trigger one reaction in one person and an entirely different one in another.

Diagnosing and Treating Underlying Causes

Every year, there are more recognized cases of allergy in the United States. In fact, statistics suggest that over half the population is affected by some form of allergy, mild or acute. With the growing legitimacy of environmental medicine and other alternative allergy therapies, the connection between allergies and headaches is beginning to get the attention it deserves. Alternative practitioners are especially prepared to deal with allergy/sensitivity problems because their holistic training equips them with tools and insights designed to make sense out of the baffling array of seemingly unrelated maladies and symptoms.

The first rule of unraveling an allergy/sensitivity headache is to pay attention to its onset. If you get headaches only after eating a chocolate bar or when you put on nail polish, you can put 2 and 2 together and eliminate these substances. However, because there are an infinite number of potentially headache-triggering foods and substances, it is not always easy to establish the allergy/headache connection. This is why it is often best to visit an alternative practitioner and take advantage of their tools and experience.

In any event, the practitioner will take a thorough history, which includes a record of past allergic reactions among you and your family members (i.e., your mother was allergic to milk), other medical problems (such as arthritis or hypoglycemia), associated symptoms (such as water retention, fatigue, joint pains), the time of day headaches occur (such as late afternoon), the circumstances before headache (such as your computer crashed), during the headache (such as eating a candy bar while driving with a smoking friend), and after the onset of your headache (such as spending three days with swollen eyes, constipation, and a dull throb in the forehead).

Once your history has been gathered, the practitioner will examine you, checking for vital signs, abnormal growths, pains, and other symptoms of discomfort.

Next comes some type of testing to determine the source of your allergy/sensitivity. This can range from do-it-yourself pulse testing and/or an elimination diet to the sophisticated but not always superior skin scratches, blood tests, and/or serum injections. An alternative practitioner may use some form of muscle testing, as in applied kinesiology or Nambudripad Allergy Elimination Technique (see page 290), to identify allergic substances.

Depending on the practitioner you see, you may be placed on an elimination diet to help break the cycle of allergy/sensitivity and to discover to which substances you react. Sometimes it takes weeks of exhaustive guessing and detective work, adding suspected foods, waiting, then trying again, before all the trigger foods can be successfully eliminated from your diet.

The process is lengthy because allergic reactions do not always come on immediately but instead can take an hour to 3 to 7 days, making it hard to know exactly which reintroduced food brought on the reaction. Finally,

Most Commonly Recognized Allergy/Sensitivity Triggers

- Dairy Products
- Salt
- Water
- Amines
- Alcohol
- Caffeine
- Chocolate
- Wheat
- Corn
- Preservatives
- Excitotoxins: Aspartame and MSG
- Chemical Residue in Produce
- Drugs
- Contactants and Molds, Dust, and Pollens
- Cigarettes, Carbon Monoxide, and Other Chemical Pollutants
- Heavy Metals

Nambudripad Allergy Elimination Technique (NAET)

One method used for the detection and desensitization of allergy/sensitivity, the Nambudripad Allergy Elimination Technique (NAET) is a remarkably simple technique that combines kinesiology's muscle response testing, acupuncture, and chiropractic to retrain the brain and nervous system and stop them from responding to allergy-causing substances.

Interestingly, NAET was discovered by chance when Dr. Devi Nambudripad, herself formerly food sensitive, accidentally kept a trigger substance in her hand as she give herself acupuncture in the middle of an intense reaction. To her astonishment, she recovered so fully that the next time she came in contact with the food it no longer bothered her.

Through subsequent trial and error, she determined that the treatment worked because she was holding the substance within her own electromagnetic field; so she gave it a name and for the last 12 years has used it to permanently eliminate the allergies of between 80 and 90% of her patients. Today over 600 practitioners—including M.D.s, acupuncturists, and chiropractors—have joined her and are using NAET with equal success.

What is unique to NAET is that through a simple, noninvasive procedure allergies can be permanently eliminated. First, the practitioner has the patient lie down on the table, and she tests the muscle strength in the patient's arm or leg as they hold a substance in a vial in one hand. Once the allergy-causing substance has been identified, the patient again holds this substance in one hand while the practioner uses acupuncture (or acupressure if the patient prefers) to reorganize the way the body responds to the substance, thereby removing the allergic charge.

For the treatment to become permanent, the patient must stay away from the offending substance for at least 24 hours, and sometimes more than one treatment is necessary.

depending upon the practitioner, you may also receive a series of desensitization treatments. Especially if you are among the few who react to nearly every food and substance you encounter, such treatments are a critical part of regaining control of your life.

Once the allergy is gone, your body can begin to repair itself, a process which can be helped considerably by the use of complementary treatment modalities. Detoxification therapies are a common choice, as are herbs, acupuncture, and nearly any therapy that clears energy blockages, restores metabolism, and aids in repair. The best defense against an allergy/sensitivity is a healthy immune and digestive system—that is, prevention. If you are well-nourished, fit, and mentally healthy, your body becomes less sensitive and more capable of withstanding the bombardment from the world around you.

ALTERNATIVE TREATMENTS

METABOLIC/ BIOENERGETIC BIOCHEMICAL-BASED THERAPIES

ACUPUNCTURE

Lawrence, a C.P.A. in his mid-for-

Reintroducing Allergic/Sensitivity Foods into Your Diet

Even if you do not opt for desensitization, you probably will not have to swear off all headache-causing foods forever. Only about 5% of all food allergies/sensitivities are permanent conditions, so it is more likely that after eliminating the offending foods and being allergy-free for at least 3 months, you will be able to reintroduce these substances into your diet on a rotational basis—meaning eating them no more than once every 4 days—without resensitizing yourself. Here are some suggestions for reintroduction offered by Dr. James Braly, M.D.:

- Make sure you allow enough time for any delayed reaction to show itself by waiting at least 3 days before reintroducing new foods. It may take months for those with many allergies to test out their foods.

- Do the pulse test before you eat the food, and make sure you eat enough of the food because too little may not give you an accurate result.

- While trying to avoid exercise or emotional outbursts, do the pulse test again, first 5 minutes after eating food, then 15, 30, and 60 minutes later. If your pulse rises 12 to 16 beats, you are still allergic to the food and should continue to avoid it.

- Even if your pulse does not rise, monitor yourself to make sure other symptoms do not arise.

- Do not eat any other food for at least 6 hours in order to devote your attention solely to the effects of the reintroduced food.

- If you are unsure of your results, test the food again at least 3 days later. If the food does not produce an allergy, rotate it into your diet and remember to eat it only in moderation.[1]

ties, came to the Milne Medical Center one morning before work because his allergies had become so bad that he had begun having severe headaches in the front of his head, starting in the center of his right eyebrow and radiating to his eye. As we interviewed him, he talked of pain that "felt like it started in his brain and then came out his eye" and told us he had stopped sleeping well at night and felt tired upon rising. He also complained of blurry and sometimes double vision, which had prompted him to visit his eye doctor the day before. The eye doctor had advised him that his eyes were fine, that he was probably suffering from a migraine headache, and that he needed to wait a few months for his vision problems to subside.

See Chapter 17, An A-Z of Alternative Medicine, for more information on each treatment method.

After full evaluation of his condition, we decided to perform acupuncture to address Lawrence's allergy and sinus problem. During the treatment, Lawrence relaxed and fell asleep, only to wake up 45 minutes later, surprised and happy: he was without pain or nasal congestion. His headaches did not come back.

COMBINATION OF DETOXIFICATION THERAPY AND MAGNETIC FIELD THERAPY

For Gina, a 45-year-old woman with high blood pressure, every day started with a headache. The narcotics her doctor prescribed helped somewhat, but she was constantly depressed and felt as if she were "out of her body."

Ceramic disk magnets like the ones used by Dr. Philpott can be purchased through Philpott Medical Services, 17171 S.E. 29th St., Choctaw, OK 73020; 405-390-3009.

When a friend suggested she see William Philpott, M.D., a psychiatrist and neurologist with a 40-year practice in Choctaw, Oklahoma, she figured she had nothing to lose, so she made an appointment.

After evaluating her, Dr. Philpott determined that Gina's headaches were food-related, so he put her on a fast. For 5 days, Gina drank only water and avoided everything she usually ate. To her surprise, for the first time in years, her headaches went away.

Gina and Dr. Philpott began the slow but rewarding journey of elimination and reintroduction. Since Dr. Philpott also practices magnetic field therapy, he was able to lessen the severity and duration of Gina's allergic reactions by teaching her how to use magnets at home. Whenever she got a headache from a newly introduced food, she would put ceramic disk magnets (1 1/2 inch across by 3/8 inch thick) on both temples, directly in front of her ears, for 10 to 30 minutes, and the headache would disappear.

Eventually, it became clear that Gina's headaches were caused by soybeans, a food she consumed so frequently that, over time, her body began rejecting it. Gina gave up soy products, and now her headaches are gone as well.

ENVIRONMENTAL MEDICINE

When 33-year-old Anika first went to see Dr. Nambudripad, she was in terrible emotional and physical pain. For 13 years, her migraines and the medications she took for them had ruled her life. During their interview, Anika told Dr. Nambudripad that she wanted to stop hating herself for her headaches and for the fact that her own body kept her from enjoying time with her children.

Dr. Nambudripad performed a physical evaluation and tested Anika for allergies using NAET. Anika lay on the table and held suspected substances in her hands while Dr. Nambudripad checked Anika's muscles to see if they became weak (indicating an allergic response). Through testing, it became clear that Anika suffered from a severe allergy to chocolate and coffee, substances she regularly consumed. Using NAET, Dr. Nambudripad desensitized Anika to these substances. In addition, because Anika's headaches were also related to her emotions, Anika and Dr. Nambudripad used NAET to uncover emotional triggers and blockages. After 9 treatments spread out over a month, Anika's headaches and depression disappeared completely.

HOMEOPATHY

Diego, a 16-year-old high school student with chronic headaches and asthma, came to the Milne Medical Center after he and his parents realized that drug therapies were only partially helpful. Having suffered from chronic bronchitis and 2 episodes of pneumonia when he was younger, Diego was always catching cold, had an irritating, burning nasal discharge, and a chronic, hacking cough. He also complained of nausea and thirst. Furthermore, tuberculosis ran in his family.

On physical examination, Diego was pale and lethargic, his nose red with a thick yellow discharge, his lungs wheezing, his skin dry and flaky. After careful evaluation, we recommended he eliminate dairy products and refined carbohydrates from his diet and increase his intake of fresh fruits and vegetables. In addition, we prescribed *Arsenicum iodatum* 3X (iodide of arsenic, a mixture of the two), 3 times daily, a homeopathic remedy primarily for lung conditions that have a chronic nature and/or are associated with a burning or irritating discharge in the lungs, and/or tuberculosis. Over 2 months, Diego's lungs gradually improved, his nasal discharge cleared up, and his headaches vanished.

NUTRITIONAL THERAPY

Charcoal tablets—While they should be used only in rare instances because they absorb "good" nutrients as well as toxins, charcoal tablets are an effective safety measure which you can use if you suspect you may

---

Heparin for Headaches

There is evidence that inhaling heparin, a natural substance the body produces to prevent blood clotting, reduces the number of cells involved in an allergic reaction associated with the incidence of headaches and helps to resume normal immune system functioning. Inhalation can raise lowered T-cell levels to normal values, thereby strengthening the immune system and protecting the body from future disease. In addition, heparin can be used to abort a headache attack in progress.

SOURCE—E. Thonnard-Neumann and L.M. Neckers. "Immunity in Migraine: The Effect of Heparin." *Annals of Allergy* 47 (1981), 328-332.

come in contact with sensitivity-causing foods. Charcoal tablets neutralize substances the body mistakes as toxins. If you encounter a situation in which it is impossible for you to control every ingredient in the dishes you are served, you can take 2-5 tablets before eating and 1-3 tablets after eating to help your digestive process.

OTHER METABOLIC/BIOENERGETIC/ BIOCHEMICAL-BASED THERAPIES

The following therapies may also be beneficial for treating allergy/sensitivity headaches:

- Ayurvedic Medicine
- Energy Medicine

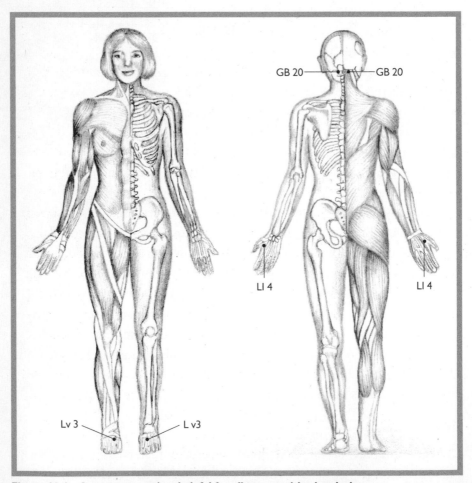

Figure 10.1—Acupressure points helpful for allergy sensitive headaches.

- Light Therapy
- Naturopathy
- Oxygen Therapy
- Traditional Chinese Medicine

STRUCTURALLY ORIENTED THERAPIES
BODYWORK

Chris, a traveling salesman in his early forties, had such uncomfortable allergy/sensitivity headaches that he was forced to quit working and go on disability for 2 years. His condition had progressed to the point where there were few things he could eat or drink, and his life was becoming limited. A friend sent him to see bodyworker, Janiece Piper, M.S.W., C.A.M.T.

After giving Chris a 90-minute, full-body acupressure treatment, she taught him specific acupressure points that he could stimulate on his own to help him detoxify his system. These included Gall Bladder 20 (GB 20) on the back of his skull, Large Intestine 4 (LI 4), and Liver 3 (Lv 3). Due to the increasing restrictions in his life, Chris was highly motivated, and since Piper's treatment had brought him relief, he applied himself and faithfully practiced self-acupressure 4 to 5 times a day. Within 2 weeks of self-acupuncture, plus 4 complete treatment sessions with Piper, Chris felt 80% better, good enough to return to work. Once back out on the road, he continued to stimulate the acupressure points and, within 2 months, his headaches disappeared entirely.

BIOLOGICAL DENTISTRY

At 12, Carla had her first filling and shortly thereafter began having headaches and chronic constipation. Digestion problems persisted throughout her teens, and she often tasted metal in her mouth. By the age of 20, she was experiencing severe migraines, but because her mother had had them when she was younger, the doctor told Carla that hers were probably inherited.

CAUTION

Mercury fillings should not be removed by just any dentist, but one experienced in the procedure, because improper removal can create further mercury leakage. In addition, a thorough detoxification program must be combined with the removal of the fillings, since residual toxins remain in the system even after the fillings are taken out.

When she was 30, she lost a tooth and had a bridge put in her mouth. From then on, she suffered from increasingly bad headaches, nausea, vomiting, light sensitivity, irritability, and depression, as her overall health deteriorated. The metal taste in her mouth also had become more pronounced.

Eventually, she became allergic to almost all foods and chemicals. She also developed insomnia, numbness down her left shoulder, and a burning sensation on the left side of her head, face, and eye. Yet, despite her many symptoms, her doctor could find nothing wrong with her, and sent her home with prescriptions.

Desperate, Carla knew she had to take her health into her own hands. She bought a diary and, after writing "search for health" on the first page, began charting her condition. Soon she noticed that her symptoms got worse after she ate or chewed gum, but it was not until she saw the "60 Minutes" television report on mercury fillings that she understood the connection. A year and a half later, thanks to the replacement of her mercury fillings, and taking vitamin supplements, juicing, massages, colonics, and homeopathic remedies, Carla has found relief.

OTHER STRUCTURALLY ORIENTED THERAPIES

Depending upon the underlying cause, the following therapies can also be useful:

- Alphabiotics
- Chiropractic
- Craniosacral Therapy
- Neural Therapy
- Osteopathy

PSYCHO/EMOTIONAL THERAPIES

The following therapies are valuable tools for dealing with the psychological effects of allergy/sensitivity headaches:

- Biofeedback
- Flower Essence Therapy
- Hypnotherapy
- Psychotherapy

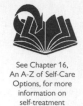

See Chapter 16, An A-Z of Self-Care Options, for more information on self-treatment methods.

SELF-CARE OPTIONS
DIETARY CHANGES

This is undoubtedly the most important factor in dealing with allergy/sensitivity headaches. A simple, if difficult, change in your eating habits can forever alter the way you feel. The best way to approach these changes is not to be too concerned about what you must give up or avoid; instead, focus on reconnecting with the foods that have been giving humans vital energy for thousands of years. Replace canned, processed, and refined foods with the foods that your body loves—fresh fruits and vegetables, whole grains, legumes, water, and sea vegetables.

Another great preventive measure is to read food and beverage labels carefully and reject anything that contains preservatives or chemicals, even those you do not immediately recognize. If you want to be certain you are not getting a mouthful of chemicals, grow your own food or buy organic whenever possible.

Taking control of your diet invites a renewed commitment to life, a sense of empowerment and energy that connects you to the fact that you do have the ability to determine how you feel and live.

EXERCISE

Exercise is more important than ever in a polluted world because it enhances oxygenation and stimulates the immune system. It also helps to metabolize and neutralize the effects of the many toxins we eat and breathe, while providing a way to work off extra calories. In fact, unlike the sedentary life, an active lifestyle actually inhibits allergic responses—which is the primary reason why athletes get away with dietary indiscretions that would cause problems for a normal person.

FOLK REMEDIES

The following folk remedies are particularly useful for allergy/sensitivity headaches:

Vinegar compresses: Soak a washcloth with vinegar and place it in

Food Headaches You Can Easily Avoid

Hangover headaches: Drink in moderation; use herbs or homeopathic remedies for liver dysfunction; drink lots of fluids to counteract dehydration; consume fructose (present in fruit juices, tomato juice, and honey) which helps to burn the chemical by-products of alcohol; avoid coffee, as it is a diuretic that depletes the body of liquids; to prevent, avoid overconsumption, drink water along with relatively pure alcoholic beverages, and drink fruit juice before going to bed.

Hypoglycemic headaches: Maintain blood sugar level with small but frequent meals and avoid sweets and refined carbohydrates. If you feel foggy or dizzy, listen to your body's warning and eat before a full-blown headache comes on; also eat regular, well-balanced meals with sufficient protein and plenty of complex carbohydrates, such as fruits, vegetables, and whole grains; supplement with B complex vitamins, vitamin C, and vitamin E.

MSG headaches: If you love Chinese food and do not want to limit yourself to MSG-free restaurants, eat a food that does not contain MSG first because MSG is especially hard to digest on an empty stomach.

Ice cream headaches: The easiest way to cure these headaches is to avoid extremely cold foods and beverages; otherwise, eat and drink slowly, letting extremely cold foods cool at the front of the mouth so the palate has time to cool gradually instead of being shocked by cold.

the refrigerator until it is sufficiently chilled. Then apply the compress to your forehead, temples, and neck. You can also inhale vinegar for even faster relief. Boil equal parts vinegar and water, pour mixture into a bowl, and place a towel over the bowl and your head as you inhale the rising steam.

Ginger compress: Cut and peel one root of fresh ginger, then boil it in 3 cups of water until the water turns cloudy. Soak a washcloth in the mixture, then apply it to the back of your neck. This helps to expand the contracted muscles and relieve dull, steady pain.

Herbal compress: Boil 3 cups of water and pour over 1 tablespoon lavender and 1 tablespoon chamomile, letting it steep 20 minutes. Soak a soft cloth in the mixture, then wring it out, and apply on the back of neck or forehead. Cold herbal compresses are also effective.

Drink a headache tonic: Fill a large pot of water and mix in small pieces of fresh ginger root, coriander seeds, diced garlic, and a little honey to taste. Boil off half the liquid and drink what is left periodically throughout the day.

Apple cider vinegar and honey tonic: To offset the causes of a digestive headache, particularly one related to excess acid production, D.C. Jarvis, M.D., in his book *Vermont Folk Medicine*, suggests taking apple cider vinegar in water and/or 2 teaspoons honey every day to help regulate the body's pH balance. Dr. Jarvis has observed that, when taken as a rescue remedy, this mixture will stop any headache, including a migraine, within a half-hour. If you do not like the taste, you can place equal parts apple cider vinegar and water in a steamer, place your face over it with your head covered with a towel, and inhale 75 breaths.

Eat 2 kiwis: This proven hangover remedy is believed to work because kiwis are loaded with potassium and thus help to replenish lost fluids and bring blood sugar back up to normal.

Li Shou **(arm swinging):** This Chinese technique uses motion to relieve headaches by creating a relaxed, meditative state and is still taught to school children to relieve stress. Swing your arms back and forth until the blood shifts from your head to your hands, reducing your swollen blood vessels. Next, use your warmed hands to stroke your face, using a circular motion, paying particular attention to the area around your eyes. Repeat the exercise several times.

Wrap rubberbands around your fingers: Take 10 rubberbands and wrap them around each of your fingers at the first joint, the one closest to your fingernail. Put them on tight, and although they may turn your fingers purplish and hurt a bit, leave them on for no more than 9 minutes to find that your headache has disappeared.

HERBAL SUPPLEMENTS

The following herbs can provide effective relief for allergy/sensitivity headaches and work well with other therapies:

Allergy/sensitivity or digestive disorders—black horehound, cayenne, chamomile, fenugreek, feverfew, ginger, nettle, passion flower, peppermint, rosemary, safflower, slippery elm, St. John's wort, wood betony

Constipation/detox—aloe, burdock, dandelion, goldenseal (root), milk thistle, nettle, Oregon grape root, senna, vervain, wood betony

Stress, anxiety, insomnia, depression, and tension—cramp bark, feverfew, hawthorn, *Ginkgo*, ginseng, lavender, linden blossom, passion flower, pennyroyal, peppermint, rosehips, skullcap, St. John's wort, valerian, vervain

Vascular imbalances—balm, basil, black willow, cayenne, elder, feverfew, garlic, ginger, *Ginkgo*, goldenrod, Jamaican dogwood, lavender, marjoram, peppermint, rosemary, rue, thyme, sage, willow bark, wood betony, wormwood

These herbal teas may also be helpful:

General headache relief—sage, rosemary, peppermint, and wood betony: mix equal parts of each herb in boiling water, and take every 2 hours until relief is obtained.

Headache prevention tea—4 tablespoons chamomile, 1 tablespoon white willow bark, 1 tablespoon valerian root: place herbs in glass tea jar and pour in 1 pint boiling water; let the mixture steep 30 minutes (a good overall self-heal tea).

Tea for digestive problems—½ teaspoon each of chamomile leaves, catnip flowers, fennel seed, and peppermint leaves: pour 1 quart of boiling water over the herbs and let them steep for 10 minutes.

Antinausea headache tea—simmer 1 teaspoon of fresh ginger in a pot of water for 7 minutes, then let it steep for another 10 minutes.

For constipation, try this laxative tea—Mix 1 teaspoon elder flowers, 1 teaspoon licorice root, 1 teaspoon peppermint leaves, and ½ teaspoon fennel seed: pour 3 cups boiling water over the herbs, and let steep 10 minutes. Strain and then add ½ cup prune juice.

OTHER SELF-CARE OPTIONS

The following self-help techniques can also be helpful for allergy/sensitivity headaches:

- Affirmations/Autosuggestions
- Aromatherapy
- Breathing Exercises
- Creative Visualization
- Ice and Heat
- Lifestyle Changes
- Massage
- Meditation
- Relaxation Exercises
- Support Groups

RECOMMENDED READING

Alternative Medicine: The Definitive Guide. Compiled by the Burton Goldberg Group. Tiburon, CA: Future Medicine Publishing, 1994.

"Arthritis Unyielding to Drugs." *Medical Advertising News* (May 1991): 26-27.

Benson, Paul, D.O. "Biofeedback and Stress Management." *Osteopathic Annals* 12 (August 1984), 20-26.

Blaylock, Russell L., M.D. *Excitotoxins: The Taste That Kills.* Santa Fe, New Mexico: Health Press, 1994.

Braly, James, M.D. and Torbet, Laura. *Dr. Braly's Food Allergy and Nutrition Revolution.* New Canaan, CT: Keats Publishing, Inc., 1992.

Carper, Jean. *Food: Your Miracle Medicine.* New York: Harper Collins, 1993.

Clark, Linda, M.A. *A Handbook of Natural Remedies for Common Ailments.* Greenwich, CT: The Devin-Adair Company, 1976.

Faber, William J., D.O. *Pain, Pain Go Away.* San Jose, CA: ISHI Press International, 1990.

Ford, Norman D. *Eighteen Natural Ways to Beat a Headache.* New Canaan, CT: Keats Publishing, Inc. 1990.

Frazier, Claude A., M.D. *Coping with Food Allergy.* New York: Quadrangle/The New York Times Book Company, 1974, 318-319.

Herzberg, Eileen. *Migraine: A Comprehensive Guide to Gentle, Safe & Effective Treatment.* Rockport, MA: Element Inc., 1994.

Hills, Hilda Cherry. *Good Food to Fight Migraine.* New Canaan, CT: Keats Publishing, Inc., 1979.

Igram, Cass, M.D. *Who Needs Headaches?* Cedar Rapids, IA: Literary Visions Publishing, 1991.

Jensen, Bernard, D.C., Ph.D. *Tissue Cleansing through Bowel Management,* 10th ed. Escondido, CA: Bernard Jensen Publishing, 1981.

Lilienthal, Samuel, M.D. *Homeopathic Therapeutics.* New Delhi: Jain Publishing Co., 1996.

Manahan, William D., M.D. *Eat for Health.* H. J. Kramer, Inc., Tiburon, CA, 1988.

Nambudripad, Devi, S., D.C., L.Ac., R.N., Ph.D. *Say Goodbye to Illness.* Buena Park, CA: Delta Publishing, 1993.

National Headache Foundation Fact Sheet. Chicago: National Headache Foundation, October 1994.

Natural Health Secrets from around the World. Boca Raton, FL: Shot Tower Books, 1996.

Rapoport, Alan M., M.D. and Sheftell, Fred D., M.D. *Headache Relief.* New York: Simon & Schuster, 1990.

Rapoport, Alan M., M.D. and Sheftell, Fred D., M.D. *Headache Relief for Women.* New York: Little, Brown, and Company, 1995.

Robbins, Lawrence, M.D. and Lang, Susan. *Headache Help.* New York: Houghton Mifflin Company, 1995.

Rogers, Sherry A., M.D. *The EI Syndrome.* New York: Prestige Publishing, 1986.

Rothschild, Peter R., M.D., Ph.D. and Fahey, William. *Free Radicals, Stress, and Antioxidant Enzymes: A guide to cellular health.* Honolulu, HI: University Labs Press, 1991.

Sacks, Oliver, M.D. *Migraine: Understanding a Common Disorder.* Berkeley, CA: University of California Press, 1985.

Simpson, Kristine, et al., eds. *The Experts Speak 1996: The Role of Nutrition in Medicine.* Sacramento: Kirk Hamilton PA-C, 1996, 121-122.

Solomon, Seymour, M.D. and Fraccaro, Steven. *The Headache Book.* Mount Vernon, NY: Consumer Reports Books, 1991.

Stromfeld, Jan and Weil, Anita. *Free Yourself from Headaches: The Natural Drug-free Program for Prevention and Relief.* Palm Beach Gardens, FL: The Upledger Institute, Frog, Ltd., 1995.

Chapter 11

Sinus Headaches

True sinus headaches, despite what television ads suggest, are rare, afflicting only 2% of headache sufferers. They begin in the sinuses, the hollow tunnels beneath the forehead, bridge of the nose, and cheekbones, and are felt as gnawing, painful pressure, tenderness, and/or swelling.

"**I** moved into a rural area for the first time when I was in my mid-thirties. I began getting headaches shortly thereafter, but, since my head was stuffy as well, I naturally assumed my headaches were sinus/allergy-related and began taking decongestants. But they only offered temporary relief, and always my pain would come back. Finally, after a couple weeks of steady sinus pressure and pain, I blew my nose and saw hints of blood in my thick mucus.

I immediately went to a naturopathic practitioner who told me I had a low-grade sinus infection that had been worsened rather than helped by the over-the-counter medications I'd been taking. Since it was still only a minor infection, the naturopath said he could treat it naturally, so he laid his hands on my face, head, neck, and stomach and gently manipulated my tissues until the blockage opened. He then gave me a homeopathic remedy, herbs, and nutritional supplements to take home. Within a week or 2, I began to feel myself again, and now, 8 months later, my sinus headaches are completely gone.
— Katherine, a massage therapist from Michigan

What Is (and Isn't) a Sinus Headache?

Thanks to the influence of television, many people mistakenly believe that if their headache is accompanied by sinus symptoms, it must be a sinus headache. True sinus headaches, however, are rare occurrences, afflicting only 2% of all headache sufferers. Most so-called chronic sinus headaches

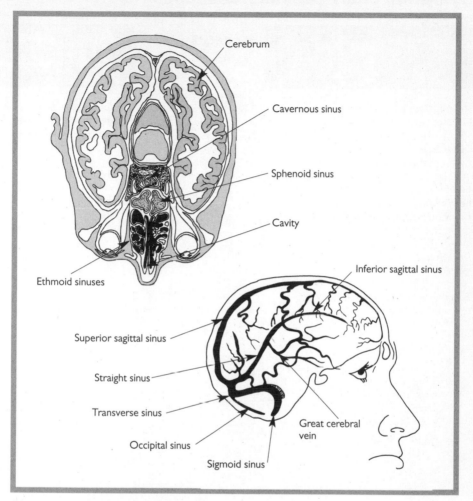

Figure 11.1—Sinuses in the head.

are really frontal headaches (digestive), mild migraines, allergy/sensitivity, cluster, or tension headaches.

A true sinus headache starts in the sinuses. The sinuses are the hollow tunnels located within layers of bone beneath the forehead, bridge of the nose, and cheekbones. These tunnels are lined with mucus-secreting membranes, which allow mucus to flow through them and down into the nose; however, if the sinuses become blocked, mucus builds up, causing the sinuses to swell and create pressure and pain. As the sinuses become more inflamed, the blood vessels in the mucous membranes become dilated,

Symptom Chart — Sinus Headaches

SYMPTOMS	HEADACHE TYPE	PAIN LOCATION
Description: gradual onset, gnawing, dull, aching pain **Other Symptoms:** pressure between eyebrows, above or below eye sockets, or in eyes, forehead, behind or above one eye, back of head and/or neck; top of head; runny nose, postnasal drip and/or fever; red, teary eye(s) **Duration:** intensifies as day goes on **Frequency:** 1 hour to all day; rarely or continuously	**SINUS HEADACHE**	forehead or face; depending on which sinus group affected, felt more intensely between or above eyebrows or behind cheekbones; (if all sinus groups affected, felt in all these areas)

Causes: inflammation and/or infection of sinus (as well as nasal polyps, deviated septum, or an anatomical deformity that affects the sinus ducts) worsened by metabolic imbalances, structural disturbances, emotional/psychological factors

Triggers: dietary (especially dairy foods) and/or or environmental sensitivity, structural disturbances, psychological stress

see medical doctor to rule out infection

Primary:
- environmental medicine
- nutritional therapy
- osteopathy
- enzyme therapy
- acupuncture
- naturopathy
- detoxification
- chiropractic

Secondary:
- Ayurvedic medicine
- bodywork
- craniosacral therapy
- energy medicine
- herbal medicine
- homeopathy
- magnetic field therapy
- traditional Chinese medicine

- aromatherapy
- affirmations
- biofeedback
- breathing exercises
- creative visualization
- exercise
- flower remedies
- folk remedies
- herbal supplements
- ice and heat
- journal writing
- lifestyle changes
- massage
- meditation
- nutritional therapy
- relaxation techniques
- support groups

Page 303

Mistaking Sinus Headaches for Migraine Headaches

Like migraines, sinus headaches can be quite painful, and since 15 to 20% of all migrainers also have sinus symptoms, migraines are often misdiagnosed as sinus headaches.

Dilated blood vessels in the face and sinuses, irritations along the head's large trigeminal nerve, allergies, weather changes, and environmental sensitivities can trigger sinus reactions in migraine sufferers. In fact, vasomotor rhinitis, the most common type of sinus discomfort, characterized mainly by a mild pressure over the sinus areas and a stuffy, runny nose, is a migraine symptom that has nothing to do with the mechanism of sinus headaches.

If you want to know if your headache is being caused by a true sinus condition, try bending over to see if the throbbing in your forehead and face is worsened; if it is, there is good chance you have a sinus infection.

adding a vascular component to an already aching head.

Sinus headaches are felt as gnawing, painful pressure, tenderness, and swelling in the temples, behind the forehead, above the eyes, beside the nose, and/or in the cheekbones, depending on which of the 3 sinus groups are involved. Sinus headaches are typically accompanied by cold-like symptoms such as low-grade fever, teary eyes, a thick, colored drainage from the nose or in the back of the throat, sneezing, pain radiating into the teeth, loss of sense of smell, and tenderness around the sinus areas. When one or both nostrils is blocked, the head pain is almost always accompanied by a fever. These headaches tend to start in the morning and worsen throughout the day; the head pain goes away when the sinus condition clears up, which usually takes 3 weeks or more.

Causes and Triggers of Sinus Headaches

Sinus headaches are caused by trapped air and pus from infected sinus tissues creating mucus buildup and pressing against tender sinus linings. These linings then swell and push against nerve endings in the sinuses, causing lots of pressure and pain in the bridge of the nose. The following are the most common causes of sinus headaches:

Cold—A cold can provide a great opportunity for bacteria or mucus to take up residence in your sinus cavities.

Sinusitis—Sinusitis is the medical term for a sinus infection that causes inflammation of the mucous membranes lining the sinuses.

Nasal Polyps—Nasal polyps are noncancerous growths in nasal areas.

Deviated septum—A deviated septum is a condition in which the wall that divides the 2 nasal cavities breaks down and disintegrates.

Anatomical deformity—Any structural problem, whether inherited or incurred through trauma, can block the sinus ducts. Examples include tissue calcification and pinched nerves.

These are the most commonly known triggers or secondary causes of sinus headaches:

Intestinal irritation—Allergies caused by foods and chemicals, especially dairy foods, can bring on heavy secretion of phlegm and mucus.

Muscular tension and structural misalignments—When pain arises from the upper chest, it reflexively produces vascular changes in the face.

Referred pain—Deep within the sinuses is a nerve control center which carries messages to and from the face, eyes, forehead, sinuses, mouth, and meninges; a strain on your forehead can therefore be felt in the sinuses.

Stress—Research has shown that, when under stress, people tend to secrete excess mucus.

Diagnosing and Treating Underlying Causes

Since sinus headaches are so easy to misdiagnose, make sure you make a note of all your symptoms and describe them in careful detail to your practitioner. Include when and where your headaches strike, their frequency, and the type of pain they produce. This will create a clearer picture, allowing the practitioner to focus more intently on identifying the underlying cause and get you on the road to wellness without leading you down assorted dead ends.

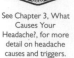

See Chapter 3, What Causes Your Headache?, for more detail on headache causes and triggers.

Although the issue is under debate, some doctors believe that antibiotics are not necessary unless the sinus condition is beyond the scope of alternative treatments. Like other conditions, a low-grade infection can easily be treated with a little help from nature's medicine chest and a qualified practitioner.

See Chapter 17, An A-Z of Alternative Medicine, for more information on each treatment method.

ALTERNATIVE TREATMENTS

METABOLIC/BIOENERGETIC/ BIOCHEMICAL-BASED THERAPIES

ACUPUNCTURE

Peg, a 35-year-old woman from Michigan, had had sinus headaches on and

NAET stands for The Nambudripad Allergy Elimination Technique. NAET is used for the detection and elimination of allergies. Developed by Devi Nambudripad, D.C., L.Ac., this simple and noninvasive method combines kinesiology's muscle response testing, acupuncture, and chiropractic to retrain the brain and nervous system. After identifying allergic substances through muscle response testing, the NAET practitioner uses acupuncture (or acupressure if the patient dislikes needles) to retrain the brain and nervous system to no longer respond allergically to a previously problem substance. For the treatment to become permanent, the patient must stay away from the offending substance for at least 24 hours, and sometimes more than one treatment is necessary.

off for about 5 years before going to see David Krofcheck, O.M.D. , D.Ac., C.A. It was spring and Dr. Krofcheck believed Peg's headaches could be allergy-related, so he performed muscle testing, which showed that Peg's muscles weakened when she came in contact with certain pollens, dust, and trees. Dr. Krofcheck then used Nambudripad Allergy Elimination Technique (NAET), performing a special series of acupuncture treatments while Peg held samples of these allergic substances in her hands, thereby retraining her nervous system not to react to them. After 3 treatments, Peg's sinus headaches never returned.

ENVIRONMENTAL MEDICINE

Charles, 53 and self-employed, suffered from sinus headaches for 8 years, waking up with pressurized congestive pain right across his face nearly every morning. He had tried beta blockers, antihistamines, and a few stronger prescriptions; he had been to medical doctors, chiropractors and acupuncturists; and he had had allergy shots. Nothing relieved his headaches and the accompanying excessive fatigue.

Then Charles found Ellen Cutler, D.C., Director of the Tamalpais Pain Clinic in Corte Madera, California. Suspecting allergies, Dr. Cutler used NAET to test Charles for many different substances and found that his worst reactions were to poultry and dairy products (especially eggs and milk), sugars, fats, and caffeine. When tests showed that caffeine was one of his worst allergens, Charles was surprised because he never drank coffee or ate chocolate. He realized, however, that he had been taking Excedrin, which contains caffeine, every day for 6 years. During the course of 2 to 3 months, Dr. Cutler prescribed enzyme therapy to help Charles digest sugars, and used NAET to desensitize him to coffee, dairy products, sugars, and fats. By the end of this period, Charles's headaches and abnormal fatigue disappeared completely.

HOMEOPATHY

The following homeopathic remedies are a sampling of those that have been used for sinus headaches. Homeopathic remedies work best, however, when prescribed by a qualified practitioner. If self-administered, these remedies should be taken only in doses of 6X or lower.

STOMACH DISORDERS—*Antimonium crudum* (inability to digest fats, especially milk); *Arsenicum album* (associated with eating foods that are too cold or fatty); *Bryonia* (acute head or eye pain accompanied by constipation); *Calcarea phosphoricum*, *Iris versicolor* (migraine-like pain on either side of head, vomiting, visual disturbances, occurring during downtime); *Ferrum phosphoricum* (congestion, vomiting, fatigue, face alternating between pale and cold to red and flushed, cold hands and feet); *Kali bichromicum* (migraine- or sinus-type pain with pain in one spot, vomiting), *Lac canium* (pain changing sides during attack or from one attack to the next); *Lac defloratum* (constipation); *Lachesis* (migraine-like pain, worse on the left side); *Lycopodium* (pain on right side, hypoglycemia, flatulence, nausea and dizziness, worse in afternoon and evening); *Magnesium phosphoricum*, *Natrum carbonicum*, *Nux vomica* (splitting pain upon waking or after overeating, sometimes with nausea, vomiting, irritability, and oversensitivity, also used as hangover remedy); *Phosphorus*, *Pulsatilla* (throbbing pain associated with indigestion of fatty foods); *Sepia* (overall digestive symptoms); *Venus merceneria* (overall digestive symptoms).

SINUS PROBLEMS—*Arsenicum album*, *Arsenicum iodatum*, *Belladonna*, *Dulcamara*, *Kali bichromatum*, *Lachesis*, *Phellandrium* (for relief from crushing head pain accompanied by burning sinuses and temples, light and sound intolerance); *Silicea* (pain in the nape of the neck associated with nervous exhaustion); *Thuja* (headaches on left side of face).

OTHER METABOLIC/BIOENERGETIC/ BIOCHEMICAL-BASED THERAPIES

The following therapies, depending upon the symptoms and conditions of the underlying sinus complaint, may be beneficial for treating sinus headaches:

- Ayurvedic Medicine
- Detoxification Therapy
- Energy Medicine
- Light Therapy

- Magnetic Field Therapy
- Naturopathy
- Nutritional Therapy
- Oxygen Therapy
- Traditional Chinese Medicine

STRUCTURALLY ORIENTED THERAPIES
BODYWORK

Marguerette, a 65-year-old historian, was seeing licensed massage therapist Jan Henry Sultan. L.M.T. of Santa Fe, New Mexico, for chronic low back pain. One day when Marguerette was suffering from a severe sinus headache, she came into Sultan's office and mentioned, "By the way, I also get these awful headaches." Her eyes were watering, her nose was dripping mucus, and she could barely function.

Sultan put Marguerette on the massage table and put her hands on Marguerette's head, discovering it to be jammed up and rock hard. Using gentle but firm pressure, Sultan began working her hands around the sutures of the skull and the neck muscles. Ten minutes later Marguerette looked up and said her headache was going away, as if someone had opened up a drain and caused the pressure to drop. She was extremely surprised, since usually nothing would relieve her sinus headaches other than lying down in a dark room and letting them run their 3- to 4-day course.

OTHER STRUCTURALLY ORIENTED THERAPIES

Depending upon the underlying cause, the following therapies can also be useful in relieving sinus headaches:
- Alphabiotics
- Chiropractic
- Craniosacral Therapy
- Neural Therapy
- Osteopathy

PSYCHO/EMOTIONAL THERAPIES
FLOWER ESSENCE THERAPY
SINUS HEADACHE FROM ALLERGY/SENSITIVITY
- **Crab Apple:** for feelings of impurity or imperfection, particularly

feeling ashamed of the physical body and its imperfections

- **Dill:** for those who are overwhelmed, hypersensitive, or overstimulated; known to enhance digestive function
- **St. John's wort:** used for headache accompanied by light sensitivity or vulnerability to environmental stress, including allergies
- **Yarrow:** strengthens the sensitivity that occurs when body tries to deal with input overload, either through the environment or through digestion
- **Yarrow Special Formula:** similar to yarrow, but more specifically geared to help one cope with the environmental hazards of modern living

GENERAL HEADACHE

- **Lavender:** good overall headache remedy, used to dispel nervousness and overstimulation, which deplete the physical body
- **Five Flower Remedy** (also called Rescue Remedy): for panic, disorientation, or loss of consciousness; used to restore calm and stability in emergencies or during intense stress

OTHER PSYCHO/EMOTIONAL THERAPIES

The following therapies can also help to relieve the tension and stress surrounding a sinus headache:

- Biofeedback
- Hypnotherapy
- Psychotherapy

SELF-CARE OPTIONS

ACUPRESSURE

The following points can be helpful to relieve the pain of sinus headaches:

- Governing Vessel 16 (GV 16)
- Governing Vessel 23(GV 23)
- *Yin Tang* point (GV 24.5)
- Stomach 3(St 3)

See Chapter 16, An A-Z of Self Care Options, for more information on self-treatment methods.

313

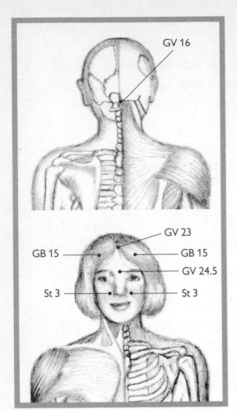

Figure 11.2—Acupressure points.

■ Gall Bladder 15 (GB 15)

AROMATHERAPY

Any one or more of the following aromatherapy techniques can provide relief from sinus headaches:

INHALATION

Sinus relief: To clear and relieve sinus congestion and sinus-related headaches, fill an aroma lamp, bowl, or diffuser with water and mix equal amounts of lavender, peppermint, and rosemary. Since all 3 of these oils have antiseptic qualities, this mixture can also help combat an underlying sinus infection.

For congestive or sinus headaches: Cajuput, geranium, niaouli, and tea tree oils; peppermint, rosemary, or eucalyptus oils are preferred when congestion is caused by a nasal infection because these also have an antiseptic effect.

MASSAGE

Temple rub: Combine lavender (a sedative) and peppermint (a stimulant) oils and rub the mixture on your temples for pain relief of painkilling drugs without the side effects.

BATHS

Aroma soak: For relief of a headache in progress, fill a bath with warm to hot water, add eucalyptus, wintergreen, or peppermint oils, and immerse yourself 20 to 30 minutes.

COMPRESSES AND STEAMS

Cold compress relief: Mix 3 drops rose, 1 drop melissa, and 1 drop lavender oils in 2 pints water. Stir thoroughly and place a towel or washcloth in the water. Let it soak for 5 minutes, then wring to remove excess water. Lie back and put the compress on the painful area. Rest. Change the compress as soon as it reaches room temperature.

Aromatherapy steam: Boil 2 pints water and pour into a large bowl; add 1 drop melissa, 2 drops peppermint, and 2 drops lavender oils. Put your head over the bowl and cover your head and the bowl with a large towel. Inhale deeply through your nose for about 10 minutes.

EXERCISE

CRANIAL STRETCH—These simple exercises help to release the sinuses by gently separating bones from each other so the joints can decompress. They should be performed at least twice a week, and used as a tool whenever relief is needed. Sit comfortably with your back straight, breathing comfortably and gently throughout.

- **Frontal Sinus Release:** Grasp your nose with one hand and your forehead hair with the other, pull the nose down and lift the forehead hair up toward the ceiling; hold for 15 to 60 seconds.
- **Maxilla Sinus Release:** Place your left thumb on the right side of the roof of your mouth and place your right thumb on the left side of the roof of your mouth, holding your other fingers together out in front of your face for support (prayer position); slowly press your thumbs out toward your fingers, feeling your upper palate widen; hold for 15 to 60 seconds.

FOLK REMEDIES

The following folk remedies have been used for sinus headaches:

Salt water nasal douching: Because salt water shrinks tissues and swollen blood vessels, this remedy is used when there is swelling or tenderness over the sinuses; add 1 tablespoon sea salt to a cup of warm water and stir until cloudy; use a tincture dropper or eye dropper and, with your head leaning back, apply 1 dropper-full into each nostril; do this 2 to 3 times a day until the swelling is relieved.

Chlorophyll nasal drops: This natural remedy is wonderful for preventing sinus complaints. Pour either oil-soluble or water-soluble (diluted with distilled water) liquid chlorophyll, which is available from health food stores, into a tincture bottle and put no more than 1 or 2 drops into each nostril twice a day, preferably upon rising and at bedtime.

Warm salt pack: To make a salt pack, roast 1 cup of salt in a dry frying pan until salt is warm to the touch, being careful that it does not overheat. Pour salt into a thin dish towel and fold it so you can apply it to your head, rubbing the painful areas rather than keeping the pack in one place.

Ginger compress: Cut and peel one root of fresh ginger and boil it in 3 cups of water until the mixture turns cloudy. Add a washcloth and let it soak; then apply it to the back of your neck. This works well to expand the contracted muscles and relieve dull, steady pain.

Herbal compress: Boil 3 cups water and pour over 1 tablespoon lavender and 1 tablespoon chamomile, letting it steep 20 minutes. Soak a soft cloth in the mixture, wring it out, and apply on the back of neck or forehead. Cold herbal compresses are also effective.

Herbal foot bath: This is an excellent way to draw blood and congestion away from your head. Place 1 tablespoon of powdered mustard or ginger in a deep basin big enough for both feet. Fill the basin with water as hot as you can bear, then sit in a comfortable chair, and slowly immerse your feet in the water. Drape a thick towel over the basin to keep in the heat, and place a cool or cold towel on your neck or forehead. Close your eyes and relax, breathing deeply for about 15 minutes.

HERBAL SUPPLEMENTS

Allergy/sensitivity or digestive disorders—cayenne, chamomile, fenugreek, feverfew, ginger, nettle, passion flower, peppermint, rosemary, safflower, slippery elm, St. John's wort, wood betony

General headache relief—angelica, feverfew, meadowsweet, willow bark

Immune system—*Echinacea*, garlic, ginger, *Ginkgo*, golden seal, nettle, rosehips

Sinus congestion—lavender, rosemary, peppermint, eucalyptus

Stress, anxiety, insomnia, and tension—feverfew, lavender, passion flower, pennyroyal, peppermint, rosehips, skullcap, St. John's wort, valerian, vervain

MASSAGE

Both of these self-massage techniques can help to relieve a sinus headache:

Carotid Artery Massage—This helps to relieve brain congestion and stimulate the stomach meridian, relieving headaches associated with digestive problems, congestion, high blood pressure, and stress. Located on both sides of the neck, the carotid arteries can be found by finding your carotid pulse, which is located at the spot between the Adam's apple and the neck muscles just below the jaw. Massage one artery at a time, by gently stroking from the jawbone down, using 4 fingers.

Sinus Massage—If your headache is accompanied by sinus-type symptoms, try this simple massage. With your thumb and index finger, using a circular motion, gently massage the bridge of your nose for about 30 seconds. Next take your thumb and press into the area along the browline where your nose meets your forehead, and hold with a steady pressure for about 15 seconds. Finally, move up a little, halfway between where you just were and the center of your forehead, and, again using a circular motion, massage for about 30 seconds.

REFLEXOLOGY

See Chapter 16, An A-Z of Self-Care Options, for directions on how to stimulate these points:

- Brain
- Head
- Sinuses
- Neck

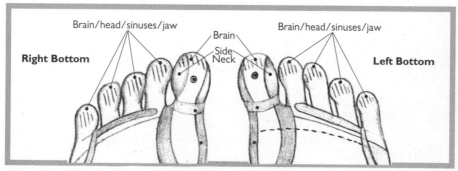

Figure 11.3—Reflexology areas of the feet.

OTHER SELF-CARE OPTIONS

The following self-help techniques can also be helpful for sinus headaches:

- Affirmations/Autosuggestions
- Breathing Exercises
- Creative Visualization
- Ice and Heat
- Lifestyle Changes
- Meditation
- Nutritional Therapy/Dietary Changes
- Relaxation Exercises
- Support Groups

RECOMMENDED READING

Alternative Medicine: The Definitive Guide. Compiled by the Burton Goldberg Group. Tiburon, CA: Future Medicine Publishing, 1994.

Braly, James, M.D. and Torbet, Laura. *Dr. Braly's Food Allergy and Nutrition Revolution.* New Canaan, CT: Keats Publishing, Inc., 1992.

Clark, Linda, M.A., *A Handbook of Natural Remedies for Common Ailments.* Greenwich, CT: The Devin-Adair Company, 1976.

Faber, William J., D.O. *Pain, Pain Go Away.* San Jose, CA: ISHI Press International, 1990.

Ford, Norman D. *Eighteen Natural Ways to Beat a Headache.* New Canaan, CT: Keats Publishing, Inc., 1990.

Igram, Cass, M.D. *Who Needs Headaches?* Cedar Rapids, IA: Literary Visions Publishing, 1991.

Ivker, Robert, M.D. *Sinus Survival.* Los Angeles: Jeremy P. Tarcher, Inc., 1992.

Jouanny, Jacques, M.D. et al. *Homeopathic Therapeutics: Possibilities in Chronic Pathology.* France: Editions Boiron, 1994.

Lilienthal, Samuel, M.D. *Homeopathic Therapeutics.* New Delhi: Jain Publishing Co., 1996.

Murray, Michael, N.D. and Pizzorno, Joseph, N.D. *Encyclopedia of Natural Medicine.* Rocklin, CA: Prima Publishing, 1991.

Nambudripad, Devi S., D.C., L.Ac., R.N., Ph.D. *Say Goodbye to Illness.* Buena Park, CA: Delta Publishing, 1993.

National Headache Foundation Fact Sheet. Chicago: National Headache Foundation, October 1994.

Natural Health Secrets from around the World. Boca Raton, FL: Shot Tower Books, 1996.

Rapoport, Alan M., M.D. and Sheftell, Fred D., M.D. *Headache Relief*. New York: Simon & Schuster, 1990.

Rapoport, Alan M., M.D. and Sheftell, Fred D., M.D. *Headache Relief for Women*. New York: Little, Brown and Company, 1995.

Rick, Stephanie. *The Reflexology Workout*. New York: Harmony Books, 1986.

Robbins, Lawrence, M.D. and Land, Susan. *Headache Help*. New York: Houghton Mifflin Company, 1995.

Stromfeld, Jan and Weil, Anita. *Free Yourself from Headaches: The Natural Drug-Free Program for Prevention and Relief*. Palm Beach Gardens, FL: The Upledger Institute, Frog, Ltd., 1995.

Solomon, Seymour, M.D. and Fraccaro, Steven. *The Headache Book*. Mount Vernon, NY: Consumer Reports Books, 1991.

Wilson, Roberta. *Aromatherapy for Vibrant Health & Beauty*. Garden City Park, NY: Avery Publishing Group, 1994.

Alternative practitioners are

especially prepared to deal

with allergy/sensitivity problems

such as headaches because

their holistic training equips them

with tools and insights

designed to make sense out of the

baffling array of seemingly

unrelated maladies and symptoms.

Chapter 12

TMJ/Dental Headaches

Jaw and dental stress can cause headaches. Tooth decay, crooked teeth, impacted wisdom teeth, gum disease, ill-fitting restorations, jaw misalignment, and low-grade infections can all irritate the jaw nerve and lead to a headache.

Eleven-year-old Tommy suffered from chronic headaches with pain so severe that he was failing school. His jaw and mouth were producing such unmanageable pain that his dentist wanted to fracture Tommy's jaw and realign it with wires to create a better bite. Tommy's parents, hoping to stave off such desperate measures, decided to try craniosacral therapy, and made an appointment with physical therapist Don Ash, R.P.T.

Craniosacral therapy refers to correcting imbalances in the relationship among breathing, the sacrum, and bones of the skull (cranium) especially the occiput. The sacrum (or hip bone) acts as a pump to propel cerebrospinal fluid up the spine to the brain; the cranial bones contract and pump it back down. Health depends on a smoothly functioning sacro-occipital pump; craniosacral work, as delivered by a chiropractor, restores the sacrum to full motion and balance with respect to the cranial bones.

Three months later, after only 4 craniosacral therapy treatments consisting of light touch equal to the weight of a nickel to gently open and release the compressed skull and jawbones, Tommy's headaches had completely disappeared, his oral surgery had been postponed indefinitely, and his grades had improved in every subject.

What Is a TMJ/Dental Headache?

Although the American Dental Association estimates that 60 million Americans may have temporomandibular joint syndrome (TMJS) symptoms—which include sore jaw joint, difficulty chewing or talking, and headaches—jaw and dental stress is an underlying contributor to headaches that is often overlooked by conventional medicine. It is logical that a mouth and jaw under continuous strain affect other parts of the body. Problems such as tooth decay, crooked teeth, impacted wisdom teeth, gum disease, muscle spasm, ill-fitting restorations, and low-grade infections from old fillings all bring stress to the lower jaw, bringing about muscular and structural compensations in the jaw.

The Temporomandibular Joint

TMJ stands for the temporomandibular joint, the joint where the temporal bone, the skull bone that descends in front of each ear, meets the mandible, the bone known as the lower jaw. The TMJ moves every time you chew or talk, making it one of the most active joints in the body. Unlike the ball-and-socket design of most other joints, the TMJ is a sliding joint, distributing the forces of chewing, swallowing, and talking over a wider joint surface that is lined by cartilage for smoother motion. The entire joint is also sheathed with supporting ligaments.

It is the lower jaw that is responsible for the opening and closing mechanism of the jaw. But the TMJ is a unique coupling of 2 inter-related parts in that move-ments on one side of the jaw must be coordinated and balanced with move-ments on the other. These movements are powered by the strong antigravity mus-cles of the jaw (the mas-seters and pterygoids), which also allow it to move sideways and up and down.

You can feel the TMJ movement by placing your fingers on the side of your face, just in front of your ears, as you open and close your mouth. Move your fingers up along your hairline and notice how the TMJ extends all the way to your temple.

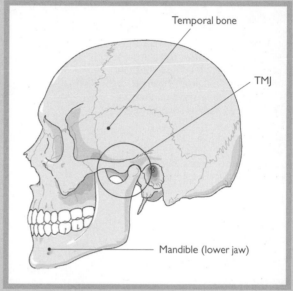

Figure 12.1—Temporomandibular joint (TMJ).

As the jaw takes on more pressure and pain, it begins to send these sensations to other areas in the skull, which in turn conveys the message to the central nervous system, thereby initiating a complex mechanism which helps to explain the headaches, depression, concentration difficul-ties, insomnia, neck and back pain, and other chronic symptoms that often accompany TMJS.

Harold E. Ravins, D.D.S., C.Ac., of Santa Monica, California, a prac-titioner of alternative dentistry, says that TMJS is a clear example of how headaches mirror the relationships between the head and other parts of the body. The jaw is designed so that the upper and lower jawbones move to-

Symptom Chart—TMJ/Dental Headaches

SYMPTOMS	HEADACHE TYPE	PAIN LOCATION
Description: similar to tension headache, with dull, steady pain usually felt as pressure on top of head, often accompanied by clicking sound	**TMJ/DENTAL HEADACHE**	most often on both sides of head or as a band-like sensation around head
Symptoms: tendency to chew on only one side; painful to chew; teeth grinding; strained smile; bleeding gums; jaw clicking; feeling tired after chewing; clenched teeth; sometimes an earache; face, head, neck, and/or shoulder pain		tenderness around jaw, within mouth, and at temporomandibular joints (where jaw meets skull)
Duration: 1 hour to all day		
Frequency: twice a week, once a month or less; chronic TMJ can occur daily		

UNDERLYING CAUSES AND TRIGGERS	PRIMARY AND SECONDARY TREATMENTS	SELF-CARE TREATMENTS	WHERE IN THE BOOK PAGE #
Causes: dysfunction of one or both temporomandibular joints due to faulty bite; teeth infections, other dentistry problems; worsened by metabolic imbalances, structural disturbances, emotional/psychological factors	**Primary:** ■ acupuncture ■ biological dentistry ■ bodywork ■ chiropractic ■ craniosacral therapy ■ detoxification ■ environmental medicine ■ homeopathy ■ neural therapy ■ osteopathy	■ aromatherapy ■ affirmations ■ biofeedback ■ breathing exercises ■ creative visualization ■ exercise ■ flower remedies ■ folk remedies ■ herbal supplements ■ ice and heat ■ journal writing ■ lifestyle changes ■ massage ■ meditation ■ nutritional therapy ■ relaxation techniques ■ support groups	Page 321
Triggers: dietary and/or environmental sensitivity, hormonal imbalance, lifestyle, structural imbalances, psychological stress	**Secondary:** ■ Ayurvedic medicine ■ energy medicine ■ herbal medicine ■ hydrotherapy ■ magnetic medicine ■ naturopathy ■ nutritional therapy, esp. enzymes ■ oxygen therapy ■ reflexology ■ traditional Chinese medicine		

gether at the temporomandibular joints located above each earlobe. When moving in harmony, the jawbones produce a pumping action as they move; when the lower jaw hits the upper one, there is a natural flow of energy, and the fluids of the brain are distributed evenly throughout the body. But if the jaws are not coming together correctly, blood flow is reduced, the brain receives the wrong message, and the entire body is thrown off balance.

TMJ problems also affect and are affected by the jaw nerve, creating a trickle-down neurological effect on the health of the body. The jaw nerve is the biggest nerve of the body—28% of your sensory cortex is devoted to it—and when it becomes inflamed or hyperactive, so does the brain. Medical literature has even dubbed the jaw the mediator of headaches. This is because two-thirds of the brain's pain-sensitive nerves receive their nerve supply from the jaw nerve.

When the jaw nerve is irritated, levels of substance P increase, which inhibits serotonin production. Because the jaw nerve is closely related to the functions that control posture and muscle tension, jaw problems affect muscle tension throughout the body. The jaw, in other words, is closely related to many cause-and-effect mechanisms of headaches and to many other parts of the body. It therefore makes sense that it is the jaw you hit when you want to knock someone out.

A Quick Look at Causes and Triggers of TMJS

faulty or uneven bite

dental infections

physical trauma

muscular imbalances

gait and postural problems

mercury amalgam fillings

hormones

vascular changes

diet and allergy

stress

The diverse symptoms associated with TMJS headaches often hide true conditions. For this reason, they have been labeled "The Great Imposter," Although frequently marked by pain that begins over the joint and radiates to the side of the head, cheek, and lower jaw, TMJS headaches can just as easily be marked by muscle spasms in the skull, face, and jaw.

Other possible symptoms include impacted teeth; gum pain; unpleasant taste in mouth (especially when biting down); red, swollen gums around the affected tooth; bad breath; difficulty swallowing; teeth marks on the outer edges of the tongue; drawn or tense facial expression; upper neck and shoulder problems; fatigue; dizziness; earache and/or ear ringing; clicking, grinding, or popping sounds that originate in the jaw; jaw locking; and pain and pressure behind the eyes.

Causes and Triggers of TMJS/Dental Headaches

Although TMJS is equally famous for producing migraine-like headaches, it is believed that it is more likely related to tension-type headaches than any other type. This is because the mechanism of TMJS is thought to be brought on by musculoskeletal imbalances that then contribute to metabolic distortions and neurovascular changes.

The following causes are most closely implicated in TMJS:

Faulty bite—Misalignments of the teeth and jaw, caused by inherited congenital defects, missing or decaying teeth, and/or bad dental work are closely connected to TMJS. Whenever the jaws and teeth are out of alignment, the entire cranium will distort in order to allow for proper chewing, since chewing is the vital mechanism by which the body gets its nutrients.

If teeth do not come together firmly, the muscles of the jaw must work even harder. Because these jaw muscles not only stabilize the upper and lower teeth while eating and talking but also control swallowing, an act you perform more than 2,000 times during a 24-hour period, any additional strain on these already overworked muscles produces pain.

Dental infections—Since bacteria from dental infections can move from teeth to gums to bloodstream in no time at all, dental infections can be a particularly serious problem, especially if these infections are hiding beneath fillings, in root canals, or in obscured gum pockets.

Trauma—A past injury or an automobile accident can produce "jaw

> *The symptoms associated with TMJS headaches can be so diverse that it has been labeled "The Great Imposter," often hiding true conditions. Although the American Dental Association estimates that 60 million Americans may have TMJS, jaw and dental stress is an underlying contributor to headaches that is often overlooked by conventional medicine.*

Health Symptom Analysis of Patients Who Eliminated Mercury Dental Fillings

The following chart summarizes the findings of 6 different studies in which a total of 1,569 patients were evaluated to determine the health effects of removing mercury dental amalgams and replacing them with non-mercury fillings.

% reporting	Symptom	No. reporting	No. improved or cured	% of cure or improvement
14	allergy	221	196	89
22	depression	347	315	91
22	dizziness	343	301	88
45	fatigue	705	603	86
34	headaches	531	460	87
15	intestinal problems	231	192	83

Source—S. Ziff, "Consolidated Symptom Analysis of 1569 Patients." *Bio-Probe Newsletter* 9:2 (March 1993), 7-8.

lash" or whiplash of the jaw. This is because the jaw and the neck are connected, so both are subject to a similar shock in an accident. Jaw lash is often ignored, however, and only the neck whiplash is treated, despite the fact that an injured TMJ throws the entire jaw out of alignment. When jaw lash is left untreated, the teeth are forced to compensate by readjusting to an unnatural position, and, over time, the muscles surrounding the joint become strained, stressing other muscles and nerves.

Muscular imbalances—In addition to those in the jaw, neck, and shoulder muscles, other muscles of the body may also contribute to TMJS. This can best be seen by likening your head and body to a grapefruit balanced atop a straw and held in place by strategically positioned rubber bands. If you strain just one of these rubberbands (such as a muscle in your jaw), the others must compensate, some by stretching, others by shortening—which is exactly what happens when the muscles in the body are called upon to keep the head balanced on top of the spinal column.

Gait and postural problems—According to Michael Gelb, D.D.S., M.S., Director of the TMJ and Facial Pain Program at the New York University College of Dentistry, an important relationship exists between the mouth and the feet. Dr. Gelb reports that before he looks into a patient's mouth, he looks at the feet because if there is a foot or ankle injury, it usually means there is a problem in the jaw as well.

This is substantiated by researchers at Tufts University in Massachusetts, who have shown that it is possible to change someone's bite by changing the way they walk and stand. Thus, if you sprain an ankle, it can affect your jaw, and vice versa. This is why improperly fitting shoes can cause gait and posture problems which lead to headaches. This is a bigger problem for women because women's fashion does not seem too concerned with the natural shape of a woman's foot.

Mercury amalgam fillings—Both the scientific and anecdotal evidence against dental mercury is overwhelming: it is highly toxic and one of the deadliest materials on earth. Yet conventional dentists continue to use it—usually without informing their patients of the dangers, leaving many unsuspecting people with headaches and other mysterious ailments.

Hormones—Although the connection has not been proven, some theories suggest that TMJS may somehow be related to hormonal imbalances because a majority of those suffering from TMJ headaches are female; this phenomenon is believed to be intertwined with the metabolic changes that are brought about by stress to the central nervous system.

Vascular changes—Stresses in the mouth and jaw cause the bones in the skull to lose their normal range of motion, generating a reduction in circulation and therefore less oxygen, causing the blood vessels to constrict and cause headache.

Diet and allergy—In the last 200 years, inherent developmental problems have become much more common in the teeth and upper jaw—a condition which researchers suggest may be due in part to the intake of processed or chemicalized foods, especially refined sugar and flour.

Stress—Habits or coping mechanisms that overwork the jaw muscles, such as teeth grinding (also known as bruxism), jaw clenching, and nail biting, are generally attributed to emotional strain; since pain makes you feel tense and uptight, stress worsens the muscle spasm and contributes to the overall cycle of pain. Doctors at the University of California at Los Angeles TMJ Clinic report that TMJS sufferers often harbor a deep, repressed anger toward someone or something. This unexpressed anger may be "biting out," producing TMJ problems.

Diagnosing and Treating Underlying Causes

Since the symptoms of TMJ/dental headaches are similar to those of oth-

See Chapter 3, What Causes Your Headache?, for more detail on headache causes and triggers.

Both the scientific and anecdotal evidence against dental mercury is overwhelming: it is highly toxic and one of the deadliest materials on earth. Yet conventional dentists continue to use it, usually without informing their patients of the dangers, leaving many unsuspecting people with headaches and other mysterious ailments.

er conditions, nearly every type of medical professional may be consulted before the patient finally turns to an alternative practitioner. Ironically, it is because of this diversity that these headaches respond well to the flexible and multidisciplinary approach of alternative medicine. Once you have found a qualified practitioner, it is usually just a matter of time before you get to the root of your problem and become headache free.

Alternative practitioners who specialize in TMJS and dental problems (such as a biological dentist, bodyworker, craniosacral therapist, neural therapist, or osteopath) will first attempt to determine the structural condition of your TMJS by looking at the symmetry and alignment of your facial features, the midline shift of your teeth, the asymmetric wear of your dental surfaces, and the asymmetric movements of your jaw. Next, they will rub and palpate your jaw, neck, shoulder, and any other relevant muscles for joint soreness and tenderness. Sometimes, the practitioner will gather additional diagnostic information from X rays, MRIs, blood tests, electroencephalograms, applied kinesiology, and electrodermal screening.

Once it is determined that your headaches are due to TMJS or dental problems, a good practitioner then goes for the total body approach. For example, biological dentists may want to fit you with a removable dental appliance, remove mercury fillings, or do restorative work on your teeth and gums to prevent further problems. Then they may treat you with chiropractic, cranial therapy, neural therapy, bodywork, and/or acupuncture (or send you to other practitioners for these therapies) to reduce spasm in the jaw, head, and neck muscles, ease circulation and energy flow, and ensure that your musculoskeletal structure is properly aligned.

As this structural work is being done, they also test for

Biological dentistry stresses the use of nontoxic restoration materials for dental work and focuses on the unrecognized impact that dental toxins and hidden dental infections can have on overall health. Typically, a biological dentist will emphasize the safe removal of mercury amalgams; in many cases, the avoidance or removal of root canals; the investigation of possible jawbone infections (cavitations) as a "dental focus" or source of bodywide illness centered in the teeth; and the health-injuring role of misalignment of teeth and jaw structures.

food allergies and incorporate nutritional therapy, to see that the body's metabolic needs are being met as well. Finally, they may recommend that you try biofeedback, hypnotherapy, exercises, meditation, psychotherapy, and/or relaxation to relieve stress and stop destructive dental habits, such as teeth grinding or jaw clenching.

Since the symptoms of TMJS cross so many boundaries, it is almost impossible for one discipline to adequately treat every case. For this reason, many dentists are crossing over into acupuncture, herbal medicine, homeopathy, nutritional therapy, neural therapy, bodywork, and craniosacral therapy. Furthermore, recognizing the need to address the emotional/ psychological component of TMJS, many dentists are employing social workers, psychologists, and biofeedback technicians as members of their staff.

See Chapter 17, An A-Z of Alternative Medicine, for more information on treatment methods.

ALTERNATIVE TREATMENTS

METABOLIC/ BIOENERGETIC/ BIOCHEMICAL-BASED THERAPIES
ACUPUNCTURE
Michael Gelb, D.D.S., M.S., uses a combination of orthopedic treatments, acupuncture, vitamin therapy, and psychotherapy to treat his patients. He frequently prescribes 400 mg of magnesium citrate, taken at night,

to control muscle spasms. He also sends about 75% of his patients to a chiropractor or physical therapist. Posture improvement and exercise are part of his treatment strategy.

ENERGY MEDICINE

A specialized field within energy medicine, dental energy medicine looks at the relationship between acupoints (treatment points on the acupunture meridians), teeth, and organs. Using electrodermal screening, a dentist examines these relationships to decipher whether bad teeth are bringing about health problems, determining how a problem in a tooth might be affecting the function of its corollary organ or system and vice versa.

Electrodermal screening is also used to detect unseen infections below the teeth that can contribute to mystery diseases and ailments with no obvious origin. Finally, it is used to screen patients for possible allergies, preventing dental toxicity by testing patients for dental materials and anesthetics before these substances are introduced into the body.

ENVIRONMENTAL MEDICINE

Yolanda, a 52-year-old music teacher from Nevada, had suffered from TMJ headaches accompanied by aching pain on both sides of her jaws for 15 years. She had been to dentists and oral surgeons; for years, she had worn a dental appliance, which, although it took away some of the pain, did not give her true relief. After her oral surgeon advised her that jaw surgery was her only hope for lasting relief, Yolanda called the Milne Medical Center.

The first day she came into our office, she was in terrible pain. Her abdomen was extremely tender to palpitation, and all of her muscles were sensitive to touch. It was obvious that she was suffering from multi-organ dysfunction. As soon as we realized that her TMJS was related to a metabolic problem, we immediately went to work to eliminate its cause.

We used electrodermal screening to test her for allergies, and then put her on a strict diet eliminating all but the safest foods. With this out of the way, we started a detoxification program that consisted of colon therapy and acupuncture for the liver and gallbladder. We then performed a series of neural therapy injections of lidocaine 1% with B12 in the painful regions of her mouth and jaw. We also gave her a Chinese herbal formula of bupleurum and peony (in powdered form, 3 grams, 3 times a day) to sedate and tone her digestion and balance her hormones.

Finally, we gave Yolanda 4 different homeopathic treatments to take 3 times daily, which consisted of *Petroleum* 6X, a remedy suited to a jaw that is easily dislocated, *Rhus tox* 6X, (poison ivy) a remedy for cracking and popping of the jaw, and *Argentum nitricum* 3X, (silver nitrate) for digestive problems, and *Cimicifuga* 3X (black cohosh) for pelvic and hormonal disturbances. Over time, her headaches and jaw pain gradually declined, until, 4 months later, she stopped suffering from headaches entirely.

HOMEOPATHY

The following homeopathic remedies are a sampling of those that have been used for TMJ/dental headaches. However, homeopathic remedies work best when prescribed by a qualified practitioner; when self-administered, these remedies should be taken only in doses of 6X or lower.

STRUCTURAL MISALIGNMENTS AND TRAUMA

Actae Racemosa, *Arnica montana* (bruise-like ache, worsened by movement, associated with physical exhaustion or trauma); *Byronia*, *Calcarea carbonica* (physical overexertion); *Colocynthis*, *Ranunculus bulbosus* (head pain associated with postural problems, pains in the back and side); *Rhus toxicodendron* (physical overexertion); *Silicea* (pain in the nape of the neck associated with nervous exhaustion).

Jaw Orthopedics

If your bite is misaligned due to missing teeth, crooked teeth, or ill-fitting restorations (fillings and crowns), a biological dentist uses various methods to correct it. For example, when necessary, some TMJ specialists will perform what is called an equilibration, in which they grind your teeth surfaces so the teeth meet properly for chewing. Others will remove ill-fitting dental work and replace it with fillings and crowns that allow you to bite down properly.

However, since the TMJ can correct itself over time, dental appliances such as mouthpieces or splints are the dental technique most often prescribed by biological dentists to speed up this process. These dental appliances are customized to your needs through the use of sophisticated computerized technology designed to analyze jaw motion to determine irregularities.

Typically, you get 2 appliances, one for day wear and one for night, because while you are awake and conscious your jaw muscles maintain one tone, but when you are sleeping they relax and lose tone, requiring a sturdier appliance that provides more muscle control. Appliances are usually made of plastic, sometimes held together by wire, and usually are very unobtrusive and easy to put in and take out.

However, as with all treatments, a balanced approach must be taken; equilibration, dental work, and dental appliances that are used to correct the bite will do little good if the underlying structural and metabolic imbalances remain untreated.

STRESS, TENSION, AND ANXIETY—

- irritability, moodiness, intellectual overwork (*Anacardium orientale*)
- craving sweets, mental exertion (*Argentium nitricum*)
- vague but distressing tension-type pain, associated with anxiety and visual disturbances, intensified with noise and movement (*Chamomilla, Gelsemium*)
- depression, suicidal thoughts, delusions, fear (*Hura Braziliensis*)
- hypersensitivity, hysterical outbursts, heavy, pressurized pain, sometimes nausea and dizziness (*Ignatia*)
- intellectual overwork, overall physical fatigue (*Kali phosphoricum*)
- developing after intense mental work, for those who are ambitious, driving, and eager to achieve (*Lachesis, Natrum muriaticum*)
- fatigue, nervous exhaustion, indifference to life (*Phosphoricum acidum*)
- migraine-like pain that travels from neck to one eye, associated with nervous exhaustion, sometimes vomiting (*Silica*)
- nervous and mental fatigue, aggravated by intellectual effort (*Staphysagria, Zincum metallicum*)

OTHER METABOLIC/ BIOENERGETIC/BIOCHEMICAL- BASED THERAPIES

The following therapies, depending upon the underlying mechanism, have also been beneficial for treating TMJ/dental headaches:

- Ayurvedic Medicine
- Detoxification Therapy
- Light Therapy
- Magnetic Field Therapy
- Naturopathy
- Nutritional Therapy
- Oxygen Therapy
- Traditional Chinese Medicine

STRUCTURALLY ORIENTED THERAPIES
BIOLOGICAL DENTISTRY

Tessa, a 71-year-old housewife from Southern California, had been suffering from 1 to 2 headaches a week for 6 1/2 years. She felt pain in her temples, across her forehead, and sometimes in the back of her head. Doctors had told her these were sinus headaches and prescribed decongestants. When she noticed she was having tooth and gum problems, yet still completely unaware of the possiblity that her dental problems could be contributing to her headaches, she went to see Dr. Harold Ravins, D.D.S., C.Ac., in Santa Monica, California.

Upon hearing that Tessa had headaches as well as dental discomfort, Dr. Ravins did a comprehensive analysis, looking not just at the infection that was expressing itself in teeth and gum problems, but also at the structure of Tessa's jaw, her diet, and other possible stressors that could be contributing to the physical, chemical, and energetic imbalances in her body. Dr. Ravins fit Tessa for a mouthpiece to reshape her jaw and referred her to a holistic practitioner who specializes in nutritional deficiencies.

Within 2 weeks, during which Tessa wore the mouthpiece and saw Dr. Ravins 3 times a week for acupuncture, Tessa's condition was 50% improved and, within 6 months, her headaches stopped and never came back. In Tessa's words, "I've learned never to let my teeth and body go again."

CRANIOSACRAL THERAPY

Janice, in her early sixties, suffered from chronic TMJ headaches that would leave her incapacitated for days. Over a period of 13 years, she had spent well over $10,000 on drugs and mouth appliances and still could not find relief. She then went to see osteopath John Upledger, D.O., of the Upledger Institute in Palm Beach Garden, Florida.

In his first few treatments, Dr. Upledger attempted to release Janice's jaw from her head by using a gentle maneuver to bring her jaw down-

Do You Have Dental Stress?

Make a fist, open your mouth as wide as you can, and insert your fist to see how many knuckles will fit into your mouth. Three or more is normal, with 2 or less indicating some kind of jaw or head injury. In addition, to determine whether you have dental stress, try answering the following questions:

- Do you favor one side of your mouth when you chew?
- Do you feel tenderness over your jaw joint?
- Do you grind your teeth?
- Do you have trouble swallowing 3 or 4 times in a row?
- Do you have a poor sense of balance?
- Do you feel fatigued after eating because of chewing?
- Do you feel strain when you smile?
- Do your gums bleed?
- Do you hear a clicking, popping, or grating sound when you open or close your mouth?

If you answered yes to any of these questions, chances are your headaches are related to or caused by some kind of dental stress.

ward, but when he realized this was not working, he decided to try a technique called Somato Emotional Release, in which the body is gently moved and rocked in order to get to stored-up emotional patterns.

During the treatment, Janice began to talk about a memory she had long since forgotten, describing a time when she was 16 years old and she was spending summer vacation on a lake. She remembered feeling a bit uptight because she was wearing a 2-piece bathing suit of which her mother did not approve, so Janice quickly dove into the water, and just as she was coming to the surface again, a young man dove in, hitting her on top of the head. This was the root of her TMJ problems 30 years later. Dr. Upledger used Janice's recovered memory to change the way he released her head, this time lifting the top of her skull to counter the impact of the injury, and, as he did, her headaches disappeared.

NEURAL THERAPY

Barbara had had terrible "migraines" since the age of 8. She had been on medication much of her life but was frustrated because these medications were keeping her from becoming pregnant. Furthermore, these drugs were also causing her to feel a terrible pain behind her eyes.

On her first visit to Joseph Schames, D.M.D., headache specialist, Director of Hollywood Community Hospital, and Codirector of the Craniofacial Pain/TMJ Clinic at White Memorial Medical Center in Los Angeles, California, Dr. Schames determined that Barbara's headaches were due to muscle tenderness in her mouth area. He injected the tender spots in her facial muscles with $1/2$% procaine and fitted her with a mouthpiece to wear at night.

He also prescribed therapeutic exercises (see "Self-Care Options" in this chapter) and had her eat a diet of only soft, blended foods. In 2 weeks, her headaches were gone, and she was gradually weaned from her medications. A year later, Barbara had a baby and named him Joseph in honor of Dr. Schames.

OSTEOPATHY

Sheila, a 61-year-old part-time office worker from Michigan, had chronic TMJS headaches, with pain so bad that she had trouble seeing and would sometimes wake up in the middle of the night thinking someone was sitting on her head. She had been to a dentist who had made her 4 different appliances, one to wear before eating, one for eating, one for after eating, one for overnight. Still her pain persisted. Then, her son, who was a dentist, sent her to the Upledger Institute in Florida to see John Upledger, D.O.

Dr. Upledger evaluated Sheila's jaw and cranial bones to detect blockages in energy, and worked his way down her back until he reached her right hip. Realizing this was the source of her pain (a fact confirmed when Shirley later explained that she had fainted and fallen on her hip before the headaches began), he released her hip using a gentle rhythmic technique, and, within 4 sessions, Shirley's headaches disappeared entirely. She no longer needed the appliances and, on Dr. Upledger's recommendation, she began swimming and using creative visualization in order to see herself further relaxed and healthy.

OTHER STRUCTURALLY ORIENTED THERAPIES

Also helpful in the treatment of TMJ/dental headaches are the following therapies:

- Alphabiotics
- Bodywork
- Chiropractic

PSYCHO/EMOTIONAL THERAPIES

FLOWER ESSENCE THERAPY

The following flower essences have been used to treat the physical and psychological tension often associated with TMJ headaches:

TRAUMA

Arnica: for severe trauma in which it feels as if you have left your body; restores conscious embodiment

Five Flower Remedy (also called Rescue Remedy): for panic, disorientation, or loss of consciousness; used to restore calm and stability in emergencies or during intense stress; contains cherry plum, clematis, impatiens, rock rose, star of Bethlehem

Queen Anne's Lace (also called wild carrot): often used to treat head trauma, as it helps to ground and stabilize

St. John's Wort: for headache accompanied by light and/or environmental

SPG Block for Orofacial Pain

The SPG (which stands for the sphenopalatine ganglion) block is used to treat and manage pain relating to the face and mouth which is often accompanied by a headache. The SPG is a nerve center of the face, particularly the sinuses. Developed by Dr. Joseph Schames, D.M.D., and his colleagues, the SPG block is a relatively noninvasive procedure which is simple to employ. In the treatment, the patient is seated in a chair, with his or her head tilted back. Two cotton tipped applicators (similar to Q-tips) that have been soaked in the anesthetic lidocaine are slid into the nasal passages and left in place for about 20 minutes. In a 1995 study, SPG was shown not only to quickly relieve facial pain, but also to reduce the frequency of headaches—even after treatments have been stopped.

SOURCE—Joseph Schames, D.M.D., "Sphenopalatine Ganglion Block: A Safe and Easy Method for the Management of Orofacial Pain," *Journal of Craniomandibular Practice* 13:3 (July 1995).

sensitivity

Self-Heal (the flower *Prunella vulgaris*): used to restore the physical body after a blow or injury, especially when damage seems overwhelming; restores a vital sense of self

STRESS AND TENSION

Dandelion: for stress and tension held in the muscles of the body; brings about dynamic, effortless energy

Fuschia: for repressed emotions that cause psychosomatic symptoms; allows the expression of genuine feelings and emotional states

Impatiens: for people who are constantly rushing, impatient, intolerant, tense; creates acceptance and patience for the flow of life

Five Flower Remedy: helps in coping with stress in general

Snapdragon: used for those who hold tension in the jaw and mouth and/or grind their teeth

GENERAL HEADACHE

Lavender: good overall headache remedy, used to dispel nervousness and over-stimulation which deplete the physical body

Five Flower Remedy (Rescue Remedy): good overall stress remedy

OTHER PSYCHO/EMOTIONAL THERAPIES

The following techniques can also be beneficial for reducing stress and releasing the emotions that may be contributing to your TMJ/dental headache:

- Biofeedback
- Hypnotherapy
- Psychotherapy

SELF-CARE OPTIONS

Although TMJ/dental headaches can be prevented and alleviated with most of the same self-help techniques that are useful for tension and migraine headaches, the following suggestions should also prove beneficial:

- Visit your dentist regularly to maintain proper dental health.
- Make sure your dentist does not use mercury fillings.
- Be sure to get adequate nutrition by eating a well-balanced diet.
- Supplement your diet with calcium, magnesium, and a multivitamin.
- Chew your foods thoroughly.
- Stretch your muscles and get some kind of moderate exercise, such as swimming, at least 3 times a week.
- Correct your posture and wear properly fitting shoes.
- Try to avoid such habits as nail-biting and teeth clenching or grinding.
- Rest your jaw as much as possible.

See Chapter 16,
An A-Z of Self-Care
Options, for more
information on
self-treatment
methods.

AROMATHERAPY

The following aromatherapy treatments have been helpful in relieving the pain associated with TMJ/dental headaches:

INHALATION

Wafting relief: Fill aroma lamp, bowl, or diffuser with water and mix in 4 drops melissa and 2 drops peppermint or Roman chamomile oil.

For aroma to go: Put 2 to 3 drops of melissa, peppermint, and lavender oils on a handkerchief or cloth and inhale throughout the day for prevention.

MASSAGE

Temple rub: Combine lavender (a sedative) and peppermint (a stimulant) oils and rub the mixture on your temples for pain relief.

Sore muscle massage: Mix 10 drops juniper (which adds heat), 8 drops rosemary, 8 drops lavender, and 2 drops lemon with 2 ounces vegetable oil and use to massage your neck and shoulders.

Additional oils for general headaches: Basil, chamomile, coriander (very small doses only), melissa, and sage can be massaged into the temples, eye sockets, and the base of the neck and shoulders.

COMPRESSES AND STEAMS

Cold compress relief: Mix 3 drops rose, 1 drop melissa, and 1 drop lavender oils in 2 pints water. Stir thoroughly and place a towel or washcloth in the water. Let it soak for 5 minutes, then wring to remove excess water. Lie back and put the compress on the painful area. Rest. Change the compress as soon as it reaches room temperature.

Compress for sore muscles: Soak clean cloth in a mixture of 1 drop ginger, 2 drops marjoram, 1 drop peppermint, and 1 drop rosemary oils added to hot water; apply to neck, shoulders, and/or jaw.

EXERCISE

JAW EXERCISE—The following therapeutic jaw exercise is good for strengthening and stretching the TMJ. Hold each thrust for 10 seconds, keeping your fist steady and immobile throughout. Repeat the entire series 6 times twice a day, preferably in the morning and in the evening:

■ Open your mouth about an inch, make a fist, and place it in front of your lower jaw; try to jut your jaw forward against it;

■ next, place your fist on one side of the jaw, and again thrust your lower jaw against the fist;

■ do this on the other side; and finally;

■ place your fist beneath your lower jaw and thrust against it.

If you have any neck, shoulder, or back condition currently under treatment by a chiropractor, osteopath, or other bodywork professional, consult with this practitioner first before doing these exercises.

HEAD, NECK, AND SHOULDER STRETCH—Joseph Schames, D.M.D., recommends the following series of exercises to his patients to help stretch the head, neck, and shoulder muscles. As each exercise is designed to work a different muscle, he recommends that they be done in sequence. Furthermore, each should be performed with a passive, non-jerking stretch, using your arm and hand as a weight. Do them once an hour while pain persists.

Exercise #1: Placing one hand against the back of your head, bend your head down as far as you can. Hold the stretch for 7 to 30 seconds while breathing deeply.

Exercise #2: Place the left hand against the back of your head, point your nose toward your right armpit, and stretch your neck while tilting the back part of your head down to the center of your chest. Hold the stretch for 7 to 30 seconds while breathing deeply. Repeat on the other side.

Exercise #3: Sitting in a chair with your back straight, your chin tucked to your chest, and your left hand holding on to the chair for support, place your left hand to your head and use it to help stretch your ear toward your left shoulder. Hold the stretch for 7 to 30 seconds while breathing deeply. Repeat on the other side.

Exercise #4: Keeping your back straight, place your left hand on your head and your right hand on your chin, and then lightly tilt your head upward and back to the left, pointing your nose up and over your left shoulder. Hold the stretch for 7 to 30 seconds while breathing deeply. Repeat on the other side.

Exercise #5: Standing with erect

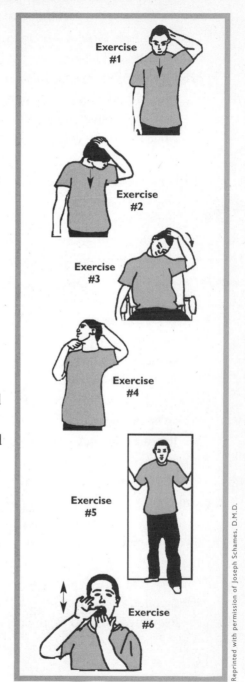

Reprinted with permission of Joseph Schames, D.M.D.

Figure 12.2—Head, neck, and shoulder stretch exercises.

posture in a doorway, pull your chin in slightly, hold both sides of the doorway with your hands, and step one leg forward so you feel the stretch. Hold for 7 to 30 seconds while breathing deeply. Repeat with the other leg.

Exercise #6: Place your right thumb on the edge of your upper teeth and your left fingers on the edge of your lower teeth and use them to stretch your mouth open. Hold the stretch for 7 to 30 seconds while breathing deeply. Repeat on the other side.[1]

FOLK REMEDIES

For TMJ relief, add the following simple technique to the folk remedies listed in Chapter 16, An A-Z of Self-Care Options.

Gentle jaw alignment—For temporary relief, hold a pencil, a straw, or other cylindrical object of a similar size crossways between your teeth, being careful not to bite down.

HERBAL SUPPLEMENTS

The following herbs are most commonly used for TMJ/dental headaches:

General headache—angelica, feverfew, meadowsweet, willow bark

Hormonal/reproductive problems—black cohosh, black haw, cayenne, chasteberry, cramp bark, lavender, passion flower, skullcap, St. John's wort, wild yam

Immune system—*Echinacea*, garlic, ginger, *Ginkgo*, golden seal, nettle, rosehips

Musculoskeletal pain and spasms—cayenne, chamomile, elder, meadowsweet, nettles, *qiyelian*, turmeric, valerian, vervain, willow bark

Stress, anxiety, insomnia, and tension—feverfew, lavender, passion flower, pennyroyal, peppermint, rosehips, skullcap, St. John's wort, valerian, vervain

Vascular imbalances—balm, basil, cayenne, elder flower, feverfew, garlic, ginger, *Ginkgo*, goldenrod, Jamaican dogwood, lavender, marjoram, peppermint, rosemary, rue, thyme, sage, willow bark, wormwood

ICE AND HEAT

For temporary relief of TMJ pain, try one of the following:

For swelling and inflammation: Apply an ice pack to the jaw region for periods of 20 to 30 minutes, making sure that you take at least a 30-

minute break between applications.

For nagging, recurring pain: Apply moist heat in the form of a compress or hot water bottle to the affected area for 20 minutes, resting for 30, and then applying heat again as needed.

MASSAGE

These 2 simples massage techniques—mouth massage and jaw massage—can be used in addition to the massage techniques outlined in Chapter 16, An A-Z of Self-Care Options.

JAW MASSAGE—This technique is helpful for relieving a tender jaw and associated head pain:

- Start by pressing your fingers around your eyes to locate the tender spots;
- As you come across a tender spot, gently but firmly press with your finger and hold the pressure for about 10 seconds;
- Next grasp your ears with your fingers and slowly pull your ears out and down, away from your head;
- Follow by massaging all around each ear, and then work your way up to the temples;
- Then, starting from the base of your neck, use downward strokes and massage your way up to the base of your skull;
- Press firmly but gently on the points where your neck and skull join, again holding the pressure for about 10 seconds; and
- Finally, use your thumbs to locate the tender parts on each side of your jaw, applying pressure and holding each spot for 10 seconds.

MOUTH MASSAGE—Although it may take several repetitions of this procedure before your pain will start to subside, it definitely works, according to Dr. Ravins. He suggests you try the following

Since the symptoms of TMJ/dental headaches are so similar to those of other conditions, just about every type of medical professional may be consulted before the patient finally turns to an alternative practitioner. Ironically, it is because of this diversity that these headaches respond so well to the flexible and multidisciplinary approach of alternative medicine.

technique whenever you feel a headache coming on:

- Wash your hands and put your thumb in your mouth on the side of the pain (or on the right side if it is generalized);
- reach up with your thumb to find your cheekbone and gently press it up and out for 30 seconds;
- repeat the process on the other side of your mouth; and
- finally, place both thumbs inside your mouth on the upper palate and gently press the sides of your palate out for 30 seconds.

OTHER SELF-CARE OPTIONS

The following self-care techniques can also be helpful for TMJ/dental headaches:

- Affirmations/Autosuggestions
- Breathing Exercises
- Creative Visualization
- Lifestyle Changes
- Meditation
- Nutritional Therapy/Dietary Changes
- Relaxation Exercises
- Support Groups

RECOMMENDED READING

Alternative Medicine: The Definitive Guide. Compiled by the Burton Goldberg Group. Tiburon, CA: Future Medicine Publishing, 1994.

Bonner, Phillip. "Looking Down in the Mouth," *Express* (June 1983), 17-18.

Braly, James, M.D. and Torbet, Laura. *Dr. Braly's Food Allergy and Nutrition Revolution.* New Canaan, CT: Keats Publishing, Inc., 1992.

Clark, Linda, M.A. *A Handbook of Natural Remedies for Common Ailments.* Greenwich, CT: The Devin-Adair Company, 1976.

Faber, William J., D.O. *Pain, Pain Go Away.* San Jose, CA: ISHI Press International, 1990.

Ford, Norman D. *Eighteen Natural Ways to Beat a Headache.* New Canaan, CT: Keats Publishing, Inc., 1990.

Graff-Radford, Steven B., D.D.S. "The Jaw Bone's Connected to the Headbone: TMJ and Headaches." *Headache.* The American Council for Headache Education, December 1993.

Igram, Cass, M.D. *Who Needs Headaches?* Cedar Rapids, IA: Literary Visions Publishing, 1991.

Jensen, Bernard, D.C., Ph.D. *Tissue Cleansing through Bowel Management,* 10th ed. Escondido, CA: Bernard Jensen Publishing, 1981.

Jouanny, Jacques, M.D. et al. *Homeopathic Therapeutics: Possibilities in Chronic Pathology.* France: Editions Boiron, 1994.

Keller, Erich. *The Complete Home Guide to Aromatherapy.* Tiburon, CA: H.J. Kramer, Inc., 1991.

Nambudripad, Devi S., D.C., L.Ac., R.N., Ph.D. *Say Goodbye to Illness.* Buena Park, CA: Delta Publishing, 1993.

National Headache Foundation Fact Sheet. Chicago: National Headache Foundation, October 1994.

"Patient Adverse Reaction Report." *DAMS* (March 1994), 93-102.

Price, W.A. *Dental Infections, Volume 1: Oral and Systemic.* Cleveland, OH: Benton Publishing, 1973.

Prudden, Bonnie. *Pain Erasure: The Bonnie Prudden Way.* New York: Ballantine Books, 1980.

Rapoport, Alan M., M.D. and Sheftell, Fred D., M.D. *Headache Relief.* New York: Simon & Schuster, 1990.

Rapoport, Alan M., M.D. and Sheftell, Fred D., M.D. *Headache Relief for Women.* New York: Little, Brown and Company, 1995.

Retzlaff, E.W. and Michael, D.K. "Cranial Bone Mobility." *Journal of the American Osteopathic Association* 74 (May 1975), 869-873.

Robbins, Lawrence, M.D. and Lang, Susan. *Headache Help.* New York: Houghton Mifflin Company, 1995.

Stromfeld, Jan and Weil, Anita. *Free Yourself from Headaches: The Natural Drug-Free Program for Prevention and Relief.* Palm Beach Garden, FL: The Upledger Institute, Frog, Ltd., 1995.

Solomon, Seymour, M.D. and Fraccaro, Steven. *The Headache Book.* Mount Vernon, NY: Consumer Reports Books, 1991.

Taylor, J. *The Complete Guide to Mercury Toxicity from Dental Fillings.* San Diego: Scripps Publishing, 1988.

Upledger, J.E. *Your Inner Physician and You, Craniosacral Therapy Somato Emotional Release.* Berkeley, CA: North Atlantic, 1992.

Wang, K. "A Report of 22 Cases of Temporomandibular Joint Dysfunction Syndrome Treated with Acupuncture and Laser Radiation." *Journal of Traditional Chinese Medicine* 12:2 (June 1992), 116-118.

Watts, P.G., Peet, K.M.S., and Juniper, R.P. "Migraine and the Temporomandibular Joint: The Final Answer?" *British Dental Journal* 161 (1986), 215-216.

*Since the symptoms of TMJ/
dental headaches are
similar to those of other conditions,
nearly every type of medical
professional may be consulted
before the patient finally turns to
an alternative practitioner.
Ironically, it is because of this diversity that these headaches
respond well to the flexible
and multidisciplinary approach of
alternative medicine.*

Chapter 13

Eyestrain Headaches

Although they're called eyestrain headaches, technically the pain you feel is not due to your eyes themselves but to the muscles around them. These muscles get overworked by frequent squinting, straining, blinking, and other visually demanding tasks, eventually resulting in a steady pain behind the eyes.

Every afternoon, like clockwork, once I hit the 6-hour mark at my computer, my eyes would start to ache and I would get a mild pressure that felt as though it was coming in through the top of my head. But I work on deadlines, so I would keep on working until the pain got so bad that I could no longer think, and by then I was really bad off—because then I had both a terrible headache and an unhappy client. —Mark, an accountant

What Is an Eyestrain Headache?

Like TMJ and sinus headaches, eyestrain headaches tend to be attributed to referred pain. In this case, a pain in the eyes gets translated by the brain as overall head pain. Although these headaches are called eyestrain headaches, technically the pain you feel is not due to your eyes themselves but to the muscles around them. These muscles get overworked by frequent squinting, straining, blinking, and other visually demanding tasks, which in turn can put pressure on the muscles across the face and scalp and eventually result in a mild but steady frontal pain, usually felt behind the eyes—in other words, a muscle contraction or tension-type headache.

The Causes and Triggers of Eyestrain Headache

As the name suggests, eyestrain headaches originate in the eyes. A number of different eye problems can bring on headaches; however, when talking about eyestrain headaches, we are referring to a general type of stress that occurs in the eyes. This can be due to reading or staring at a computer monitor for prolonged periods of time, especially if the light is inadequate; it can be brought on by not wearing glasses or by wearing incorrect

See Chapter 5, Organic Headaches, for more information on headaches related to eye problems.

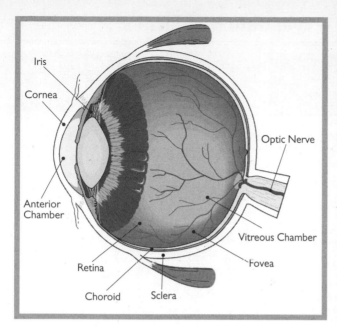

Figure 13.1—The eye.

Visual Conditions and Eyestrain Headaches

The following are 3 common vision conditions that often trigger eyestrain headaches:

- PRESBYOPIA— progressive decrease in the ability to focus on objects at close range

- REFRACTIVE DISORDERS— depending on the type of disorder, blurred vision or an inability to clearly see objects that are either near or far

- ASTIGMATISM— irregularity in the curvature of the lens of the eye which results in blurred vision

ones. Basically, eyestrain headaches are brought on by nearly any event that forces your eyes to struggle to see the world around you.

To exacerbate the situation, many eyestrain headaches are not caused by visual disorders, such as far- or near-sightedness per se, but to the eyes' inability to work together as a team, or postural problems, in which case stronger and stronger lenses may not correct the underlying cause. For example, in an effort to self-correct a minor visual disturbance, people often tilt their heads to achieve focus. In addition to straining the neck, this maneuver turns the world askew, putting greater stress on your eyes.

Other postural problems, such as sitting bent over at a desk all day, especially if you are doing close work like writing or bookkeeping, can also contribute to eyestrain headaches. Unnatural postures cause your head to sit heavy on your shoulders, further contracting your muscles, which further strains your eyes.

If you wear contact lenses, your eyestrain headaches may be due to an improper fit or to leaving the lenses in too long, especially in the case of extended-wear lenses. You should always clean lenses carefully, remembering to use an enzymatic or heat cleaner once a week to remove protein

Symptom Chart—Eyestrain Headaches

SYMPTOMS	HEADACHE TYPE	PAIN LOCATION
Description: can resemble tension headache, with mild steady pain usually felt as pressure on top of head or around head **Symptoms:** similar to tension headache; if digestion-related, burping and belching; teary or reddened eyes; sometimes aggravated by movement **Duration:** 1 hour to all day **Frequency:** occurs when reading or doing other close activities, particularly in the afternoon or on weekends; rarely or continuously	**EYESTRAIN HEADACHE**	forehead and face sometimes with pain at back of head and/or neck

UNDERLYING CAUSES AND TRIGGERS	PRIMARY AND SECONDARY TREATMENTS	SELF-CARE TREATMENTS	WHERE IN THE BOOK PAGE #

Causes: overuse of eyes; worsened by metabolic imbalances, structural disturbances, emotional/psychological factors

Triggers: lifestyle factors (uncorrected faulty vision, astigmatism, excessive frowning or squinting, long periods of reading or close work, constant use of computer, TV, or VCR, inadequate nutrition); dietary and/or environmental sensitivity, hormonal imbalance, autoimmune disturbances, structural disturbances (poor posture), psychological stress

Primary:
- acupuncture
- behavioral optometry
- bodywork
- environmental medicine
- homeopathy
- nutritional therapy
- osteopathy

Secondary:
- chiropractic
- craniosacral therapy
- energy medicine
- herbal medicine
- naturopathy
- neural therapy
- oxygen therapy
- traditional Chinese medicine

- affirmations
- aromatherapy
- biofeedback
- breathing exercises
- creative visualization
- exercise
- flower remedies
- folk remedies
- herbal supplements
- ice and heat
- journal writing
- lifestyle changes
- massage
- meditation
- nutritional therapy
- relaxation techniques
- support groups

Page 347

A Quick Look at Eyestrain Triggers

- uncorrected faulty vision
- excessive frowning or squinting to see clearly
- reading or doing close work for long periods of time without rest
- constant use of video display terminal (VDT)
- poor posture
- poor lighting, especially flickering neon or overhead fluorescent lighting
- prolonged exposure to television, video monitors, and computer screens

Behavioral optometry is a speciality within optometry. With 3000 American practitioners, it understands vision problems within a holistic framework, involving the mind, body, and behavior. Its principles were first outlined in the 1920s by A. M. Skeffington who explained that the purpose of vision is to process information and requires the entire visual system from eye to brain. A behavioral optometrist uses special lenses, exercises, nutrition, and corrective measures to retrain the eyes and enable the person to permanently relearn how to see.

buildup; however, be careful when choosing the solutions and cleaners you use, since many of them contain preservatives to which you may be sensitive or allergic. To be safe, use contact solutions that are made without the chemical thimerosal, or other solutions made specifically for sensitive eyes. Furthermore, contacts should not be replaced only when you happen to lose one; like everything else, they wear out.

See Chapter 3, What Causes Your Headache? for more detail on headache causes and triggers.

Diagnosing and Treating Underlying Causes

The best way to treat an eyestrain headache is, first, to have your eyes examined. Vision changes over time, so even if you already wear glasses, a visit to an optometrist or ophthalmologist should be the first step you take. If your headaches are due to a simple visual disturbance, you will find relief when you are fitted with the necessary corrective lenses.

Although eyeglasses often eliminate the need to tilt the head, they may not always be enough to stop the stress in your eyes. If this is the case—or if your headaches eventually come back—you might want to do postural exercises or eye exercises (listed under "Self-Care Options" at the end of this chapter) to retrain and strengthen both your body and your eyes. In addition, you should also keep in mind that, according to traditional Chinese medicine, the eyes are under the influence of the liver, meaning that many eye problems go away when the condition of the liver improves.

If you prefer to skip all other steps and get directly to the root of your vision problem, it is wise to see a behavioral optometrist first, since this is where you will be able to correct your vision, the way you use your eyes, and your posture under the guidance of one practitioner. A behavioral optometrist not only will prescribe corrective lenses but also will teach you the physiology of your headaches and show you how to prevent them by retraining your eyes and body.

For example, a behavioral optometrist views the type of headache that comes on whenever you try to read as a communication problem occurring between the way your eyes focus and the way your eyes work together as a team. What this means is that even when your eyes try to focus at one distance, the mechanism that controls their ability to work as a team and sustain this focus stops functioning properly, forcing your eyes to compensate in order to see. Behavioral exercises, similar to those outlined later in the chapter, can help you learn to coordinate these systems again, thus improving the overall health of your eyes.

ALTERNATIVE TREATMENTS

METABOLIC/BIOENERGETIC/BIOCHEMICAL-BASED THERAPIES

BEHAVIORAL OPTOMETRY

Nancy, an avid reader and poet in her mid-fifties, could not read or write for longer than 15 minutes without getting a dull headache that would last the next 24 hours. Convinced her headaches were caused by eyestrain, she went to an optometrist, who fitted her with corrective lenses, but, even with the glasses, her headaches persisted. Finally, after months of suffering, she heard about Anne Barber, O.D., an optometrist specializing in behavioral optometry in Santa Ana, California, and

Signs of Imbalances in the Visual-Perception System

According to behavioral optometrists, these are some of the signs that your headaches are related to a visual perception system that is not working as it was intended:

Problems with eye teaming or focusing—closing one eye to focus, one or both eyes that cross in or out, frequent squinting while concentrating or in bright light, misaligning numbers when working across a column, difficulty determining where objects are in space;

Problems or soreness in eyes themselves—red, burning, or itching eyes, swollen eyelids, blurred or double vision, a thin coating or film over the eyes, excessive blinking;

Problems with hand-eye coordination—slow printing and difficulty writing on printed lines or marking the circles on multiple choice tests, avoiding tasks that require hand-eye coordination, such as softball or catch;

Problems with form and perception—confusing or misreading similar shapes, letters, words, and numbers, difficulty using a dictionary;

Problems with spatial and perceptual abilities—confusing left and right, mixing up spatial words such as north and south and out and in, easily frustrated when reading maps or interpreting directions, transposing letters, getting lost even if traveling to a familiar site.

SOURCE—Richard Leviton, *Brain Builders* (New York: Simon & Schuster, 1995).

decided to give her a try.

After the initial evaluation, Dr. Barber determined that Nancy's headaches were being caused by visual habits, more specifically an eye system that did not work as a team, making reading and close work difficult. Dr. Barber put Nancy on a retraining schedule that included weekly office sessions and 15 to 20 minutes a day of home practice.

Unlike others, Nancy was an especially difficult case. She had to work so hard to keep her eyes focusing as a team that even the retraining exercises gave her a headache. However, since both Nancy and Dr. Barber were determined, they were able to work through these headaches after a couple of weeks and, 4 weeks later, Nancy was reading and writing without eyestrain headaches.

See Chapter 17, An A-Z of Alternative Medicine, for more information on treatment methods.

HOMEOPATHY

A behavioral optometrist will not only prescribe corrective lenses but also will teach you the physiology of your headaches and show you how to prevent them by retraining your eyes and body.

Andrew, a 24-year-old college student working for his master's in biochemistry, came to the Milne Medical Center complaining of eyestrain headaches that came on whenever he studied for more than 2 or 3 hours. Andrew had visited his optometrist and was given eyeglasses, and when they did not help, his mother suggested he try alternative medicine.

Upon evaluation, it was obvious that his condition was due to a straightforward case of eyestrain, so we gave him the homeopathic eyestrain remedy, *Ruta graveolens* 3X (rue or bitter herb), 4 to 6 times daily as needed. Within a few days, Andrew found that he was able to study for longer periods of time without pain and, within a week, was able to devote the time necessary to pass his final exams without the added burden of eyestrain headaches.

The following homeopathic remedies are a sampling of those that can be useful for eyestrain headaches. Homeopathic remedies work best when prescribed by a qualified practitioner; when self-administered, these therapies should be taken only in doses of 6X or lower.

Eyestrain or Visual Disturbances—*Aurum, Gelsemium, Glonoinum, Natrum muriaticum, Onosmodium, Physostigma* (worsening of myopic sight); *Phosphorus* *prunus, Ruta graveolens, Spigelia* (left-sided eye pain, fatigue, and general disability)

Stress, Tension, and Anxiety

- irritability, moodiness, intellectual overwork (*Anacardium orientale*)
- mental exertion (*Argentium nitricum*)
- vague but distressing tension-type pain, associated with anxiety and visual disturbances, intensified with noise and movement (*Chamomilla, Gelsemium*)
- depression, suicidal thoughts, delusions, fear (*Hura Braziliensis*)
- hypersensitivity, hysterical outbursts, heavy, pressurized pain, sometimes nausea and dizziness (*Ignatia*)
- intellectual overwork, overall physical fatigue (*Kali phosphoricum*)
- developing after intense mental work, for those who are ambitious, driving, and eager to achieve (*Lachesis, Natrum muriaticum*)
- fatigue, nervous exhaustion, indifference to life (*Phosphoricum acidum*)
- migraine-like pain that travels from neck to one eye, associated with nervous exhaustion, sometimes vomiting (*Silica*)
- nervous and mental fatigue, aggravated by intellectual effort (*Staphysagria, Zincum metallicum*)

> *Within a few days of taking a homeopathic remedy for his eyestrain headaches, Andrew found that he was able to study for longer periods of time without pain and, within a week, was able to devote the time necessary to pass his final exams without the added burden of headaches.*

OTHER METABOLIC/ BIOENERGETIC/ BIOCHEMICAL-BASED THERAPIES

The following therapies, depending upon whether other associated conditions are contributing to the eyestrain problem, may be beneficial for treating eyestrain headaches:

- Acupuncture

- Ayurvedic Medicine
- Detoxification Therapy
- Energy Medicine
- Environmental Medicine
- Herbal Medicine
- Homeopathy
- Light Therapy
- Magnetic Field Therapy
- Naturopathy
- Nutritional Therapy
- Oxygen Therapy
- Traditional Chinese Medicine

STRUCTURALLY ORIENTED THERAPIES
BODYWORK

See Chapter 17, An A-Z of Alternative Medicine, for information on specific types of bodywork.

Since eyestrain headaches are often associated with tight, contracted muscles, bodywork is a useful therapeutic. It helps you to relax and become more aware of the way you hold and move your body. All the bodywork methods are helpful; choosing one is a matter of individual preference.

OTHER STRUCTURALLY ORIENTED THERAPIES

Depending upon the underlying cause, the following therapies can also be useful:

- Alphabiotics
- Biological Dentistry
- Chiropractic
- Craniosacral Therapy
- Neural Therapy
- Osteopathy

PSYCHO/EMOTIONAL THERAPIES

As the mind is involved in all healing processes, it is often useful to incorporate some type of emotional/psychological modality just to help you release stress and relax. Any one of these therapies can be effective. You might try learning a biofeedback technique to learn how to relax contracted muscles in the face and neck. Flower essences may help you to let go of emotional issues that are contributing to your eyestrain.

FLOWER ESSENCE THERAPY

The following flower essences can be useful for eyestrain headaches:

ALLERGY/SENSITIVITY

St. John's Wort: used for headache accompanied by light sensitivity or vulnerability to environmental stress, including allergies

See Chapter 16, An A-Z of Self-Care Options, for more information on self-treatment methods.

Yarrow: strengthening; eases the sensitivity that occurs when the body tries to deal with input overload, either from the environment or through digestion

TRAUMA

Self Heal (the flower *Prunella vulgaris*): used to restore the physical body after a blow or injury, especially when damage seems overwhelming; restores a vital sense of self

STRESS AND TENSION

Dandelion: stress and tension held in the muscles of the body; brings about dynamic, effortless energy

Iris: tension, especially in the neck region; unable to feel inner freedom

Lavender: releases high-strung, nervous tension, allows full relaxation in order to receive the benefits of the healing work

Mimulus: for those who are frequently in fear of their next headache attack

Five Flower Remedy (also called Rescue Remedy): for coping with stress in general; contains cherry plum, clematis, impatiens, rock rose, star of Bethlehem

GENERAL HEADACHE

Lavender: good overall headache remedy, as it used to dispel nervousness and overstimulation which deplete the physical body

OTHER PSYCHO/ EMOTIONAL THERAPIES

Other helpful therapies that can relieve the stress and tension of eyestrain headaches include:

- Biofeedback
- Hypnotherapy
- Psychotherapy

SELF-CARE OPTIONS
ACUPRESSURE

The following points can be helpful to relieve the pain of eyestrain headaches:

- Bladder 2 (B 2)
- *Yin Tang* point (GV 24.5)
- Stomach 36 (St 36)
- Large Intestine 4 (LI 4)
- Liver 3 (Lv 3)
- Liver 14 (Lv 14)
- Gall Bladder 1 (GB 1)

AROMATHERAPY
INHALATION

Wafting relief: Fill aroma lamp, bowl, or diffuser with water and mix in 4 drops melissa and 2 drops peppermint or Roman chamomile oil.

MASSAGE

Temple rub: Combine lavender (a sedative) and peppermint (a stimulant) oils and rub the mixture on your temples to get the relief of painkilling drugs without the side effects.

Additional oils for general headaches: Basil, chamomile, coriander (small doses only), melissa, and sage can be massaged into the temples, eye sockets, and base of the neck and shoulders.

BATHS

Aroma soak: For relief of a headache in progress, fill a bath with warm to hot water and add eucalyptus, wintergreen, or peppermint oils and soak 20 to 30 minutes.

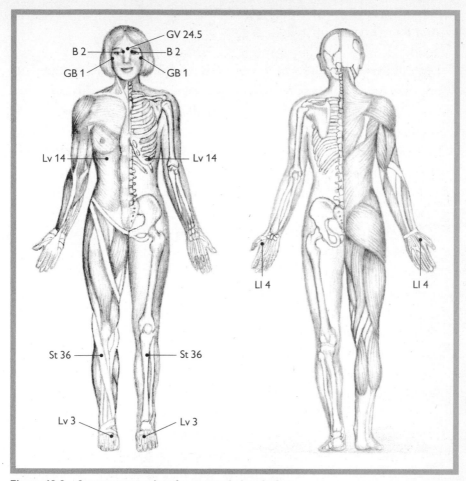

Figure 13.2—Acupressure points for eyestrain headaches.

COMPRESSES AND STEAMS

Compress for eyestrain headache: Lie down in a darkened room with a cool compress made with chamomile, rosemary, or parsley oils over your closed eyes.

EXERCISE

Not only can eye exercises relieve eyestrain, but also they can strengthen your eyes and help to prevent future vision problems. These exercises are particularly helpful if you are working with your eyes for long periods of time, since they give your eyes a chance to change focus from close- to long-range, helping to prevent your eye muscles from straining. An easy exercise is simply remembering to look up from close work and change your focus every 15 minutes.

Eyeball Stretch—These exercises are intended to improve eyesight and relax the mind. Do these exercises in seated position as you breathe comfortably and rhythmically. Do this series 10 times, moving your eyes as far as you can in the direction indicated (but don't strain). Take a long breath in between each set. When you are finished with all 10 cycles, close your eyes and take 3 relaxing breaths.

1. Move your eyes up toward the ceiling, then down toward the floor.
2. Move your eyes from the left side to the right side.
3. Move your eyes diagonally, going from upper left to lower right, then from lower left to upper right.
4. Rotate your eyes, first clockwise, then counterclockwise.

Thumb Rotations—Anne Barber, D.O., recommends this exercise to anyone interested in keeping their eyes healthy and strong regardless of whether they have visual problems. This exercise gets the circulation in the eyes flowing and helps the eyes to work together as a team.

1. Ball your hand into a fist but leave your thumb out so it sticks straight up and extend your arm out in front of you.
2. With your thumb pointing upward, move your arm in a wide circle, following your thumb with your eyes without moving your head.
3. Repeat 5 times.
4. Repeat steps 1 through 3 using the other arm.

Pencil Push-ups—Dr. Barber also recommends this exercise to improve the ability of your eyes to come together and focus as one.

1. Use both hands to clasp a pencil and extend your arm directly out in front of you, at the level of your nose.
2. Slowly bend your arms and pull the pencil back toward you until you see 2 pencils. (This should be just about at the point where the pencil touches your nose.)
3. Repeat 5 to 10 times.

HERBAL MEDICINE

In addition to the herbs listed in Chapters 16 and 17, bilberry is especially helpful for eye-related conditions, including eyestrain headaches. Bilberry is known for its ability to scavenge and neutralize free radicals. It contains anthocyanidins, powerful flavonoids which support the long-term health of the eyes by improving capillary permeability and circulation.

LIFESTYLE CHANGES

Here are some everyday steps you can take to prevent eyestrain:

- Make sure work or reading area is well lit.
- Have eyes checked regularly and wear glasses if needed.
- Take breaks from close work, letting your eyes look up and focus across the room every 15 minutes.
- Replace fluorescent lights with full-spectrum bulbs.
- Rest eyes when they feel fatigued.
- VDT users should monitor the clarity of the screen, and, if necessary, purchase a glare-reducing screen.
- Wear polarized, tinted, or dark glasses and a wide-brimmed hat in bright sunlight.
- Don't tilt your head to achieve focus.
- Blink regularly.
- Be aware of your posture.
- Incorporate eye exercises and massage into your day.

MASSAGE

Giving yourself a gentle massage can bring about temporary relief from eyestrain. This can be done by massaging your forehead and temples, rubbing gentle circles around your eyes (but never directly on your eyes), and pressing up on the eyebrow ridge with your thumbs, going from the top of your nose to the edge of your eyebrows.

Another easy eye-relaxing technique that you can do anywhere is known as palming. Although it is preferable to do this exercise without contact lenses, sometimes it is inconvenient to remove them, so just be careful not to put pressure on your eyes:

1. Remove your glasses, and sit or lie down comfortably, turning down the lights if possible.

2. Place your hands, palm side down, gently but firmly over your eyes so they block out the light.

3. Keep your eyes open and stare into the blackness for 30 to 60 seconds.

4. Close your eyes and lower your hands.

5. Keep your eyes shut for a few seconds, then open them slowly.

REFLEXOLOGY

See Chapter 16, An A-Z of Self-Care Options, Reflexology, for an illustration of these points and directions on how to stimulate them.

BRAIN—all headaches, circulation, and overall body function

HEAD—all headaches, stress, shoulder and neck tension

EYES—vision, stress

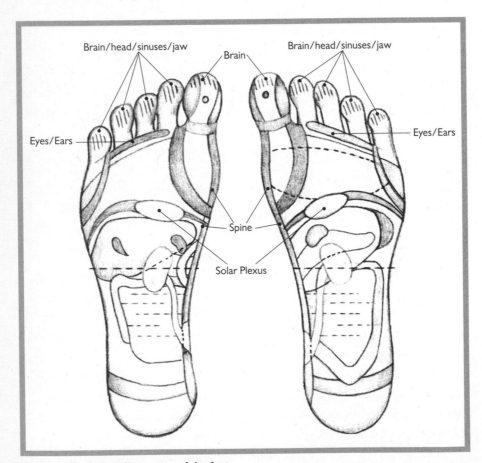

Figure 13.3—Reflexology areas of the feet.

SPINE—all headaches, trauma, stress, tension, digestion

SOLAR PLEXUS—stress, anxiety, digestion

OTHER SELF-CARE OPTIONS

The following self-care techniques can also be helpful for eyestrain headaches:

- Affirmations/Autosuggestions
- Breathing Exercises
- Creative Visualization
- Folk Remedies
- Ice and Heat
- Meditation
- Nutritional Therapy/Dietary Changes
- Relaxation Exercises
- Support Groups

See Chapter 16,
An A-Z of Self-Care
Options, for more
information on
self-treatment
methods.

RECOMMENDED READING

Alternative Medicine: The Definitive Guide. Compiled by the Burton Goldberg Group. Tiburon, CA: Future Medicine Publishing, 1994.

Bates, W.H. *The Bates Method for Better Eyesight without Glasses*. New York: Henry Holt & Co./Owl Books, 1981.

Clark, Linda, M.A. *A Handbook of Natural Remedies for Common Ailments*. Greenwich, CT: The Devin-Adair Company, 1976.

Claire, Thomas. *Bodywork—What Type of Massage to Get and How to Make the Most of It*, New York: William Morrow & Co., 1995.

Faber, William J., D.O. *Pain, Pain Go Away*. San Jose, CA: ISHI Press International, 1990.

Ford, Norman D. *Eighteen Natural Ways to Beat a Headache*. New Canaan, CT: Keats Publishing, Inc., 1990.

Igram, Cass, M.D. *Who Needs Headaches?* Cedar Rapids, IA: Literary Visions Publishing, 1991.

Lilienthal, Samuel, M.D. *Homeopathic Therapeutics*. New Delhi: Jain Publishing Co., 1996.

National Headache Foundation Fact Sheet. Chicago: National Headache Foundation, October 1994.

Natural Health Secrets from around the World. Boca Raton, FL: Shot Tower Books, 1996.

Peachey, G.T. "Perspective on Optometric Visual Training." *Journal of Behavioral Optometry* 1:3 (1990), 65-70.

Rapoport, Alan M., M.D. and Sheftell, Fred D., M.D. *Headache Relief.* New York: Simon & Schuster, 1990.

Rapoport, Alan M., M.D.. and Sheftell, Fred D., M.D. *Headache Relief for Women.* New York: Little, Brown and Company, 1995.

Rick, Stephanie. *The Reflexology Workout.* New York: Harmony Books, 1986.

Robbins, Lawrence, M.D. and Lang, Susan. *Headache Help.* New York: Houghton Mifflin Company, 1995.

Stromfeld, Jan and Weil, Anita. *Free Yourself from Headaches: The Natural Drug-Free Program for Prevention and Relief.* Palm Beach Gardens, FL: The Upledger Institute, Frog, Ltd., 1995.

Solomon, Seymour, M.D. and Fraccaro, Steven. *The Headache Book.* Mount Vernon, NY: Consumer Reports Books, 1991.

Wilson, Roberta. *Aromatherapy for Vibrant Health & Beauty.* Garden City Park, NY: Avery Publishing Group, 1994.

Zaba, J.N. and Johnson, R.A. "Literacy: The Vision, Learning and Volunteer Connection." *Journal of Behavioral Optometry* 3:5 (1992), 128-130.

Chapter 14

Rebound
Headaches

If head pain is a message from your body, then the steady, generalized throbs of a rebound headache are a shout. Caused by the roller-coaster effects that result from the consumption and withdrawal of stimulants, these chronic headaches are a sign that the medications or caffeinated substances you are ingesting are causing your body more trouble than good.

J enny, a 34-year-old mother of 3 was at the end of her rope. Over a period of 2 years, her condition had progressed from a monthly migraine to almost daily headaches. While her headaches were not as excruciating as her migraines, she realized that it was taking more and more prescription medication to get relief, and even then her headaches seemed to come back as soon as the medication wore off, forcing her to start the cycle all over again. Frightened by her growing reliance on drugs, Jenny tried to stop taking her medications, but her headache then came on so ferociously that she soon went back to taking drugs.

When she came to the Milne Medical Center she was desperate for a way out of this no-win situation. During her initial interview, we discovered that Jenny's chronic head pain was being caused by overreliance on pain medications, so we immediately started her on a detoxification program consisting of a 2-day raw juice fast (using a carrot, celery, apple, and spinach combination) and a single colon therapy treatment.

We then treated her with neural therapy, in which we injected 1% lidocaine and B12 into acupuncture points to relieve the muscle tension accompanying her headaches. Finally, for metabolic balancing and repair, we prescribed a special blend of herbs, which included feverfew, milk thistle, valerian root, hops, and the herbs magnetite and cinnabar (6 pills, 3 times a day). Within 10 days, Jenny's system was free of painkillers, and her rebound headaches went away.

What Is a Rebound Headache?

If head pain is a message from your body, then the steady, generalized throbs of a rebound headache are a shout. Caused by the roller-coaster effects that result from the consumption and withdrawal of stimulants, these chronic headaches are a sign that the caffeinated substances or medications you are ingesting are causing your body more trouble than good. Far from bringing you extra energy or relief, these substances are actually creating additional pain and fatigue.

Like many others in the same position, you may be unaware that your problem is related to the substances that you believe are helping you. As you continue to medicate your system, you worsen an already desperate state. Furthermore, even if you, like Jenny, recognize the connection, you may be so paralyzed by pain when you try to stop drinking coffee or taking medications that you feel you have little choice but to continue—since at least the pain these substances cause is both familiar and manageable.

You may be unaware that your rebound headaches are related to the substances that you believe are helping you. As you continue to medicate your system, you worsen an already desperate state.

According to a 1995 study published in *Modern Medicine*, 50 of 90 headaches evaluated involved the rebound effect. Other data shows that up to 80% of all headache sufferers unknowingly experience rebound headaches at one time or another. One factor that makes people so prone to rebound headaches is that pain unfolds gradually with steady use of a substance, subtly building in intensity and frequency until, a year or 2 into the cycle, the headache sufferer is in constant pain and does not know why.

Once the problem is pointed out, however, the reason becomes obvious: When you stop taking medication or a caffeine-containing substance, you develop a headache from the withdrawal; then, as soon as you take it again, the headache disappears, but the cycle simply begins anew.

In the past, such headaches were blamed on tension or stress. Generally, rebound headaches come on between 12 and 24 hours of the last intake of

Symptom Chart—Rebound Headaches

SYMPTOMS	HEADACHE TYPE	PAIN LOCATION
Description: throbbing, generalized headache; steady jolts of pain; can be similar to migraine **Other Symptoms:** anxiety, restlessness, nervousness, irritability, depression, fatigue, mood swings; nausea; intolerance for light, noise, or movement; tender scalp; stiff neck; flu-like feelings; insomnia **Duration:** 1 hour to all day **Frequency:** usually occurs in morning after waking; rarely or continuously	**REBOUND HEADACHE**	one or both sides of the head, often felt as total head pain; can begin at back of neck and spread to entire head or side of head

UNDERLYING CAUSES AND TRIGGERS	PRIMARY AND SECONDARY TREATMENTS	SELF-CARE TREATMENTS	WHERE IN THE BOOK PAGE #
Causes: overuse of narcotics, caffeine, or other stimulants; worsened by metabolic imbalances, structural disturbances, emotional/psychological factors **Triggers:** dietary and/or environmental sensitivity, hormonal imbalance, auto immune disturbances, lifestyle factors, structural disturbances, psychological stress	**Primary:** ■ acupuncture ■ bodywork ■ detoxification ■ environmental medicine ■ homeopathy ■ neural therapy ■ nutritional therapy **Secondary:** ■ Ayurvedic medicine ■ energy medicine ■ herbal medicine ■ magnetic field therapy ■ naturopathy ■ oxygen therapy ■ traditional Chinese medicine	■ affirmations ■ aromatherapy ■ biofeedback ■ breathing exercises ■ creative visualization ■ exercise ■ flower remedies ■ folk remedies ■ herbal supplements ■ ice and heat ■ journal writing ■ lifestyle changes ■ massage ■ meditation ■ nutritional therapy ■ relaxation techniques ■ support groups	Page 365

coffee or medication, beginning with a feeling of fullness in the head, peaking within 20 to 48 hours, and finally decreasing progressively over the next 5 to 6 days. These headaches can last anywhere from a day to a week and, because everyone has a different tolerance level, it is impossible to say what quantity of the drug or caffeinated substance will bring one on.

Although the overall symptoms of rebound headaches are generally the same, the mechanism of rebound headaches is more easily understood when they are separated into subcategories based on the specific prevailing trigger. The following are the most commonly recognized types of rebound headaches:

ANALGESIC REBOUND HEADACHE

Do you take aspirin or other painkillers (either over-the-counter or prescription) more than 2 or 3 times a week? If so, you may be suffering from analgesic rebound headaches in addition to the problem that put you on medications in the first place. Sometimes referred to as CDH, for "chronic daily headache," these headaches affect people who take medication so frequently that their bodies become addicted to it.

If habituated, whenever you miss a day (or even an hour) of the drug you are taking, the body demands, by creating a headache, to be returned to its medicated state. Ironically, over time, you actually end up medicating a headache caused by the very medication you are using to get rid of it.

Analgesic rebound headaches often strike those with migraine, cluster, tension, or other types of headaches because the drugs prescribed by conventional doctors to treat many headache conditions contain either caffeine or other highly habit-forming substances. Therefore, what may have started out as mild or infrequent pain later becomes amplified by medication withdrawal.

In the early 1980s, researchers examined 100 chronic headache sufferers taking analgesics frequently or daily and discovered that those who gave up analgesics and instead took sugar pills felt much more relief than those who took the antidepressant amitriptyline in addition to an analgesic. Another study conducted at approximately the same time discovered that 75 to 80% of chronic daily headache sufferers started taking drugs for periodic migraines as teenagers, the majority of whom took larger than recommended amounts of medication, and that the frequency of their attacks increased until, by the age 30, they had become daily.

The overuse of medications is more than just a headache hazard, as analgesic medications become even more toxic when taken in higher doses. Aspirin and ibuprofen, for example, can upset the stomach and cause peptic ulcers or intestinal bleeding; large amounts of acetaminophen can damage the liver; and all of them can cause kidney damage.

CAFFEINE WITHDRAWAL HEADACHE

Caffeine is one of the most widely used drugs in the world. Coffee, black tea, soft drinks (especially colas and Mountain Dew), diet pills, energy supplements, diuretics, cold medicine, pain relievers, and allergy tablets all contain caffeine, and, when taken in excess and then withdrawn, can lead to rebound headaches.

One study found that 52% of patients who were deprived of their regular intake of coffee came down with a headache, while 13% got such bad headaches that they broke from the study and resumed consumption of caffeine.

These headaches can come on whether or not you are intentionally giving up caffeine, especially in the morning, since your body may be reacting to a night without caffeine. If you do not give your body what it craves, the physiological dependence on caffeine disappears as soon as the headache subsides, but, if you satisfy the craving, the dependence returns the minute caffeine is reintroduced into the system.

While there is no strict rule as to how much caffeine is a threat, it is believed that any amount, from a couple of sips to 5 cups of coffee a day can bring on a rebound reaction, typically striking those who average 1 or 2 cups a day or the caffeine equivalent. However, if coffee is taken with over-the-counter pain relievers, many of which contain as much as 100 to 200 mg of caffeine per dose, caffeine consumption can skyrocket among even moderate coffee drinkers.

A rebound headache usually comes on within 12 to 24 hours of the last caffeine fix, and studies have shown that sufferers classify these headaches as painful, migraine-like headaches. In a study conducted by the Johns Hopkins University School of Medicine, 52% of the patients who were deprived of their regular intake of coffee came down with a headache, while another 13% got such bad headaches that they broke from the study and resumed consumption of caffeine.

Plant Products That Stimulate the Central Nervous System

Whether you are drinking caffeine as a beverage, eating it as chocolate, or taking it as a pill, these are the most common plant sources of caffeine:

COFFEA ARABICA—Caffeine is a component of its dried, ripened seeds, which we commonly call coffee beans; 1 cup of beverage contains 40 to 125 mg of caffeine, brewed coffee 75 to 125 mg, and instant approximately 40 mg per cup.

COLA NITIDA—Caffeine is the active ingredient of embryonic leaves of the cola plant; 1 cup contains approximately 40 to 50 mg of caffeine.

CAMELLIA SINENSIS—Although caffeine can come from many different types of tea leaves and leaf buds, this is the most common type of black tea; 1 cup contains 30 to 50 mg.

THEOBROMA CACAO—This is the roasted seed of the cacao tree, otherwise known as cocoa; 1 cup contains 10 to 50 mg of caffeine, or 1 to 15 mg per ounce of bar chocolate.

PAULLINIA CUPANA—Otherwise known as guarana, the crushed seeds of this plant are often used in herbal energy drinks and stimulants; usually contain up to 100 mg per serving.

As we mentioned in Chapter 3, What Causes Your Headache?, caffeine can also elevate blood pressure, exacerbate PMS symptoms, bring on stress, trigger food/allergy sensitivities, cause insomnia, and disrupt healthy digestion.

WEEKEND, HOLIDAY, OR TRAVEL HEADACHE

These headaches most commonly affect people who drink coffee, tea, or soda during the week but abstain, drink less, or change their consumption time on weekends, holidays, or when they travel. People who have high-pressure weekdays are most susceptible to this type of rebound headache because stress acts as an additional trigger.

POSTSURGERY HEADACHE

Recent studies are reshaping the way doctors view headaches that come on after surgery. Initially, it was believed that these headaches were somehow related to the administration of general anesthesia; however, evidence is beginning to demonstrate that postsurgical headaches are often related to caffeine withdrawal because, in abiding by the "no eating or drinking 12 to 24 hours before surgery" rule, patients miss their regular dose of caffeine.

Causes and Triggers of Rebound Headaches

Rebound headaches occur because the body is trying to balance itself again after getting thrown off course by caffeine and or addictive medications. This means returning to the painful state the body was in before the caffeine or drug entered the bloodstream and suppressed the headache mechanism. Although the headache mechanisms of painkillers and caffeine are almost identical (sometimes literally identical), it is easier to look separately at drugs and their influence on analgesic rebound headache and caffeine and its influence on caffeine withdrawal headache.

DRUGS—Few people who take painkillers realize that all it takes to change the pain threshold is 1 regular tablet. Taking any more has no effect on pain, but may have the side effect of a couple of cups of coffee. Most painkillers, whether prescription or OTC, are generally absorbed by the system within 20 minutes of consumption and will continue to elevate the pain threshold for 2 to 4 hours thereafter.

CAFFEINE—Caffeine is a nervous system stimulant which speeds up the heart, elevates blood pressure, acts as a diuretic, and inhibits relaxation. It is also a vasoconstrictor which is capable of calming painfully dilated blood vessels and hastening the absorption through the bloodstream of other medications. Interestingly enough, those who consume more caffeine experience a less pronounced rebound reaction. This is especially true when caffeine is taken throughout the day because this allows caffeine to stay in the bloodstream longer, reducing headache-inducing highs and lows.

Is Your Headache a Rebound Headache?

If you answer yes to 3 or more of the following questions, you are probably suffering from rebound headaches.

- Do you regularly drink caffeinated products or take OTC or prescription medications?
- Do your headaches occur daily or almost daily?
- Do you feel irritable, anxious, or depressed?
- Do you have trouble sleeping?
- Do you have occasional or periodic attacks of a more severe type of headache, such as migraines or clusters?
- Do headaches run in your family?

See Chapter 3, What Causes Your Headache?, for more detail on headache causes and triggers.

Diagnosing and Treating Underlying Causes

Once a rebound headache has been identified, the most important treatment is to eliminate the drug or caffeinated substance that is triggering it. This is not, however, always as easy as it sounds. For instance, you may be reluctant to give up your morning ritual of drinking a pot of coffee while reading the newspaper, or you may be afraid to stop taking your medications based on your previous attempts. Even when you manage to convince yourself to give withdrawal a try, you may again experience so much pain

Drugs That Cause Headaches

Although many conventional drugs on the market today list headaches as a possible side effect, the following drugs are known to trigger rebound headaches if overused, which means used more than 2 or 3 days a week:

- painkillers, such as aspirin, acetaminophen, or ibuprofen
- painkillers that contain caffeine in addition to aspirin or acetaminophen, such as Anacin and Excedrin
- nasal sprays and decongestants, such as Entex
- barbiturate-based drugs, such as Fiorinal, Fioricet, and Esgic
- narcotic-based drugs, such as Tylenol #3, Vicodin, Percocet, Tylox, Darvon, Demerol, Dilaudid, morphine, and cocaine
- calcium channel blockers, such as verapamil
- vasodilators, such as sumatriptan
- antidepressents, such as amitriptyline or fluoxetine
- ergotamine tartrate, such as Cafergot, Wigraine, Ergostat, Ergomar, Medihaler, DHE 45
- cold medicines and antibiotics
- appetite suppressants and diuretics
- oral contraceptives
- heart medications, such as nitroglycerin
- medications prescribed for hearing problems
- medications used to treat high blood pressure
- arthritis medications[1]

that you rethink your decision.

However, there are ways to make this withdrawal process more manageable, including:

- Don't quit medications or coffee abruptly. It is much better to gradually wean yourself from the substance over a few weeks; by not jarring your system any more than you have to, your headaches will be less intense.
- Depending upon how much you drink, try to cut back a half to a whole cup every couple of days, dilute it, and wait until your symptoms subside before cutting back more; apply the same technique to medications.
- As you taper off your coffee consumption, switch from the drip method to percolated or instant coffee because these have less caffeine, or mix a barley herbal roast such as Inka, Postum, or Caffix (available at health food stores) with your regular to bring down the caffeine content even further; dilute each cup with additional water; also remember to avoid chocolate and drink only caffeine-free sodas.
- Complement your willpower with alternative therapies, such as switching to a more energizing natural diet, or using homeopathy or flower essences to help you overcome your emotional addiction to caffeine or medications.

Rebound headaches normally disappear once the body rids itself of the side effects of the substance, but do not be surprised if it takes several weeks or a month before your rebound headaches fully subside. An alternative practitioner can help you through this painful withdrawal process.

A practitioner might put you on a detoxification program, prescribe nutritional supplements such as magnesium, calcium, and B complex or herbs such as ginseng and feverfew, use acupuncture to relieve your pain and quicken the detoxification process, or give you an intravenous infusion of vitamins and minerals if your symptoms persist. In all, as in treating other types of head pain, it is best to approach rebound headaches from a perspective of detoxification and repair.

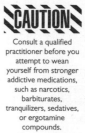

CAUTION

Consult a qualified practitioner before you attempt to wean yourself from stronger addictive medications, such as narcotics, barbiturates, tranquilizers, sedatives, or ergotamine compounds.

ALTERNATIVE TREATMENTS

METABOLIC/BIOENERGETIC/ BIOCHEMICAL-BASED THERAPIES

DETOXIFICATION THERAPY

Years of processing drugs can overburden and weaken the liver, leading to associated symptoms of fatigue and mental fog. Detoxification therapy, particularly when accompanied by supplements to support liver function, is an effective way to begin to eliminate medication dependencies. The following are the detoxification methods that are most helpful in the treatment of rebound headaches:

- Colon Therapy
- Enemas
- Fasting
- Herbal Bowel Cleansers
- Special Detoxification Diets

ENVIRONMENTAL MEDICINE

Mara, a 41-year-old nurse from La Mirada, California, started getting migraine headaches when she was a nursing student in India. She drank pot after pot of coffee to keep up her studies, and soon she found herself need-

Why Getting the Toxins Out of Your Body Can Help You Become Headache Free

If there is one thing that most alternative medicine doctors agree on, it is that too many toxins in the body produce illness. Increasingly, a toxic body is identified as the predisposing factor in a long list of acute and chronic degenerative illnesses. Signs and symptoms of the toxic body can include headaches, excess weight, bloating, intestinal gas, constipation, insomnia, nausea, bad breath, asthma, tension, depression, stress, allergies, and menstrual problems.

Where do all the toxins come from? They come from a polluted environment (air, water, and food), lack of water, overconsumption, a nutritionally inadequate diet, lack of exercise, accumulated stress, excess antibiotics, and chronic constipation and poor elimination.

"When was the last time you cleaned your liver, your heart, your lungs, or your body's sewage system?" asks nutritionist Lindsey Duncan, C.N., founder of Home

Nutrition Clinic in Santa Monica, California, and Nature's Secret, a specialty health products company in Boulder, Colorado. In case you've never "cleaned" your organs, Duncan has a practical solution in a series of inner detoxification products—Super Cleanse, Ultimate Fiber, and A.M./P.M. Ultimate Cleanse.

The latter is a 2-part vegetarian detoxification formula, containing 29 cleansing herbs, amino acids, antioxidants, digestive enzymes, vitamins and minerals, and 5 kinds of fiber. Signs that the program is working can include a flu-like feeling, a cold, runny nose, transient pimples, headaches, brain-fog, or fatigue. These symptoms will pass in 1-2 days, says Duncan.

"The goal is to stimulate, feed, and detoxify the complete internal body, not just the bowel," states Duncan. "My objective is to address

For information and products, contact: Nature's Secret, 4 Health, Inc., 5485 Conestoga Court, Boulder, CO 80301; tel: 303-546-6306; fax: 303-546-6416.

all 5 channels of elimination, as well as the vital organs and tissues." At the end of the program, a person should be having 2-3 bowel movements every day. Once the internal system is cleaned out, nutrient absorption is more efficient.

One user, who had endured chronic constipation and bloating for 25 years and only 2-3 bowel movements per week, lost 16 pounds on the program and started moving her bowels up to 3 times daily after being on the formula for 3 weeks.

Another user reported that persistent acne (38 years duration), fatigue, and depression cleared up by the time he completed the internal cleansing program. Another client with lifelong migraine headaches learned that her chronic constipation was a major factor; both were resolved as a result of taking A.M./P.M. Ultimate Cleanse.

ing coffee all the time or she became grouchy. Her headaches worsened until, eventually, she was getting a headache every day. She went to doctors and was given prescription medications which provided only temporary relief.

Then she consulted Devi S. Nambudripad, D.C., L.Ac., R.N., Ph.D., of Buena Park, California, who recognized that Mara's headaches were a rebound response to all of the coffee she consumed. Dr. Nambudripad performed allergy testing on Mara and discovered she reacted to caffeine, sugar, and her own hormones. After Dr. Nambudripad performed 4 Nambudripad Allergy Elimination Technique (NAET) treatments to detoxify Mara's body and desensitize her to these substances, Mara's headaches went away. Although she no longer has the craving for it, Mara is now able to drink 1 or 2 cups of coffee a day without a problem.

NUTRITIONAL THERAPY

Besides the recommendations presented under Nutritional Supplements in the Nutritional Therapy section of Chapter 16, it is important to note that studies have shown that drinking caffeinated beverages can increase the urinary excretion of calcium and magnesium for up to 3 hours after consumption. Since this effect is proportionate to the amount of coffee consumed, it is especially important that coffee drinkers supplement their diet with additional sources of calcium and magnesium. Vitamin C, which aids in detoxification and the absorption of calcium, and B-complex vitamins, especially B6, can help ease the withdrawal process.

OTHER METABOLIC/ BIOENERGETIC/ BIOCHEMICAL-BASED THERAPY

Depending on the symptoms and conditions of the rebound mechanism, the following therapies may be beneficial for treating rebound headaches:

- Acupuncture
- Ayurvedic Medicine
- Energy Medicine
- Homeopathy
- Light Therapy
- Magnetic Field Therapy
- Naturopathy

See Chapter 17, An A-Z of Alternative Medicine, for more information on treatment methods.

NAET. The Nambudripad Allergy Elimination Technique, is used for the detection and elimination of allergies. Developed by Devi Nambudripad, D.C., L.Ac., R.N., Ph.D., this simple and noninvasive method combines kinesiology's muscle response testing, acupuncture, and chiropractic to retrain the brain and nervous system. After identifying allergic substances through muscle response testing, the NAET practitioner uses acupuncture (or acupressure if the patient dislikes needles) to retrain the brain and nervous system to no longer respond allergically to a previously problem substance. For the treatment to become permanent, the patient must stay away from the offending substance for at least 24 hours, and sometimes more than one treatment is necessary.

- Oxygen Therapy
- Traditional Chinese Medicine

STRUCTURALLY ORIENTED THERAPIES

Depending on the underlying cause, the following therapies can also be useful for relieving the rebound headache mechanism generated by the reliance on medication or caffeinated stimulants:

- Bodywork
- Chiropractic
- Craniosacral Therapy
- Neural Therapy
- Osteopathy

PSYCHO/EMOTIONAL THERAPIES

Drug withdrawal, whether it be from medications or caffeine, can be a scary process. If you have been taking medications for a long time, suddenly stopping them can make you feel helpless. Likewise, abstaining from caffeine can expose a psychological dependence on the extra boost of enthusiasm provided by caffeine, leaving you feeling incapable of sustaining the energy needed to accomplish your daily tasks.

All of the psycho/emotional therapies covered in detail in Chapters 16 and 17 can help you adjust to the new feelings and anxieties that can arise when you change the way you live. Simple and subtle techniques such as aromatherapy or flower essence therapy can gently help you to integrate your feelings. Biofeedback and hypnotherapy can be used to self-medicate your pain responses and the stress that withdrawal may produce. Finally, psychotherapy can give you the opportunity to understand and work out your feelings.

FLOWER ESSENCE THERAPY

The following flower essences can be helpful for relieving emotional as well as physical dependence on drugs and caffeine.

ALLERGY/SENSITIVITY

Dill: for those who are overwhelmed, hypersensitive, or overstimulated; known to enhance digestive function

St. John's Wort: used for headache accompanied by light sensitivity or vulnerability to environmental stress, including allergies

Yarrow: strengthening; eases the sensitivity that occurs when the body tries to deal with input overload, either from the environment or through digestion

STRESS AND TENSION

Dandelion: for stress and tension held in the muscles of the body; brings about dynamic, effortless energy

Impatiens: for people who are constantly rushing, impatient, intolerant, tense; creates acceptance and patience for the flow of life

Lavender: releases high-strung, nervous tension, allows full relaxation in order to receive the benefits of the healing work

Mimulus: for those who are frequently in fear of their next headache attack

Nicotiana: for those who cope with tension by using addictive substances, especially but not exclusively tobacco

GENERAL HEADACHE

Lavender: good overall headache remedy, to dispel nervousness and overstimulation, which deplete the physical body

Five Flower Remedy (Rescue Remedy): helps in coping with stress in general; contains cherry plum, clematis, impatiens, rock rose, star of Bethlehem

OTHER PSYCHO/EMOTIONAL THERAPIES

The following therapies can be helpful for alleviating the symptoms associated with rebound headaches:

- Biofeedback
- Hypnotherapy
- Psychotherapy

See Chapter 16, An A-Z of Self Care Options, for more information on self-treatment methods.

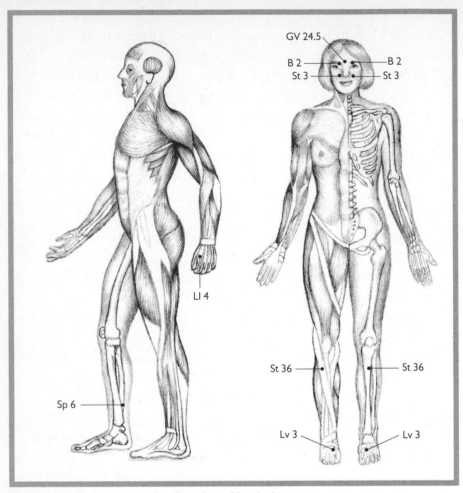

Figure 14.1—Acupressure points for rebound headaches.

SELF-CARE OPTIONS

ACUPRESSURE

Stimulating the following acupressure points can help to relieve and prevent of rebound headaches, by aiding in restoring energy flow through your body and speeding up the elimination of toxins. See the Acupressure section of Chapter 16, for information on applications.

- Bladder 2 (B 2)
- *Yin Tang* point (GV 24.5)
- Stomach 3 (St 3)

- Stomach 36 (St 36)
- Liver 3 (Lv 3)
- Large Intestine 4 (LI 4)
- Spleen 6 (Sp 6)

AROMATHERAPY
The following oil blends can help to relieve and prevent the occurrence of rebound headaches:

According to a 1995 study published in Modern Medicine, 50 of 90 headaches evaluated involved the rebound effect. Other data shows that up to 80% of all headache sufferers unknowingly experience rebound headaches at one time or another.

INHALATION
For aroma to go: Put 2 to 3 drops of melissa, peppermint, and lavender oils on a handkerchief or cloth and inhale throughout the day for prevention.

MASSAGE
Temple rub: Combine lavender (a sedative) and peppermint (a stimulant) oils and rub the mixture on your temples for pain relief.

Good oils for vascular-type headaches: Anise, basil, chamomile, coriander, eucalyptus, lavender, lemon, marjoram, melissa, onion, peppermint oils, and rosemary

BATHS
Aroma soak: For relief of a headache in progress, fill a bath with warm to hot water; add eucalyptus, wintergreen, or peppermint oils, and soak 20 to 30 minutes.

COMPRESSES AND STEAMS
Lavender and peppermint compress for vascular headache: At first sign of headache, make 2 compresses, a lavender and peppermint compress for the forehead and a hot marjoram (a vasodilator, stretches blood vessels) for the back of the neck; this combination provides relaxing, stimulating, and vasodilating effects.

Aromatherapy steam: Boil 2 pints water and pour into a large bowl; add 1 drop melissa, 2 drops peppermint, and 2 drops lavender oils.

Put your head over the bowl and cover your head and the bowl with a large towel. Inhale deeply through your nose for about 10 minutes.

DIETARY CHANGES

While it may be difficult to give up caffeine, this may be the only way to end the cycle of headaches that are leaving you in chronic pain. Fortunately, the switch to caffeine-free drinking need not deprive you of the flavors and tastes you have grown to love.

For example, health food stores carry natural and caffeine-free alternatives to coffee: dark roast herbal teas, such as those made with roasted barley, roasted chicory root, roasted carob and/or roasted dandelion, and instant beverages like Caffix.

While they do not taste like coffee, many other herbal teas (especially those containing the herbs listed in the herbal section following) can speed up your detox and repair process, helping you to feel better faster. In any event, try to avoid substituting your coffee intake with "decaffeinated" coffee beverages unless they are organic, since the harsh chemicals that are used to process out the caffeine tend to linger.

EXERCISES

CIRCULATING ENERGY—The following is a simple exercise that can be done by almost everyone, regardless of age or state of health, to restore the natural flow of energy throughout the body.

Tracing the energy pathways to circulate the life force: Making sure to breath in a smooth and natural rhythm, rub your hands together as you would if you were warming them over a fire. Once you can feel the heat in your palms, stroke them across your cheeks, eyes, and forehead as if you are washing your face. Continue to move your hands up over the top and sides of your head, down the back of your neck, and along your upper back to your shoulder joint.

Next, move your palms underneath your arms and down the sides of your body to your lower rib cage and, from here, move your palms around to the back and down your buttocks and legs and out the sides of your feet. Finally, trace up the inside of your feet and legs, to the front-side of the torso and back to your face again. This ends the first round. Repeat.

FOLK REMEDIES

The following remedies have been used to relieve rebound headaches.

Vinegar compresses: Soak a washcloth with vinegar and place it in the refrigerator until it is sufficiently chilled. Then apply the compress to your forehead, temples, and neck. You can also inhale vinegar for even faster relief. Boil equal parts vinegar and water, pour mixture into a bowl, then place a towel over the bowl and your head as you inhale the rising steam.

Warm salt pack: To make a salt pack, roast 1 cup of salt in a dry frying pan until salt is warm to the touch, being careful that it does not overheat. Pour salt into a thin dish towel, fold it so you can apply it to your head, and rub the painful areas rather than keeping the pack in one place.

Herbal compress: Boil 3 cups water and pour over 1 tablespoon. lavender and 1 tablespoon chamomile; steep for 20 minutes. Soak a soft cloth in the mixture, wring it out, and apply to the back of neck or forehead. Cold herbal compresses are also effective.

Epsom salt bath: Pour 2 to 4 cups of Epsom salts into the bathtub and fill with warm water. Soak for 15 to 30 minutes. Epsom salts are good for removing toxins from your system.

Drink a headache tonic: Fill a large pot of water and mix in small pieces of fresh ginger root, coriander seeds, diced garlic, and a little honey to taste. Boil off half the liquid and drink what is left periodically throughout the day.

Try 12 almonds: Because they contain the natural aspirin salicin, almonds can offer headache relief. This remedy is used in areas of North Africa and Asia where almond trees are common.

Li Shou (arm swinging): This Chinese technique uses motion to relieve headaches by creating a relaxed, meditative state and is taught to school children to relieve stress. Swing your arms back and forth until the blood shifts from your head to your hands, reducing your swollen blood vessels. Next, use your warmed hands to stroke your face, using a circular motion, paying particular attention to the area around your eyes. Repeat the exercise several times.

Wear a headband: In Korea, people tie cloths snugly around their heads, just above the eyebrows. This remedy has been somewhat validated by Western science: according to one study, wearing snug elastic headbands helped about a quarter of participants obtain relief of 50% or more, possibly because the headband may restrict blood flow and prevent the dilation of blood vessels.

Wrap rubberbands around your fingers: Take 10 rubberbands and wrap them around each of your fingers at the first joint, the one closest to your fingernail. Put them on tight, and although they may turn your fingers purplish and hurt a bit, leave them on for no more than 9 minutes to find that your headache has disappeared.

HERBAL SUPPLEMENTS

Try herbal remedies for stress, anxiety, insomnia, and tension instead of sleeping pills or antianxiety medications. Similarly, if caffeine-free living leaves you feeling like you need an extra energy boost, try taking herbs for brain function instead. Ginseng is especially helpful because it brings about both mental and physical stimulation, and helps your body to assimilate vitamins and minerals—unlike caffeine, which actually robs your body of these nutrients. The following herbs may be beneficial in treating your headache:

Brain function: *Ginkgo*, ginseng, rosemary

Constipation/toxicity: dandelion, milk thistle, nettle, senna, vervain, wood betony

General headache: angelica, feverfew, meadowsweet, willow bark

Stress, anxiety, insomnia, and tension: feverfew, lavender, passion flower, pennyroyal, peppermint, rosehips, skullcap, St. John's wort, valerian, vervain

Vascular imbalances: balm, basil, cayenne, elder, feverfew, garlic, ginger, *Ginkgo*, goldenrod, Jamaican dogwood, lavender, marjoram, peppermint, rosemary, rue, thyme, sage, willow bark, wormwood

REFLEXOLOGY

Similar to acupressure, stimulating the following foot and hand reflexology areas provides proven relief and prevention of rebound headaches, by restoring energy flow through your body, speeding up the elimination of toxins, and facilitating your body's repair process. See the Reflexology section of Chapter 16, for instructions on how to stimulate the areas.

BRAIN: all headaches, circulation, and overall body function

HEAD: all headaches, stress, shoulder and neck tension

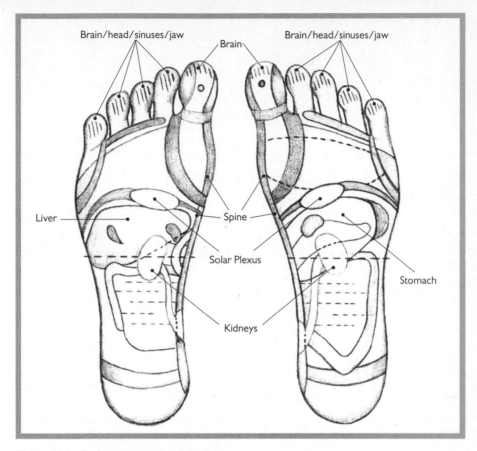

Figure 14.2—Reflexology areas of the feet.

SPINE: all headaches, trauma, stress, tension, digestion
SOLAR PLEXUS: stress, anxiety, digestion
STOMACH: digestion, sensitivity/allergy, migraine
KIDNEY: vascular, allergy/sensitivity, toxicity, migraine
LIVER: digestion, circulation, toxicity

OTHER SELF-CARE OPTIONS

The following self-care techniques can also be helpful for rebound headaches:

- Affirmations/Autosuggestions
- Breathing Exercises
- Creative Visualization
- Exercise

- Ice and Heat
- Lifestyle Changes
- Meditation
- Relaxation Exercises
- Support Groups

RECOMMENDED READING

Carper, Jean. *Food—Your Miracle Medicine*. New York: HarperCollins Publishers, 1993.

Diamond, Seymour, M.D. and Still, Bill and Cynthia. *The Hormone Headache*. New York: Macmillan, 1995.

National Headache Foundation Fact Sheet. Chicago: National Headache Foundation, October 1994.

Robbins, Lawrence, M.D. and Land, Susan. *Headache Help*. New York: Houghton Mifflin Company, 1995.

Stromfeld, Jan and Weil, Anita. *Free Yourself from Headaches: The Natural Drug-Free Program for Prevention and Relief*. Palm Beach Gardens, FL: The Upledger Institute, Frog, Ltd., 1995.

Rapoport, Alan M., M.D. and Sheftell, Fred D., M.D. *Headache Relief*. New York: Simon & Schuster, 1990.

Rapoport, Alan M., M.D. and Sheftell, Fred D., M.D. *Headache Relief for Women*. New York: Little, Brown and Company, 1995.

Solomon, Seymour, M.D. and Fraccaro, Steven. *The Headache Book*. Mount Vernon, NY: Consumer Reports Books, 1991.

Tyler, Varro E., Ph.D., Sc.D. *Herbs of Choice: The Therapeutic Use of Phytomedicinals*. New York: Pharmaceutical Products Press, 1994.

Chapter 15

Exertion Headaches

Exertion headaches, which may be caused by the increased energy demands of exercise, sex, or coughing, are usually harmless, short-lived, and only rarely the sign of a more serious condition. They are equally common in men as in women, typically occur in those over the age of 40, and generally last about 20 minutes.

"Not tonight dear" was once a joke my husband and I shared. Then his headaches started, and it was no longer a laughing matter. After a while, his pain became so tied into our lovemaking that we didn't know what else to do but to stop sleeping in the same bed. He wasn't the only one who suffered.

— Mary, a frustrated wife

What Is an Exertion Headache?

Although their sudden appearance and violent disposition make these headaches appear quite frightening, exertion headaches are usually harmless and only rarely the sign of a more serious condition. Generally, these headaches fall into one of 3 subcategories:

EXERCISE HEADACHE

Exercise-induced headaches tend to hit people 40 and older who have just begun an exercise program for the first time or who are out of shape and rarely push their bodies. Equally common in men and women, these headaches generally come on during or after strenuous exercise such as running or aerobics, sports in which the head is hit, such as soccer or diving, and activities that incorporate heavy lifting, such as weight training and moving furniture. These headaches can last from a few minutes to all day, but most commonly last 15 to 20 minutes.

SEXUAL HEADACHE

Also called benign orgasmic cephalgia or benign coital headaches, sexual headaches are triggered by the exertion of lovemaking or masturbation. More common in men than women, these headaches are marked by sudden, moderate to severe head pain that peaks just moments before or during orgasm, although they have been known to come on any time from the moment sex is considered to hours after the sexual act is completed. The pain, which may be described as someone clobbering you on the back of the head with a baseball bat, generally subsides within moments but sometimes can last hours.

COUGHING HEADACHE

This type of exertion headache refers to brief but intense head pain that comes on either during or after passive exertion, such as sneezing, coughing, crying, laughing, or straining one's bowels. A rare type of headache that predominately hits middle-aged men, coughing headaches tend to hurt all over or in the back of the head, although sometimes they can occur on one side of the head. Generally, they go away after a few dramatic minutes and remain dormant until the body's next physical outburst; however, an unfortunate few have physical conditions that keep them in a steady state of passive excrtion and thus a constant headache.

Although not always chronic, exertion headaches tend to be repetitive, the number of times they strike varying from person to person. In one study of sex headaches, more than 50% of the participants responded that they got headaches 2 out of 3 times they had sex, 15% reported they got headaches 1 in 5 times, while for the remaining 35% it was every time they had sex.[1] On a more positive note, research suggests that approximately half of those who experience exertion headaches—sexual or otherwise—on a regular basis report that these headaches subside on their own after about 6 months.

CAUTION

Because exertion headaches are associated with elevated blood pressure, if you experience them frequently, it is a good idea to visit a doctor to rule out neurological problems, such as meningitis, brain hemorrhages, or strokes, that can be induced by increased pressure in the head.

Causes and Triggers of Exertion Headaches

People with preexisting headache conditions, such as migraines, allergy/sensitivity, cluster, or mixed headaches (a combination of migraine and tension) seem more prone to exertion headaches. Considering the rapid increase in muscular and vascular activity that occurs in both the muscles and head during physical exertion, it makes sense that people already under muscular and vascular stress are at a higher risk.

This suggests that, although in their own category with a particular set of recognizable symptoms, exertion headaches are not different from other

Symptom Chart—Exertion Headaches

SYMPTOMS	HEADACHE TYPE	PAIN LOCATION
Description: sharp, throbbing headache with either generalized or localized pain **Duration:** brief to 5 minutes, but can last 15 minutes to all day **Frequency:** during or following physical or passive exertion	**EXERTION HEADACHE**	anywhere on or all over head

UNDERLYING CAUSES AND TRIGGERS	PRIMARY AND SECONDARY TREATMENTS	SELF-CARE TREATMENTS	WHERE IN THE BOOK PAGE #
Causes: lactic acid accumulation, worsened by metabolic imbalances, structural disturbances, emotional/psychological factors **Triggers:** structural disturbances, running, aerobics, sexual intercourse, sneezing, coughing, moving bowels, psychological stress	**Primary:** ■ acupuncture ■ detoxification ■ environmental medicine ■ homeopathy ■ naturopathy ■ neural therapy ■ nutritional therapy ■ traditional Chinese medicine **Secondary:** ■ bodywork ■ chiropractic ■ craniosacral therapy ■ energy medicine ■ herbal medicine ■ osteopathy ■ oxygen therapy	■ affirmations ■ aromatherapy ■ biofeedback ■ breathing exercises ■ creative visualization ■ exercise ■ flower remedies ■ folk remedies ■ herbal supplements ■ ice and heat ■ journal writing ■ lifestyle changes ■ massage ■ meditation ■ nutritional therapy ■ relaxation techniques ■ support groups	Page 387

headaches in that they are a symptom of an underlying condition that pre-disposes the body to head pain. Although they can be related to any of the conditions listed in Chapter 3, What Causes Your Headache?, exertion headaches are believed to be most closely related to the following causes:

Valsalva maneuver—Any time you exert yourself physically, whether in lifting a friend's piano or coughing uncontrollably, your body goes through a reactive process called the valsalva maneuver, in which you automatically hold your breath and bear down, as if preparing for a great weight to fall into your hands. This action blocks the even flow of energy, backing up blood and rushing pressure into your head, thereby stretching headache-causing blood vessels.

> *Although in their own category, with a particular set of recognizable symptoms, exertion headaches are not different from other headaches in that they are a symptom of an underlying condition that predisposes the body to head pain.*

Vascular changes—Linked to migraines (sometimes even called a secondary migraine disorder) and other vascular-type headaches, these headaches can be caused or worsened by metabolic conditions, especially circulation problems, hormonal imbalances (see below), digestive disorders, and other conditions that disrupt the central nervous system and bring about the dilation and contraction of blood vessels in the head, both of which can lead to headaches.

Hormonal changes—The bursts of energy needed to sustain exertion are closely related to the stress hormone adrenalin. When adrenalin is released into your bloodstream during physical activity, your heart speeds up, your pulse quickens, and your blood vessels constrict, elevating your blood pressure and tightening your muscles. When these changes are coupled with a preexisting metabolic, structural, or emotional imbalance, the impact of adrenalin is amplified, upsetting the delicate balance of your system. This effect is especially potent in the case of emotional stress, which prompts a double dose of adrenalin.

Structural abnormality—Some researchers suggest that congenital anatomical dysfunctions, structural misalignments, and/or postural problems may be at the root of exertion headaches because these conditions can disrupt the normal functioning of the central nervous system and the overall musculoskeletal system.

Muscle tension—Headaches that occur during physical exertion, whether during lovemaking, lifting heavy boxes, or sneezing uncontrollably, are marked by intense muscle contractions throughout the body. These contractions are especially pronounced around the head, neck, and shoulders, muscles which are often already strained and overburdened. Existing muscle tensions may also be aggravated by the buildup and release of lactic acid in the muscles.

Unexpressed or hidden emotions— While any kind of psychological stress can trigger or worsen a headache, the emotional connection appears to be particularly pronounced in those with sexual headaches, especially when headaches occur before or during sex. Despite the so-called sexual revolution, most people still have unresolved issues around sex; for some people, intercourse and masturbation can bring up feelings of shame and guilt, unwanted feelings that are only reinforced by a headache. Others may be nervous about their performance, unsure about their partner, or preoccupied by secret fantasies or past infidelities. In some cases, simply thinking of sex or preparing to lie down is enough to trigger a painful headache.

Additional Triggers of Exertion Headaches

- Poor cardiovascular fitness: Being overweight, or out of shape means that your body has to work twice as hard.
- Hyperventilation or panting breaths change the oxygen/carbon dioxide balance in your blood.
- Abrupt or sudden movements to which your body is unaccustomed can throw your alignment out of balance and put more pressure on already tired muscles.
- Exerting yourself too suddenly or ending exertion too abruptly does not allow your body enough time to warm up and cool down.
- Ignoring early warning signs and not resting when your body starts to become fatigued can also trigger a headache.

Diagnosing and Treating Underlying Causes

Since about 5% of ruptured blood vessels are brought on by exertion, any practitioner you see will first want to screen you with a series of tests to ensure you are not suffering from a more serious condition. Once organic causes are ruled out, the practitioner will then go about treating you in much the same way as you would be treated for a tension or a migraine headache:

See Chapter 3, What Causes Your Headache?, for more detail on headache causes and triggers.

identifying metabolic, structural, and emotional causes and triggers; removing them; and repairing your body.

ALTERNATIVE TREATMENTS

Because they are similar in nature, exertion headaches respond to many of the same treatments and techniques that are helpful for migraine or tension headaches.

METABOLIC/BIOENERGETIC/
BIOCHEMICAL-BASED THERAPIES
HOMEOPATHY

The following homeopathic remedies are a sampling of those that can be useful for exertion headaches. However, homeopathic remedies work best when prescribed by a qualified practitioner; when self-administered, these remedies should be taken only in doses of 6X or lower.

Circulatory Disorders—*Belladonna* (sudden and violent, throbbing pain, restlessness, congestion, red-flushed face); *Ferrum metallicum* (hammering, throbbing pain, red face, cold feet, usually associated with anemia); *Glonoinum* (throbbing, intolerance to heat and motion); *Gelsemium* (visual disturbances, eyeball pain, mental difficulties); *Sanguinaria canadensis* (throbbing, burning, shooting pain accompanied by redness in the cheeks, also migraine-like pain associated with menses); *Serotoninum* (sudden headaches accompanied by throbbing and sensations of heat), *Sulphur* (vascular-type headaches); *Veratrum viride* (headache with hypertension, red face, bloodshot eyes, heavy head)

Hormonal Imbalances—*Actae racemosa* (headaches proportionate to menses); *Cyclamen* (headaches associated with menstruation, accompanied by vertigo, and aggravated by fresh air); *Lachesis mutus* (premenstrual headaches); *Melilotus* (pain improved at onset of menstrual bleeding); *Pulsatilla* (throbbing headaches in women with light and less frequent periods); *Sepia* (nervous and uterine headaches)

Structural Misalignments and Trauma—*Actae racemosa, Arnica montana* (bruise-like ache, worsened by movement, associated with physical exhaustion or trauma); *Byronia, Calcarea carbonica* (physical overexertion); *Colocynthis, Ranunculus bulbosus* (head pain associated with postural problems, pains in the back and side); *Rhus toxicodendron* (physical overexertion); *Silicea* (pain in the nape of the neck associated with nervous exhaustion)

Stress, Tension, and Anxiety—*Anacardium orientale* (irritability, moodiness, intellectual overwork); *Argentium nitricum* (mental exertion); *Chamomilla, Gelsemium* (vague but distressing tension-type pain, associated with anxiety and visual disturbances, intensified with noise and movement); *Hura Braziliensis* (depression, suicidal thoughts, delusions, fear); *Ignatia* (hypersensitivity, hysterical outbursts, heavy, pressurized pain, sometimes nausea and dizziness); *Kali phosphoricum* (intellectual overwork, overall physical fatigue); *Lachesis, Natrum muriaticum* (developing after intense mental work, for those who are ambitious, driving and eager to achieve); *Phosphoricum acidum* (fatigue, nervous exhaustion, indifference to life); *Silicea* (pain in the nape of the neck associated with nervous exhaustion); *Staphysagria, Zincum metallicum* (nervous and mental fatigue, aggravated by intellectual effort)

For Headaches without Symptoms Characteristic of a Particular Remedy—*Aconitum nappellus* (taken at onset of any acute headache); *Apis mellifica* (migraines accompanied by swelling); *Secale cornutum* (migraines); *Serotoninum* (congestive headaches, particularly with unstable blood pressure)

OTHER METABOLIC/ BIOENERGETIC/ BIOCHEMICAL-BASED THERAPIES

The following therapies, depending upon the underlying mechanism, can also be beneficial for treating and preventing chronic exertion headaches:

- Acupuncture
- Ayurvedic Medicine
- Detoxification Therapy
- Energy Medicine

- Environmental Medicine
- Light Therapy
- Magnetic Field Therapy
- Naturopathic Medicine
- Nutritional Therapy
- Oxygen Therapy
- Traditional Chinese Medicine

STRUCTURALLY ORIENTED THERAPIES

Depending upon the underlying cause, the following therapies can be useful in the treatment of exertion headaches:
- Alphabiotics
- Bodywork
- Chiropractic
- Craniosacral Therapy
- Neural Therapy
- Osteopathy

PSYCHO/EMOTIONAL THERAPIES

Because exertion headaches, particularly sex headaches, often have an underlying emotional cause, all of the following therapies can be useful.

BIOFEEDBACK

Biofeedback is especially good for sex headaches because it can help you become more aware of the way you are holding your body and thus help you to relax when you sense yourself tightening. Both thermal and electromyogram (EMG) biofeedback techniques can be effective.

FLOWER ESSENCE THERAPY

Flower essences can alleviate the emotional strain that sometimes accompanies sex headaches. They work on subtle levels, so can actually bring about a change that allows you to see and resolve worries, anxieties, and guilts—even if you were not consciously aware of what they were about. Rescue Remedy, Crab Apple and Fuschia are particularly helpful for these headaches.

For more information about thermal and EMG biofeedback, see Chapter 17, An A-Z of Alternative Medicine, Biofeedback.

Allergy/Sensitivity—Crab Apple, Dill, Yarrow

Stress and Tension—Dandelion, Fuschia, Impatiens, Five

Flower Remedy (Rescue Remedy; contains Cherry Plum, Clematis, Impatiens, Rock Rose, Star of Bethlehem)
General Headache—Lavender

PSYCHOTHERAPY

Sex headaches can be related to a difficulty within a relationship. If this is the case, couples counseling or marital therapy may be an effective way to air feelings and resolve issues which may be creating a barrier that manifests itself physically as a headache. Therapy also provides a safe place to discuss fantasies and other sexual issues that you may feel uncomfortable discussing with friends and family members.

SELF-CARE OPTIONS
AROMATHERAPY

If you have sex headaches, put on some relaxing music and ask your partner to give you a massage using a relaxing oil such as lavender, or try a muscle relaxant bath before initiating sexual activity. You can also fill the room with an oil that comforts you. If you get a headache after exertion of any kind, apply compresses or take an aroma or muscle relaxant bath.

INHALATION

Wafting Relief: Fill aroma lamp, bowl, or diffuser with water and mix in 4 drops melissa and 2 drops peppermint or Roman chamomile oil.

MASSAGE

Temple rub: Combine lavender (a sedative) and peppermint (a stimulant) oils and rub the mixture on your temples for pain relief.

BATHS

Muscle relaxant bath: Fill the bath with warm water and add 3 drops chamomile, 3 drops lavender, 2 drops marjoram, 2 drops thyme, and 1 drop coriander oils.

See Chapter 16, An A-Z of Self-Care Options, for more information on self-treatment methods.

COMPRESSES AND STEAMS

Cold compress relief: Mix 3 drops rose, 1 drop melissa, and 1 drop lavender oils in 2 pints water. Stir thoroughly and place a towel or washcloth in the water. Let it soak for 5 minutes, then wring to remove excess water. Lie back and put the compress on the painful area. Rest. Change the compress as soon as it reaches room temperature.

Lavender and peppermint compress for vascular headache: At the first sign of headache, make 2 compresses, a lavender and peppermint compress for the forehead, and a hot marjoram (a vasodilator, stretches blood vessels) for the back of the neck; this mixture provides a combination of relaxing, stimulating, and vasodilating effects.

BREATHING EXERCISES

Breathing is essential to any physical activity, and the quality of your breath affects your ability to sustain periods of exertion. Never hold your breath or pant while exerting yourself; instead, breath as smoothly as possible, pulling the air deep into your diaphragm and fully releasing each breath before you take another.

EXERCISE

Before initiating any physical activity, be sure to warm up properly by stretching your arms, legs, shoulders, and neck completely. This helps to loosen your muscles and prepare them for the more demanding requirements of exertion. Also, give your body ample time to adjust by allowing your heartbeat to rise slowly, then building to a steady accelerated rhythm, and finally tapering off your effort gradually. If you feel inklings of a headache during any of these stages, stop immediately.

HERBAL SUPPLEMENTS

Depending on the severity of the headache, herbal medicine can be used either alone or as an adjunct to other therapies to relieve symptoms and strengthen the body. Although other herbs are also used to deal with associated symptoms and underlying or preexisting conditions, the following herbs can be particularly effective in cases of exertion headaches:

Circulation—feverfew, garlic, rosemary

General headache—angelica, feverfew, meadowsweet, willow bark

Hormonal/reproductive problems—black cohosh, black haw, cayenne, chasteberry, cramp bark, lavender, passion flower, skullcap, St. John's wort, wild yam

Musculoskeletal pain and spasms—cayenne, chamomile, elder, meadowsweet, nettles, *qiyelian*, turmeric, valerian, vervain, willow bark

Stress, anxiety, insomnia, and tension—feverfew, lavender, passion flower, pennyroyal, peppermint, rosehips, skullcap, St. John's wort, valerian, vervain

Vascular imbalances—balm, basil, cayenne, elder, feverfew, garlic, ginger, *Ginkgo*, goldenrod, Jamaican dogwood, lavender, marjoram, peppermint, rosemary, rue, thyme, sage, willow bark, wormwood

OTHER SELF-CARE OPTIONS

The following self-help techniques are also effective in the relief and prevention of exertion headaches:

See Chapter 17, An A-Z of Alternative Medicine, Herbal Medicine, for specific dosages and more information on how to use medicinal herbs. See Chapter 16, An A-Z of Self-Care Options, for details on folk remedies and other self-care therapies.

- Affirmations/Autosuggestions
- Creative Visualization
- Folk Remedies (especially vinegar and/or herbal compresses)
- Ice and Heat
- Lifestyle Changes
- Massage
- Meditation
- Nutritional Therapy/Dietary Changes
- Relaxation Exercises
- Support Groups

RECOMMENDED READING

Alternative Medicine: The Definitive Guide. Compiled by the Burton Goldberg Group. Tiburon, CA: Future Medicine Publishing, 1994.

Benson, Paul, D.O. "Biofeedback and Stress Management." *Osteopathic Annals* 12 (August 1984), 20-26.

Clark, Linda, M.A. *A Handbook of Natural Remedies for Common Ailments*. Greenwich, CT: The Devin-Adair Company, 1976.

Diamond, Seymour, M.D., and Still, Bill and Cynthia. *The Hormone Headache*. New York: Macmillan, 1995.

Faber, William J., D.O. *Pain, Pain Go Away*. San Jose, CA: ISHI Press International, 1990.

Ford, Norman D. *Eighteen Natural Ways to Beat a Headache*. New Canaan, CT: Keats Publishing, Inc., 1990.

Herzberg, Eileen. *Migraine: A Comprehensive Guide to Gentle, Safe & Effective Treatment*. Rockport, MA: Element, Inc., 1994.

Igram, Cass, M.D. *Who Needs Headaches?* Cedar Rapids, IA: Literary Visions Publishing, 1991.

Keller, Erich. *The Complete Home Guide to Aromatherapy*. Tiburon, CA: H.J. Kramer, Inc., 1991.

Lilienthal, Samuel, M.D. *Homeopathic Therapeutics*. New Delhi: Jain Publishing Co., 1996.

Lipton, Richard B., M.D. and Stewart, Walter F., M.P.H., Ph.D. "Migraine in the United States: A Review of Epidemiology and Health Care Use." *Neurology* 43 Suppl 3 (1993), S6-S10.

National Headache Foundation Fact Sheet. Chicago: National Headache Foundation, October 1994.

Natural Health Secrets from around the World. Boca Raton, FL: Shot Tower Books, 1996.

Rapoport, Alan M., M.D. and Sheftell, Fred D., M.D. *Headache Relief*. New York: Simon & Schuster, 1990.

Rapoport, Alan M., M.D. and Sheftell, Fred D., M.D. *Headache Relief for Women*. New York: Little, Brown and Company, 1995.

Robbins, Lawrence, M.D. and Lang, Susan, *Headache Help*. New York: Houghton Mifflin Company, 1995.

Solomon, Seymour, M.D. and Fraccaro, Steven. *The Headache Book*. Mount Vernon, NY: Consumer Reports Books, 1991.

Stang, P.E. and Osterhaus, J.T. "Impact of Migraine in the United States: Data from the National Health Interview Survey." *Headache* 33 (1993): 29-35.

Stromfeld, Jan and Weil, Anita. *Free Yourself from Headaches: The Natural Drug-Free Program for Prevention and Relief*. Palm Beach Gardens, FL: The Upledger Institute, Frog, Ltd., 1995.

Wilson, Roberta. *Aromatherapy for Vibrant Health & Beauty*. Garden City Park, NY: Avery Publishing Group, 1994.

Part Three

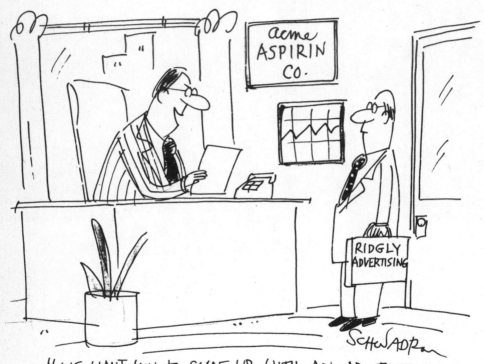

"WE WANT YOU TO COME UP WITH AN AD THAT WILL GIVE PEOPLE HEADACHES, RIDGLY."

Chapter 16

An A-Z of Self-Care Options

Once you've found the appropriate therapy for your type of headache, prevention and self-care are your keys to lifelong freedom from headaches. In this A-Z of self-help options, you may choose from many practical approaches, including aromatherapy, nutritional therapy, aerobics and stretching exercises, herbs, relaxation techniques, acupressure, and reflexology.

"**H**ealing ... is not a science, but the intuitive art of wooing nature," wrote poet W. H. Auden. This is particularly true when caring for yourself, which involves having a say in your body's processes and taking responsibility for your health. Often, this is easier said than done. The purpose of this chapter is to provide you with practical techniques to help you fulfill your commitment to health.

Prevention is the key to pain-free living, and prevention only happens when you make your health a priority. In addition to the techniques provided here, there are hundreds of healthy things you can do to feel good, ranging from laughing with your children, sleeping under the stars, and hiking in the woods to paying attention to your breathing, keeping your shoulders back when you stand, and expressing your emotions when they arise. Once you get started on the path of healing yourself, it becomes difficult to stop. And once your headaches are gone, you can continue the methods you have learned here or developed on your own to keep your headaches away for good.

ACUPRESSURE

Acupressure is an easy technique to practice on yourself. Once you learn a few simple acupoints you can give yourself immediate relief no matter where you are when your headache strikes. Always begin acupressure with a series of deep, relaxing breaths, because breathing loosens you up and makes you more receptive to the technique; you might also want to gently rub your scalp and neck to get rid of stiffness.

Finger pressure is applied with the flat parts of your fingers, not the tips, and should always be steady and firm, with about 7 pounds of force. Apply pressure for 20 seconds to 1 minute unless otherwise instructed; press the other side if applicable. Keep in mind that it is not necessary to use all of these points; instead pick 1 or 2 that seem most suited to your overall symptoms.

Bladder 2 (B 2)—Called "drilling bamboo" or "bamboo gathering," these 2 points are located in the upper hollows of the eye socket, where the eyebrow meets the bridge of the nose. Good for frontal headache, vascular, tension, eyestrain, sinus conditions.

Bladder 60 (B 60)—Called "high mountains," it is in the hollow behind the bony bump of the ankle. Good for pain at the back of the head, neck, or base of the skull, and for lower-back pain.

Gall Bladder 20 (GB 20)—Referred to as "the gates of consciousness" or "wind pool," these are 2 points located underneath the base of your skull, with one on either side of the vertical neck muscles. It is good for vascular or tension pain on the sides or the back of the head, especially when associated with digestive upset, vomiting, dizziness, tooth pain, stiff neck, irritability, and neuromotor coordination problems.

Gall Bladder 41 (GB 41)—Also called "overlooking tears" or "above tears," these 2 points are located on top of each foot, in the groove between the bones one inch above the webbing of the fourth and fifth toes. Good for tension, the vascular system, water retention, muscle pain, and shoulder tension.

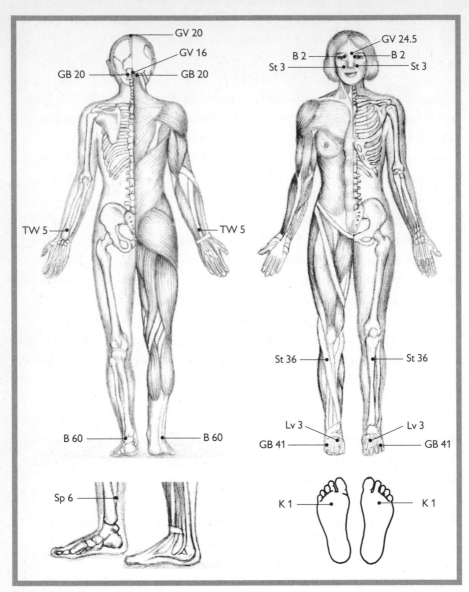

Figure 16.1—Acupressure points.

Governing Vessel 16 (GV 16)—Known as "the wind mansion," this point is located in the center of your head, just underneath the base of your skull. It is good for vascular conditions and relieves pain in the eyes, ears, nose, and throat, unclogs the nose, and relieves stiff necks.

Governing Vessel 20 (GV 20)—Known as "the hundred convergences," this point is located at the top of the head, at the mid-point of an imaginary line drawn from ear to ear. It is good for pain on top of the head, also vomiting, dizziness, memory lapse, and hemorrhages.

Governing Vessel 24.5 (GV 24.5)—Also called *Yin Tang* point, "the third eye," or "the hall of impression," this point is located midway between the eyebrows; use index finger to apply pressure as with the other points. Good for frontal headaches.

Kidney 1 (K 1)—Known as "bubbling spring," it is located on the sole of the foot in the middle of the ball where the 2 mounds come together. Good for pain on top of the head.

Liver 3 (Lv 3)—Known as "supreme surge" or "bigger rushing," these are 2 corresponding points, each located in the depression between the first and second toes at the sensitive spot about an inch above the web. Good for the vascular system, liver dysfunction, digestion, eyestrain, allergies, hangovers, and irritability.

Spleen 6 (Sp 6)—Known as "the 3 yin intersection," these 2 corresponding points are located 3 fingers up from the ankle bone on the inside of the leg; use both thumbs and press hard and deeply for about 7 to 10 seconds; do this 3 times. (Refrain from stimulating this point during pregnancy because it could cause a miscarriage.) Good for digestion, PMS, and pelvic disorders.

Stomach 3 (St 3)—Called "facial beauty" or "great bone hole" these 2 points are located at the bottom of each cheekbone, directly beneath

Headache Relief with G-Jo #13 (Li 4)

G-Jo, which translates as "first-aid," is a type of acupressure that can be used under nearly every painful circumstance. Although there are more than 20 different G-Jo acupressure points, G-Jo #13 (also called Hoku, Joining the Valley, or Large Intestine 4) is probably the best general acupoint for just about any headache (although not for pregnant women).

Using the thumb and index finger of your left hand, press the area located in the fleshy web between your thumb and index finger on the backside of your right hand. Experiment with it until you find the tender spot, and, once there, hold it firmly down toward the bone, pressing as deeply as is comfortable. Do this for 20 seconds to a minute and then reverse hands.

As you do this, you should feel some warmth or a slight flush of perspiration across your forehead, neck, or shoulders. Most people find that they feel immediately relaxed, and others say G-Jo "erases" their headache.

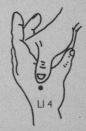

LI 4

Affirmations to Release Headaches

It is best to chose 1 or 2 affirmations that feel most comfortable and memorize them so you can say them whenever a negative or "headachy" thought enters your mind.

I feel healthy, relaxed, and free of pain.

I love myself, and I deserve to feel healthy and alive.

I approve of myself, and I am safe to be who I am.

I am flexible, open, and loving toward myself and the world around me.

Every day I feel better and better.

I am in the flow of life, and I am grateful for the gift of life.

In every way, I am healing and learning to accept the joy life offers.

My life is my own and I easily resolve my conflicts.

the pupils of the eyes when they are focused straight ahead; using a circular motion, massage this spot for 20 seconds to a minute, stimulating both points simultaneously. Good for TMJ/facial pain, toothaches, eyestrain, eye twitch and sinus, cluster, and vascular conditions.

Stomach 36 (St 36)—Known as "leg 3 li," these 2 corresponding points are located on the top of the shin bone, 3 fingers below the outside of the bottom of the kneecap; use index finger to apply firm pressure, then massage in a circular fashion for 30 to 45 seconds; repeat on other side. Good for constant headache of any variety, especially digestive.

Triple Warmer 5 (TW 5)—Called "outer gate," this point is located on the back of the arm about an inch above the wrist crease. Good for migraines in the early stages, temple or side-of-the-head headaches, or headaches accompanying a cold and sore throat.

AFFIRMATIONS/ AUTOSUGGESTIONS

Affirmations, also known as autosuggestions, are positive statements that you can use to change the way you think about yourself and your headaches. The body cannot tell the difference between a real or imagined idea, so it responds to whatever you give it. By repeating an affirmation every time a negative, self-defeating thought comes to mind, you can retrain your mind and learn to respond more confidently to the world around you. Over time, the old thoughts and mind patterns that used to make you anxious or stressed lose their charge until, eventually, they stop arising altogether.

Making affirmations doesn't mean, however, suppressing any thought that is not a good one. Instead, affirmations should be used as a reshaping tool that you can call on to rid yourself of thoughts that serve no purpose. For example, let's say your mind keeps informing you that you haven't had a headache in a while, telling you that you are due for one any minute now. Instead of giving in and feeding the destructive thought, you can overpower it by replacing it with the affirmation: "I am headache free and I deserve to stay that way." At first, it may seem silly or as if you are fooling yourself, but if you pay attention and keep repeating the affirmation, the day will come when you say it and mean it.

In France, medical doctors routinely use aromatherapy to treat infectious diseases, and, in England, hospital nurses massage their patients with essential oils to relieve pain and induce relaxation and sleep.

AROMATHERAPY

A relative of herbal medicine, aromatherapy is a healing modality that uses the essential oils of various plants and herbs to treat conditions such as immune deficiencies, circulation problems, sinus disorders, skin conditions, muscular disorders, arthritis, and stress. In France, medical doctors routinely use it to treat infectious diseases, and, in England, hospital nurses massage their patients with essential oils to relieve pain and induce relaxation and sleep. Thanks to research in Europe, some doctors in the U.S. are beginning to recognize the therapeutic value of aromatherapy.

CAUTION

Essential oils are sometimes ingested, but this method should be used only under the supervision of a knowledgeable practitioner.

Essential oils, or the plant's essence, are extracted from the flowers, stems, leaves, or roots through steam distillation or cold-pressing processes. Although the term aromatherapy suggests that these oils are used primarily for their aroma, this is not the case, as the oils themselves contain powerful pharmacological healing properties, such as antibacterial, antiviral, antispasmodic, diuretic, stimulating, relaxing, detoxifying, and/or vasodilating (stretching the blood vessels). Oil molecules are small, so their healing agents easily penetrate body tissues and begin work immediately, affecting stress level, hormonal balance, digestive processes, blood pressure, breathing, and heart rate.

One way aromatherapy is delivered is through external application. This can be done by bathing in bath water mixed with oils, massaging oils into your skin, or applying hot or cold compresses that have been soaked in oil-infused water. Another way to use the oils is to inhale them as they waft through the air around you. An inexpensive and easy way to do this is with an aroma lamp, which is a simple bowl with a built-in candle base. To use the lamp, fill the bowl with water and a few drops of essential oil. As the candle heats the water, the oil's aroma is released into the air. Even more economically, a bowl of oiled water can be placed on a furnace, wood stove, or range to produce the same effect. You can also use an electric diffuser which more actively circulates the aroma.

Aromatherapy is therapeutic for headaches, as the right oils not only help you relax physically and emotionally but also work on underlying conditions such as candidiasis, constipation, digestive disorders, eyestrain, high blood pressure, PMS, and sinus problems. When buying oils for therapeutic use, it is best to choose 100% pure essential oil, as these are concentrated, high-quality oils, and their superior healing properties are well worth the extra cost. Because they are very strong, you generally need to use only a few drops at a time.

Essential oils used for general headaches include basil, chamomile, coriander, eucalyptus, ginger, helichrysum, jasmine, lavender, lemon, marjoram, melissa, peppermint, rose, rosemary, rosewood, sage, and thyme. The following aromatherapy blends are suggested for headache prevention and relief:

Inhalation

Wafting relief: Fill aroma lamp, bowl, or diffuser with water and mix in 4 drops melissa and 2 drops peppermint or Roman chamomile oil.

Sinus relief: To clear and relieve sinus congestion and sinus-related headaches, fill an aroma lamp, bowl, or diffuser with water and mix in equal amounts of lavender, peppermint, and rosemary; because all 3 of these oils have antiseptic qualities, this mixture can also help combat any underlying sinus infection.

Aroma to go: Put 2 to 3 drops of melissa, peppermint, and lavender oils on a handkerchief or cloth and inhale throughout the day for prevention.

For congestive or sinus headaches: Cajuput, geranium, niaouli, and tea tree oils; peppermint, rosemary, or eucalyptus are preferred when congestion is caused by a nasal infection because these also have an antiseptic effect.

Massage

Temple rub: Combine lavender (a sedative) and peppermint (a stimulant) oils and rub the mixture on your temples for pain relief.

Sore muscle massage: Mix 10 drops juniper (which adds heat), 8 drops rosemary, 8 drops lavender, and 2 drops lemon with 2 ounces vegetable oil and use to massage your neck and shoulders.

Additional oils for general headaches: Basil, chamomile, coriander (small doses only), melissa, and sage can be massaged into the temples, eye sockets, base of the neck, and shoulders.

Good oils for vascular-type headaches: Anise, basil, chamomile, coriander, eucalyptus, lavender, lemon, marjoram, melissa, onion, peppermint, and rosemary.

Baths

Aroma soak: for relief of a headache in progress, fill a bath with warm to hot water and add eucalyptus, wintergreen, or peppermint oil and soak for 20 to 30 minutes.

Hangover headache bath: Add a few drops of an invigorating oil such as pepper or juniper to warm bath water.

Muscle relaxant bath: Fill the bath with warm water and add 3 drops chamomile, 3 drops lavender, 2 drops marjoram, 2 drops thyme, and 1 drop coriander oils.

Compresses and Steams

Cold compress relief: Mix 3 drops rose, 1 drop melissa, and 1 drop lavender oils in 2 pints water. Stir thoroughly and place a towel or washcloth in the water. Let it soak for 5 minutes, then wring to remove excess water. Lie back and put the compress on the painful area. Rest. Change the compress as soon as it reaches room temperature.

Icy migraine compress: Add 2 drops peppermint, 1 drop ginger, and 1 drop marjoram oils to 1 quart ice water; soak a clean cloth and apply to head, forehead, or neck at first inkling of an approaching migraine; if desired, apply an icepack over the compress to keep it from heating up. Avoid contact with your eyes.

Lavender and peppermint compress for vascular headache: At the first sign of headache, make 2 compresses, a lavender and peppermint compress for the forehead, and a hot marjoram compress (a vasodilator, stretches blood vessels) for the back of the neck; this combination provides relaxing, stimulating, and vasodilating effects.

Compress for eyestrain headache: Lie down in a darkened room with a cool compress made with chamomile, rosemary, or parsley oils over your closed eyes.

Compress for sore muscles: Soak clean cloth in a mixture of 1 drop ginger, 2 drops marjoram, 1 drop peppermint, and 1 drop rosemary oils added to hot water; apply to neck and shoulders.

Aromatherapy steam: Boil 2 pints water, pour into a large bowl, and add 1 drop melissa, 2 drops peppermint, and 2 drops lavender oils. Put your head over the bowl and cover your head and the bowl with a large towel. Inhale deeply through your nose for about 10 minutes.

BREATHING EXERCISES

CAUTION

During breathing exercises, you may experience dizziness as a result of breathing differently than you normally do or mistakenly hyperventilating. If you feel dizzy, stop the exercise. Gradually building up to the number of repetitions recommended may be a way to avoid dizziness.

More than just another function that your body performs automatically, breathing is the life-giving wind that feeds your body with vital oxygen. Breath has the power to alter consciousness, and the quality of your breath affects your emotional and physical health. Breathing practitioners in other countries have been known to use their breath to quicken metabolism, quiet their minds, and even to keep their naked bodies warm in frigid temperatures.

Many of us pay little attention to the way we breathe. Somehow, in the course of our lives, we have lost touch with this important function. As if there were a shortage of supply, we take short, shallow breaths, releasing the air we inhale before it comes close to reaching the bottoms of our lungs, and sometimes, particularly when overwhelmed by pain or stress, we forget to breathe altogether.

Fortunately, once you recognize the influence your emotions and thoughts have on your breath, you can begin to use your breath to influence these states. By remembering how to breath deeply, you can reconnect with the natural flow of life. Deep breathing allows more oxygen into the head, bringing about a reflex constriction of the blood vessels of the skin, as well as a slight drop in blood pressure and a slowing of peripheral blood flow—all events that are helpful for relieving and preventing headaches.

It is important to breathe through your nose not just during these exercises but always because the nose is lined with air purifying hairs (called cilia) which the mouth does not have. When you breathe in, initiate the action from deep inside your diaphragm to allow your lungs a full range of motion, and allow your belly to lift like a balloon filling with air.

By practicing one or more of these exercises on a regular basis, you will become more aware of the breaths you take and will find it easier to take deeper, more fulfilling breaths that nourish both body and mind. Before you start, either lie flat on your back or sit in a comfortable position; make sure you are wearing comfortable, nonrestrictive clothing. Always begin by emptying your lungs with a complete exhalation. Your eyes may be open or closed, depending on what feels best to you.

Three-part Breath

This technique is designed to draw air deep into the diaphragm so it can oxygenate the entire system. For this, you divide a deep inhalation into 3 parts, the first part lifting the belly, the second part filling the lungs, and the third part extending into the upper chest. Hold for 3 seconds, and release in one long exhalation. Repeat 5 times.

Twenty-cycle Breath

This simple breathing method can be performed anywhere, and it can be a pleasant way to change your state of mind while sitting in traffic. It is done by taking 4 short continuous breaths, followed by a long breath (5 seconds to inhale, 5 seconds to exhale), repeating this 4 times in rapid sequence.

Wu Breathing Exercise

Wu is a Chinese breathing technique known to relieve headaches. Lie down in a relaxed position with your head on a low pillow and your arms resting at your sides, your feet a little more than hip-width apart. Place the tip of your tongue on the roof of your mouth, just behind the place where the front teeth meet the gums, and breathe naturally but deeply through your nose. Imagine the breath coming through your nose to the top of your head and down to the center of your belly. Continue this for about 20 to 30 minutes, concentrating on the breath coming in through your head. Do this in the morning and at night.

Pulse Breathing

This technique involves using diaphragm breathing and a pulsed, hard exhalation—much like a karate expert yells when hitting a brick. To start, take a deep breath and exhale, then inhale and exhale forcefully (called a pulse breath). Then take 2 deep-breathing cycles and a pulse; 3 breathing cycles and a pulse; 4 breathing cycles and a pulse; 5 breathing cycles and a pulse. Perform this exercise twice daily and any time you are under stress.

CREATIVE VISUALIZATION

Also known as guided imagery or self-hypnosis, creative visualization uses the power of the imagination to elicit a positive healing response by programming your unconscious thoughts and attitudes in order to create peace and well-being rather than pain and illness. A wonderful adjunct to other therapies, creative visualization can be used to bring about greater awareness of emotional attitudes, to enhance creativity, to change mental and emotional patterns, even to affect physiological functioning.

Furthermore, it is a proven method of pain relief, and it can be used to overcome seemingly insurmountable odds, as in the cases of individuals who have won the battle against so-called terminal illnesses by envisioning armies of T-cells marching through the body destroying cancerous or other invaders.

Creative visualization takes practice, motivation, and concentration. While some people respond better than others, most who use it report the benefits of improved coping skills and better pain management. The following techniques work best when they are performed in a deeply relaxed state, so it is a good idea to do 1 or 2 breathing or relaxation exercises before you start:

- **Give your headache pain a shape, texture, or even a voice.**
  Then use your imagination to change it, soften it, reduce its power, eliminate it (turn it into a rocket and send it to outer space; imagine it growing smaller and smaller until it disappears); you might even look for an image you can call on to help you relax

whenever you feel a headache coming on (a cool, dark cave, for example).

- **Picture your body being filled with rays from the sun.** Once the healing energy is spread throughout your body, focus on your head pain and imagine it being engulfed by warm sunshine. Breathe with the feeling and imagine this sunshine stimulating your body's natural painkillers and infusing every cell in your body with well-being.

- **Try color therapy healing.** Use either green, blue, or purple. Green: Imagine the color green radiating from the center of your heart to fill your entire body; see it soothing and balancing your nervous system. Blue: Picture blue radiating from your throat and the back of your neck until your entire being is bathed in blue; see it erasing pain and encouraging you to talk about whatever is bothering you. Purple: Visualize purple pouring into your body through the top of your head and spreading into every cell, balancing your blood pressure and filling your cells with vital energy.

- **Imagine the pain draining from your head.** Then it goes down your shoulders and arms, and out through your fingertips.

- **Give your headache a name and ask it questions.** Ask: What do you represent? What are you helping me to avoid? What do you want from me? How can I help you?

- **Imagine yourself lying in the clouds with all of your worries far away.** You are surrounded by soft blue and your favorite music is the air you breathe.

- **Create your own healing journey.** Make something up that soothes you, whether you are floating through beautiful trees or gazing into a glassy lake at dusk. You can even write it down and record it or ask a friend with a pleasant voice to record it for you, so you can listen to it during times when you unable to think.

EXERCISE

Ranging from gentle stretching to aerobic movement, exercise is a valuable component of any wellness program. Offering both preventative and therapeutic benefits, exercise reduces stress, stabilizes hormones and blood pressure, strengthens internal organs, eliminates constipation, promotes vascular and muscle tone and relaxation, improves breathing, and produces pain-relieving brain chemicals such as endorphins. It also makes you more aware of your posture, normalizes your weight, and gives you a sense of being at home in your body. Research has shown that consistent exercise can also reduce the severity and frequency of headaches.

Most studies suggest that 20 to 30 minutes of moderate exercise 3 or more days a week brings the most relief to headache sufferers. In one such study, researchers at the University of Wisconsin Biodynamics Laboratory discovered migrainers were able to cut the frequency of their migraines in half through a regular aerobic training program. Over a course of 15 weeks, participants exercised, either running or walking, 3 days a week for 30 minutes, at the end of which, it was determined that exercise helped to reduce their sensitivity to other triggers.[1]

It is best to begin any exercise program slowly, working up to your goal over a period of time so as not to overexert yourself. In addition, be sure to start and end your exercise routine with gentle stretching, as this can prevent injury by giving your body a chance to gradually warm up and cool down. Do not push yourself unnecessarily; instead try to find your own middle ground—and whatever you do, relax and enjoy your body. Also remember, no exercise more strenuous than gentle stretching should ever be attempted during a headache attack.

The following techniques are just a few of the many exercise options to explore.

Aerobic Exercise

Whether biking, swimming, walking, dancing, tennis, skating, or mountain climbing, aerobic exercise is a great way to release tension, stimulate endorphins, and promote an overall sense of well-being. Regardless of which exercise you choose, be aware of your breath and how you are holding your body. Notice if you are stiffening your neck or hunching your shoulders, and try to keep everything as relaxed and aligned as possible.

Be particularly careful if you are doing sit-ups or other isometric exercises, as it is easy to compress parts of your body and cause kinks in your alignment. One way to make sure you are maintaining proper form while you exercise is to get help from a friend or a personal trainer.

Therapeutic Martial Arts

Considered preventative as well as therapeutic, the Eastern martial arts disciplines such as Qigong (pronounced CHEE-gung), combine movement, breath, and meditation to enhance the flow of energy throughout the body. When practiced regularly, they improve circulation, calm the mind, enhance inner peace and resolve, and strengthen the immune system. Therapeutic martial arts continue to evolve with the practitioner, stimulating ever greater awareness of both inner and outer environments.

Qigong is especially useful for those who suffer from chronic and acute headache pain, since even the seriously incapacitated can practice it. The following is a simple exercise that can be performed by almost everyone, regardless of their age or state of health.

Tracing the energy pathways to circulate the life force:
1. Making sure to breathe in a smooth and natural rhythm, rub your hands together as if you were warming them over a fire. Once you can feel the heat in your palms, stroke them across your cheeks, eyes, and forehead as if washing your face. Continue to move your hands up over the top and sides of your head, down the back of your neck, and along your upper back to your shoulder joint.
2. Next, move your palms underneath your arms and down the sides of your body to your lower rib cage, and, from there, move your palms around to your back, down your buttocks and legs, and out the sides of your feet.
3. Finally, trace up the inside of your feet and legs, to the front of your torso, and back to your face again. This ends the first round. Repeat.

Yoga

Yoga is among the world's oldest health-care systems and continues today to influence research in therapeutic bodywork and mind/body medicine. A combination of postures, breathing, and meditation, yoga is an expansive self-care system which can increase physical and mental awareness, reduce stress, regulate the heart rate and blood pressure, alleviate migraines, PMS, arthritis, asthma, and allergies, and improve overall body functioning.

Cranial Stretch

Developed by bodyworker Rick Williams, N.M.T., B.S., of Fairfax, California, cranial yoga is a gentle, therapeutic technique designed to bring back the natural range of motion in the cranial region; you could call it, hatha yoga for the 27 bones and 67 joints of the skull. In addition to obvious trauma, minor bumps and falls, emotional stress, and even birth, can knock the cranial bones out of alignment without your knowing it. Over time, these interlocking bones get jammed or stuck, causing the entire system to stop working as it should—often resulting in headaches.

Based on Williams' work in biomechanics and neuromuscular therapy, these exercises work often neglected bones and joints, loosening and opening them in order to keep them flexible. They should be done at least twice a week, and used any time relief is needed. Perform them while sitting comfortably with your back straight. Hold each posture for 15 to 30 seconds, breathing comfortably and gently throughout.

Hair Grasp #1: Start at the forehead along the hairline on the right side of the head; make a fist and grasp your hair, squeezing your fingers until you feel mild discomfort, and hold. Continue this exercise all the way around your hairline to the back of your head, then return to the forehead, and start again, this time 2 inches from your hairline. When you have finished, use your left hand to do the same steps on the left side.

Hair Grasp #2: Using your right hand over your right ear and your left hand over your left ear, grasp your hair with both hands, keeping the right elbow low and the left elbow high. Then slowly lower your left elbow and raise your right elbow until you feel mild discomfort, hold, and wait for release. Do this several times, and then repeat the above steps using the reverse motion, starting with your left elbow low and your right elbow high.

Hair Grasp #3: Keeping your elbows high, grasp the hair above your forehead with your left hand and grasp the hair at the base of the neck with the right hand; slowly bring the elbows down until you feel mild discomfort, then hold, and wait for release. Do this several times, and then follow the same steps on other side, with your left hand in back and your right hand in front.

Osteopathic Exercises

The following osteopathic self-treatment exercises can help you to improve

Flower Essences for Headaches

Although flower essence practitioners target the emotional conditions underlying a headache rather than the headache itself, a few remedies are often associated with headaches. The following list was compiled by Patricia Kaminski, flower essence practitioner, teacher, author of *Flower Essence Repertory*, and director of Flower Essence Services.

Allergy/Sensitivity

- Crab Apple: for feelings of impurity or imperfection, particularly shame of the physical body and its imperfections

- Dill: for those who are overwhelmed, hypersensitive, or overstimulated; known to enhance digestive function

- St. John's Wort: for headache accompanied by light sensitivity or vulnerability to environmental stress, including allergies

- Yarrow: strengthens the sensitivity that occurs when body deals with environmental or digestive overload

- Yarrow Special Formula: similar to yarrow but more specifically geared to help one cope with the environmental hazards of modern living

Trauma

- Arnica: for severe trauma in which it feels as if you have left your body; restores conscious embodiment

- Five Flower Remedy (also called Rescue Remedy): for panic, disorientation, or loss of consciousness; used to restore calm and stability in emergencies or during intense stress; contains cherry plum, clematis, impatiens, rock rose, star-of-Bethlehem

- Queen Anne's Lace (also called wild carrot): often used to treat head trauma, as it helps to ground and stabilize

- St. John's Wort: see above

- Self Heal (the flower *Prunella vulgaris*): used to restore the physical body after a blow or injury, especially when damage seems overwhelming; restores a vital sense of self

Stress and Tension

- Dandelion: for stress and tension held in the muscles of the body; brings about dynamic, effortless energy

- Fuschia: for repressed emotions that cause psychosomatic symptoms; allows the expression of genuine feelings and emotional states

- Impatiens: for people who are constantly rushing, impatient, intolerant, tense; creates acceptance and patience for the flow of life

- Iris: for tension, especially in the neck region, and inability to feel inner freedom

- Lavender: releases high-strung, nervous tension, allows full relaxation in order to receive the benefits of the healing work

- Mimulus: for those who are frequently in fear of their next headache attack

- Nicotiana: for those who cope with tension by using addictive substances, especially, but not limited to, tobacco

- Five Flower Remedy: helps to cope with stress in general (see above)

PMS and Menopause

- Alpine Lily: used especially for women to rebalance energy flows between the upper and lower parts of the body by grounding femininity deep in the body

- Hibiscus: for repressed feminine sexuality; allows for feminine warmth and responsiveness

- Tiger Lily: for overly aggressive, hostile attitude; brings about cooperative service with others and grounds feminine forces

General Headache

- Lavender: good overall headache remedy; used to dispel nervousness and overstimulation, which deplete the physical body

- Five Flower Remedy: good overall stress remedy

mobility and lesson the stiffness and pain that often accompany a low range of motion. Move only as far as is comfortable. Do not strain to do these exercises, and always be sure to breathe fully and naturally.

- Sit with your elbows resting on a table and your head resting in your open hands. As you hold this position, breathe in and tilt your head sideways against your right hand, exerting pressure with your head using about a fourth of your muscle strength. Hold your breath as you exert this pressure for about 5 to 7 seconds, then relax the pressure and your breath simultaneously. Repeat this 2 times, and then tilt to the left and perform the same movement 3 times.

- Place your hands together over your forehead and let your head rest in your hands, with your neck flexed. Take a deep breath, and push your hands against your forehead and your forehead against your hands, hold the contraction for 7 seconds, and then release slowly as you breathe out. Repeat 2 times.

- Flex your neck, gently tuck your chin to your chest, and place both hands against the back of your head. Breathe in and push your head backward against the weight of your hands, hold for 5 to 7 seconds and release as you breathe out. Repeat 2 times.

- Carefully tilt your head backward and look up at the ceiling. Press your hands on your forehead using only about 10% of your strength (any more could cause discomfort) while slowly attempting to push your head back into upright position. Repeat 2 times.

- Sit upright and pull your chin toward the back of your neck as if you were trying to make a double chin. Breathe in and place a hand on your chin, trying to keep it from returning to its original position. Hold the contraction for 5 to 7 seconds. Release as you breath out. Repeat twice.

- Place your left hand on your left check and use it as resistance as you breathe in and try to turn your head to the left. Again hold the contraction for 5 to 7 seconds. Repeat the exercise on the right side.[2]

For more information on **flower essences**, contact: Flower Essence Services, P.O. Box 1769, Nevada City, CA 95959; tel: 800-548-0075 or 916-265-0258; fax: 916-265-6467; or Ellon USA, Inc. (formerly Ellon Bach USA), 644 Merrick Road, Lynbrook, NY 11563; tel: 516- 593-2206.

FLOWER ESSENCES

Flower essences are available at health food stores. They can be taken directly under the tongue, diluted with drinking water, rubbed on the temples, or added to massage oil or lotion. To make a tincture for long-term use, combine 2 to 5 drops of essence with 3 parts water and 1 part brandy (substitute vegetable glycerin or apple cider vinegar if you prefer not to use alcohol).

FOLK REMEDIES

In medieval times, home headache remedies consisted of such substances as beaver testes, reptile skin, cow's brains, live toads, and leeches, and headache treatments might include placing a hot iron directly on the forehead, inserting garlic or dill inside an open cut on the head, or hanging a dead buzzard's head around your neck. Contemporary folk remedies for headache remedies are tame by comparison, but many can offer quick relief, most often with common ingredients you already have at hand.

Hair brushing: Brushing your hair and scalp with a downward motion every day is an effective way to improve blood circulation in the head and keep headaches from occurring. Using a natural bristle brush with rounded tips, begin at your temples and move the brush in tiny circles as you work your way down your scalp, doing the left side, the right side, then returning to the middle of your scalp and finishing with the same strokes, first to the left, then to the right of center.[3]

Salt water nasal douching: Because salt water shrinks tissues and swollen blood vessels, this remedy is used when there is swelling or tenderness over the sinuses. Add 1 tablespoon sea salt to a cup of warm water and stir until cloudy; use a tincture dropper or eye dropper and, with your head leaning back, apply 1 dropper full into each nostril; do this 2 to 3 times a day until the swelling is relieved.

Hanna Somatics For Headaches

Eleanor Criswell Hanna, Ed.D., reports that headache sufferers can learn to soften tight muscles and release neck and shoulder tension by incorporating these easy exercises into their daily routines. Do these exercises while in a seated position, breathing smoothly and completely throughout, making sure you feel each contraction before you release.

- Starting on the right side, bring the shoulder back a little and lift it while bringing the ear down to meet it, feel the contraction, then slowly release. Do this 3 times, and then do the same on the left side. (This is especially helpful for releasing the muscle most often used to cradle the phone.)

- Turn your head and neck to the left, away from the right shoulder; then bring your right shoulder up, and tip your head back so the head is tilting back toward the right shoulder. Slowly release. Do this 3 times and then repeat on the other side.

- Gently tilt your head back a little and let your shoulders rise at the same time; then slowly return your head and shoulders to their normal position. Do this 3 times.

- Put your palm against your forehead and bend your head down a little, then come slowly back up. Do this 3 times.

Ease Your Headaches with Feverfew

According to Oregon naturopathic physician Deborah Frances, N.D., the herb feverfew can be effective against migraines and headaches, as the following examples show.

When a young woman, aged 14, complained of sudden flashing lights in her eyes followed by head pain, Dr. Frances prescribed feverfew at the rate of 30 drops every 15 minutes for 1 hour. The symptoms went away after only 2 doses.

A woman, aged 33, had complained of daily dull headaches for 2 months, with a severely painful one every 2 weeks. Dr. Frances had her take feverfew at the rate of 30 drops twice daily for the dull headaches, and 60 drops every 15 minutes for the acute headaches. In addition, Dr. Frances prescribed *Naturum Muriaticum* (homeopathic salt), which is often used for headaches, and a liver support formula. The woman reported that her headaches had decreased to once every 4 days; when the headaches occurred, taking feverfew at 60 drops every 15 minutes (3 doses total) gave her complete relief.

Both *Naturum Muriaticum* and feverfew are widely available as over-the-counter remedies. Feverfew's use as a migraine headache remedy was described in European herbals as early as 1772 while a 1983 survey showed that 70% of 270 people suffering from migraines reported that feverfew taken daily decreased the frequency and intensity of their headaches. A 1988 British study showed that daily intake of 82 mg of feverfew over 4 months led to fewer headaches and those that occurred were of milder intensity. No side effects were reported.

SOURCE—Deborah Frances, N.D., "Feverfew for Acute Headaches: Does It Work?" *Medical Herbalism: A Clinical Newsletter for the Clinical Practitioner* 7:4 (Winter 1995-1996), 1-2.

Chlorophyll nasal drops: This natural remedy is a wonder for preventing sinus complaints. Pour either oil-soluble or water-soluble (diluted with distilled water) liquid chlorophyll, which is available from health food stores, into a tincture bottle and put no more than 1 or 2 drops into each nostril twice a day, preferably upon rising and at bedtime.

Vinegar compresses: Soak a washcloth in vinegar and place it in the refrigerator until it is sufficiently chilled. Then apply the compress to your forehead, temples, and neck. You can also inhale vinegar for even faster relief; boil equal parts vinegar and water, pour mixture into a bowl, and place a towel over the bowl and your head as you inhale the rising steam.

Warm salt pack: To make a salt pack, roast 1 cup of salt in a dry frying pan until salt is warm to the touch, being careful that it does not overheat. Pour salt into a thin dish towel, fold it so you can apply it to your head, rubbing the painful areas rather than keeping the pack in one place.

Ginger compress: Cut and peel one root of fresh ginger and boil it in 3 cups of water until the mixture turns cloudy. Add a washcloth, let it soak, and then apply it to the back of your neck. This works well to expand the contracted muscles and relieve dull, steady pain.

Herbal compress: Boil 3 cups

of water and pour over 1 tbsp. of lavender and 1 tbsp. of chamomile; steep for 20 minutes. Soak a soft cloth in the mixture, wring it out, and apply on the back of neck or forehead. Cold herbal compresses are also effective.

Herbal foot bath: This is an excellent way to draw blood and congestion away from your head. Place 1 tablespoon of powdered mustard or ginger in a deep basin big enough for both feet. Fill the basin with water as hot as you can bear, sit in a comfortable chair, and slowly immerse your feet in the water. Drape a thick towel over the basin to keep the heat in, and place a cool or cold towel on your neck or forehead. Close your eyes and relax, breathing deeply for about 15 minutes.

Icy foot bath: Fill a basin with ice water (refrigerated water with ice) and soak your feet. Believe it or not, your feet will actually start to feel warm after a few minutes. When you are finished, dry off, get under the covers of your bed, and relax.

Cold hip-sitz bath: Fill a tub with 2 inches of warm water. Sit in the tub, turn on the cold water, and let it run until it covers your hips. Dry off with a coarse towel and cover up. A muscle massage is especially beneficial after this treatment.

Epsom salt bath: Pour 2 to 4 cups of Epsom salts into the bathtub and fill with warm water. Soak for 15 to 30 minutes. Epsom salts are good for removing toxins from your system.

Alternating hot and cold showers: To improve blood circulation, try alternating hot and cold showers once a day for 2 or 3 months; this remedy also works to abort vascular-type headaches because the heat causes the blood vessels to dilate (which may temporarily cause pain) while the cold makes them contract.

Cold water and hot water wrist baths: If you feel a headache coming on while you are away from familiar territory, look for a sink and run cold and then hot water on your wrists, alternating until you feel the headache pass.

Drink a headache tonic: Fill a large pot with water and mix in small pieces of fresh ginger root, coriander seeds, and diced garlic with a little honey to taste. Boil off half the liquid and drink what is left periodically throughout the day.

Apple cider vinegar and honey tonic: To offset the causes of a digestive headache, particularly one related to excess acid production, D.C.

Jarvis, M.D., in his book *Vermont Folk Medicine*, suggests taking apple cider vinegar in water and/or 2 teaspoons of honey every day to help regulate the body's pH balance. Dr. Jarvis reports that when taken as a rescue remedy this tonic will stop any headache, including a migraine, within a half-hour. If you do not like the taste, you can place equal parts apple cider vinegar and water in a steamer, place your face over it with your head covered with a towel, and inhale 75 breaths.

Try 12 almonds: Because they contain the natural aspirin salicin, almonds can offer headache relief. This remedy is used in areas of North Africa and Asia where almond trees are common.

Eat 2 kiwis: This proven hangover remedy is believed to work because kiwis are loaded with potassium and thus help to replenish lost fluids and bring blood sugar back up to normal.

Have a cup o' Joe: While not recommended for those with caffeine sensitivities, a cup of coffee or black tea constricts the blood vessels in the head and stops the headache. Beware, however, because the relief may be temporary: caffeine can also cause a rebound headache when it wears off.

A spoonful of honey: A tablespoon of raw honey at first inkling of an impending headache can abort a vascular headache; wait a half-hour, and, if it has not worked, take another tablespoon with 3 glasses of water.

Li Shou (arm swinging): This Chinese technique uses motion to relieve headaches by creating a relaxed, meditative state and is taught it to school children to relieve stress. Swing your arms back and forth until the blood shifts from your head to your hands, reducing your swollen blood vessels. Next, use your warmed hands to stroke your face, in a circular motion, paying particular attention to the area around your eyes. Repeat the exercise several times.

Wear a headband: In Korea, locals tie cloths snugly around their heads, just above the eyebrows. This remedy has been somewhat validated by Western science: according to one study, wearing a snug elastic headband helped about a quarter of participants obtain relief of 50% or more, possibly because the headband may restrict blood flow and prevent the dilation of blood vessels.[4]

Wrap rubberbands around your fingers: Take 10 rubberbands and wrap them around each of your fingers at the first joint, the one closest to your fingernail. Put them on tight, and although they may turn your fingers purplish and hurt a bit, leave them on for no more than 9 minutes to find that your headache has disappeared.

Bite your tongue: This remedy is not about watching what you say; instead, stick your tongue out about ½ inch, then bite on it *gently* for about 9 minutes (not more than 11 minutes), keeping pressure on your tongue the entire time.

The paper bag trick: Because your exhaled breath is largely made up of carbon dioxide (CO_2), and carbon dioxide is known to dilate the cerebral arteries, some say breathing into a bag and rebreathing your expired air at the earliest sign of a vascular headache can abort the approaching attack. This works especially well if classic migraine sufferers try it the minute they see a warning aura. Try breathing into the bag for 15 to 20 minutes and then lying down for 20 minutes. If the headache has not gone away, repeat the breathing cycle one more time.[5]

Blinking red light: While too high-tech to be a true folk remedy, this may be the home cure of the future. Developed by John Anderson. M.D., of England, this treatment involves a pair of goggles that blink red light at different speeds before your eyes. In one study, 72% of those who used the treatment reported that their migraines stopped within an hour of beginning the treatment; those who reported the most success credited some of it to their ability to adjust the speed and brightness of the light to a level they found soothing.[6] (Similar light goggles can be purchased through A Sharper Image or Tools for Exploration, listed in Appendix A.)

HERBAL SUPPLEMENTS

Many herbal supplements can be purchased in health food stores and self-administered according to the dosage recommended on the label. Even so, for maximum effectiveness, particularly for chronic conditions, it is preferable to take herbs and herb combinations under the guidance of an alternative practitioner.

See Chapter 17, An A-Z of Alternative Medicine, Herbal Medicine, for more information on the herbs listed in this section.

Specific Health Conditions and the Herbs that Can Help

Allergy/sensitivity or digestive disorders—black horehound, cayenne, chamomile, fenugreek, feverfew, ginger, nettle, passion flower, peppermint, rosemary, safflower, slippery elm, St. John's wort, wood betony

Directions for Making Herb Tea

There are 2 types of tea: infusions, from the steeping method; and decoctions, from the boiled method. Infusions are best for fresh or dried green plant parts, such as leaves, flowers, or stems, and powdered herbs, while decoctions are the preferred way to prepare hard, woody, brown plant parts, such as roots, bark, nuts, and seeds. Unless otherwise noted, both methods make teas that can be taken hot, cold, or iced, and they can be sweetened with honey if desired.

INFUSION METHOD:

Put 1 to 2 tsp. herb mixture into a teapot.

Add 1 or 2 cups boiling water and cover.

Let the mixture steep for 5 to 20 minutes.

DECOCTION METHOD:

Put 1 tsp. dried herb and 3 tsp. fresh herb into a pot or saucepan.

Add a cup of water for each tsp. of herb.

Bring the mixture to a boil and let simmer for 10 to 20 minutes.

Brain function—ginseng, *Gingko*, rosemary

Circulation—cayenne, feverfew, hawthorn, garlic, rosemary

Constipation/detox—aloe, burdock, dandelion, goldenseal (root), milk thistle, nettle, Oregon grape root, senna, vervain, wood betony

General headache—angelica, feverfew, meadowsweet, willow bark

Head trauma and swelling—coriander, skullcap, St. John's wort,

Hormonal/reproductive problems—black cohosh, black haw, cayenne, chamomile, chasteberry, cramp bark, *dong quai*, lavender, Jamaican dogwood, passion flower, skullcap, St. John's wort, wild yam

Immune system—*Echinacea*, garlic, ginger, *Gingko*, ginseng, golden seal, nettle, rosehips

Musculoskeletal pain and spasms—cayenne, chamomile, elder, meadowsweet, nettles, *qiyelian*, turmeric, valerian, vervain, willow bark

Sinus congestion—lavender, rosemary, peppermint, eucalyptus

Stress, anxiety, insomnia, depression, and tension—cramp bark, feverfew, hawthorn, *Gingko*, ginseng, lavender, linden blossom, passion flower, pennyroyal, peppermint, rosehips, skullcap, St. John's wort, valerian, vervain

Vascular imbalances—balm, basil, black willow, cayenne, elder, feverfew, garlic, ginger, *Gingko*, goldenrod, Jamaican dogwood, lavender, marjoram, peppermint, rosemary, rue, thyme, sage, willow bark, wood betony, wormwood

Herbal Teas for Headaches

Many of these herbs work better when taken in combination because some are calming (such as lavender) and others stimulating (such as peppermint). When combined, herbs can produce the effects of many over-the-counter and some prescription medications. For example, a chronic headache that is accompanied by tension gets the most relief from a combination of a sedative herb (passion flower, St. John's wort, valerian), an anti-inflammatory herb (feverfew, meadowsweet, willow bark), and an antispasmodic herb (cramp bark, wild yam, passion flower). Vascular headaches respond well to stimulants (*Gingko*, nettle, peppermint) combined with anti-inflammatories.

General headache relief: Sage, rosemary, peppermint, and wood betony; steep equal parts of each herb in boiling water and take every 2 hours until relief is obtained.

Relaxing headache relief tea: Skullcap, valerian, rosemary, chamomile, and peppermint; a cup of tea should be taken every hour.

Hormonal headache relief: 3 parts lemon balm, 3 parts chamomile, 1 part skullcap, 1 part passion flower; combine these herbs to make a total of 2 to 4 tablespoons. Place herbs in a glass tea jar and pour one quart boiling water over them; steep for 20 minutes. Strain and drink ¼ cup every 30 minutes until headache is gone.

Headache prevention tea: 4 tbsp. chamomile, 1 tbsp. white willow bark and 1 tbsp. valerian root; place herbs in glass tea jar and pour one pint of boiling water over them; steep for 30 minutes (a good overall self-heal tea).

Migraine tea: Use equal parts black horehound, meadowsweet, and chamomile; make as an infused tea and drink to relieve vascular headaches accompanied by vomiting.

Tea for digestive problems: ½ tsp. each of chamomile leaves, catnip flowers, fennel seed, and peppermint leaves. Pour 1 quart of boiling water over the herbs; steep for 10 minutes.

Anti-nausea headache tea: Simmer 1 tsp. fresh ginger in a pan of water for 7 minutes; steep for another 10 minutes.

For constipation, try this laxative tea: Mix 1 tsp. elder flower, 1 tsp. licorice root, 1 tsp. peppermint leaves, ½ tsp. fennel seed, and pour 3 cups boiling water over the herbs; steep for 10 minutes. Strain and then add ½ cup prune juice.

Mind Your Sleeping Habits

Since irregular or disrupted sleep patterns are known to trigger headaches, becoming aware of your sleeping patterns is a vital tool in any headache treatment strategy. The following guidelines should help.

Make sure you get enough sleep each night, whether your body needs 6, 8, or 10 hours.

Get up at the same time each day and avoid the temptation to wake up early or sleep late, especially on weekends and holidays.

Avoid daytime naps.

If you grind your teeth at night, consult a dentist to see about wearing a bite plate while you are sleeping at night and consult your practitioner regarding digestive problems and/or parasites.

Exercise during the day helps reduce your stress and contributes to better sleep.

Eat a healthy diet and avoid substances that affect serotonin levels, such as chocolate, caffeine, alcohol, and cheese.

Make sure to record your sleeping habits in your headache diary so you can learn more about the relationship between your headaches and your sleeping patterns.

In addition, be sure to watch the positions in which you sleep, since lying on your stomach or using too high a pillow can cause neck tension and spasm. You can purchase a special neck posture pillow or a sleeping bean, or combine a flat pillow for your head and a small, soft, rolled-up towel placed under your neck and lie on either your back or side.

Since many headaches go away within 8 hours, a good night's sleep may provide the relief you are looking for. Sleep relaxes you and eases your tense muscles, giving your blood vessels a break—that is, as long as you do not get too much of it.

HOMEOPATHY

The following are homeopathic remedies for various health problem categories, all of which can be contributing factors in headaches. Homeopathic remedies work best when prescribed by a qualified practitioner; when self-administered, these remedies should be taken only in doses of 6X or lower.

Stomach disorders—*Antimonium crudum* (inability to digest fats, especially milk); *Arsenicum album* (associated with eating foods that are too cold or fatty); *Bryonia* (acute head, eye, or forehead pain, especially on the left side, aggravated by movement, accompanied by nausea, constipation and irritability); *Calcarea phosphoricum, Iris versicolor* (migraine-like pain, vomiting, on either side of head, visual disturbances, occurring during downtime), *Ferrum phosphoricum* (congestion, vomiting, fatigue, face alternating between pale and cold to red and flushed, cold hands and feet); *Kali bichromicum* (migraine- or sinus-type pain, with pain in one spot, vomiting); *Lac canium* (pain changing sides during or from one attack to the next);

Notice Your Posture

The classic description of bad posture, slouching, round-shouldered, with a protruding belly, is only one type of postural distortion. Holding yourself rigidly upright can be just as hard on the body and contribute to just as many headaches, because it also requires a great deal of muscular tension. Since poor posture is a major cause of chronic muscle pain, correcting the way you hold your body can go a long way in preventing and relieving headaches.

Healthy posture features a spine with slight, front-to-back curvature and well-toned back muscles that are capable of maintaining and supporting this curve. Envision an invisible line coming down from the sky, and imagine that it passes from the top of your head, through the middle of your shoulders and down the center of your chest and pelvis.

It is important to stand upright and tall, yet relaxed, breathing steadily, with your head forward, your shoulders lowered and pulled back slightly, your belly and pelvis tucked in, and your knees slightly bent. Deviation from this position for prolonged periods can bring about muscle strain and headache.

The way you hold your body when you sit is also important, particularly if you spend many hours at a desk. Keep your weight on the points of the sitting bones (the pelvic bones that protrude through your buttocks while sitting), with your feet flat on the floor, your lower back pressed against the chair, shoulders lowered, and belly and pelvis tucked in. Imagine a string connecting your head, trunk, and pelvis in a straight line.

It may take time to correct your posture, but with commitment, you will soon start to notice that your energy is clearer, your body more relaxed and alert. Other things you can do to improve your posture include:

TAKING BREAKS: Whenever you are in the same position for many hours at a time, such as sitting at a computer all day, incorporate 2 minutes of stretching every couple of hours to prevent muscle strain.

DOING NECK AND SHOULDER ROLLS: Whether you are driving, sitting, or standing, this helps to relax tight muscles and rebalance posture.

EXERCISING.

EATING A HEALTHY DIET.

Lac defloratum (constipation); *Lachesis* (migraine-like pain, worse on the left side); *Lycopodium* (pain on right side, hypoglycemia, flatulence, nausea, and dizziness, worse in afternoon and evening); *Magnesium phosphoricum, Natrum carbonicum, Natrum sulphuricum* (throbbing head pain with diarrhea); *Nux vomica* (splitting pain upon waking or after overeating or drinking, sometimes with nausea, vomiting, irritability, and oversensitivity, also called the hangover remedy); *Phosphorus, Pulsatilla* (throbbing pain associated with indigestion of fatty foods); *Sepia* (overall digestive symptoms); *Venus merceneria* (overall digestive symptoms).

Circulatory Disorders—*Belladonna* (sudden and violent, throbbing pain, restlessness, congestion, red-flushed face); *Ferrum metallicum* (hammering, throbbing pain, red face, cold feet, usually associated with anemia); *Glonoinum* (throbbing, intolerance to heat and motion); *Gelsemium* (visual disturbances, eyeball pain, mental difficulties); *Sanguinaria canadensis* (throbbing, burning, shooting pain accompanied by redness in the cheeks, also migraine-like pain associated with menses); *Serotoninum* (sudden headaches accompanied by throbbing and sensations of heat); *Sulfur* (vascular-type headaches); *Veratrum viride* (headache with hypertension, red face, bloodshot eyes, heavy head).

Hormonal Imbalances—*Actae racemosa* (headaches proportionate to menses); Cyclamen (headaches associated with menstruation, accompanied by vertigo, and aggravated by fresh air); *Lachesis mutus* (premenstrual headaches, menopause); *Melilotus* (pain improved at onset of menstrual bleeding); *Natrum muriaticum* (headaches associated with menstruation, before, during, or after); *Pulsatilla* (throbbing headaches in women with light and less frequent periods); *Sepia* (overall digestive symptoms).

Allergy/Sensitivity or Toxicity Headaches—*Apis Mel* (puffy face); *Coca* (sudden climate, environmental, or lifestyle changes); *Natrum arsenicosum* (sensitivity to cigarette or tobacco smoke); *Gronoine* (throbbing pain that becomes intensified by heat or sun exposure).

Structural Misalignments and Trauma—*Actae racemosa*; *Arnica montana* (bruise-like ache, worsened by movement, associated with physical exhaustion or trauma); *Byronia*, *Calcarea carbonica* (physical overexertion); *Colocynthis*, *Natrum sulphuricum* (headache after injury); *Ranunculus bulbosus* (head pain associated with postural problems, pains in the back and side); *Rhus toxicodendron* (physical overexertion); *Silicea* (pain in the nape of the neck associated with nervous exhaustion).

Eyestrain or Other Eye Disturbances—*Aurum, Euphrasia* (watery, irritated eyes); *Gelsemium, Glonoin, Magnesia phosphorica* (blurred vision with dizziness); *Natrum muriaticum* (pain that comes after reading); *Onosmodium, Physostigma* (worsening of myopic sight); *Phosphorus prunus, Ruta grav, Sanguinaria* (dry, burning eyes); *Spigelia* (left-sided eye pain, fatigue and general disability).

Sinus Problems—*Allium cepa* (runny eyes and clear nasal discharge); *Arsenicum album, Belladonna, Dulcamara, Kali bichromatum, Lachesis, Phellandrium* (for relief from crushing head pain accompanied by burning sinuses and temples, light and sound intolerance); *Silicea* (pain in the nape of the neck associated with nervous exhaustion), *Thuja* (headaches on left side of face).

Mental Stress, Tension, and Anxiety—*Aconite* (at onset or when pain is severe); *Ammonium muriaticum* (depression, especially when exaggerated or unconsolable, restlessness, craving for sweets); *Anacardium orientale* (irritability, moodiness, intellectual overwork); *Argentium nitricum* (mental exertion); *Chamomilla, Coffea* (pain that feels like a nail driven through the back of the head, sometimes insomnia); *Gelsemium* (vague but distressing tension-type pain, associated with anxiety, droopy eyes, and visual disturbances, intensified with noise and movement); *Hura Braziliensis* (depression, suicidal thoughts, delusions, fear); *Ignatia* (hypersensitivity, highly emotional state, grieving, heavy, pressurized pain, sometimes nausea and dizziness); *Kali phosphoricum* (intellectual overwork, overall physical fatigue); *Lachesis, Natrum muriaticum* (developing after intense mental work, for those who are ambitious, driving and eager to achieve); *Nux vomica* (type-A personality, irritability and anxiety, overwork, too little sleep); *Phosphoricum acidum* (fatigue, nervous exhaustion, indifference to life); *Silica* (migraine-like pain that travels from neck to one eye, associated with nervous exhaustion, sometimes vomiting); *Staphysagria, Tuberculinum* (chronic tension headaches); *Zincum metallicum* (nervous and mental fatigue, aggravated by intellectual effort).

Migraine Specific—*Natrum mur* (general migraine); *Ignatia* (general

Your Carpets May Give You a Headache

Many people who are chemically-sensitive, highly allergic, or laid out with chronic fatigue syndrome often tell their physicians that they suspected that common household items, including carpets, were somehow poisoning them. Often doctors dismiss these associations as purely psychosomatic—in the patient's head. Now there is substantial scientific data to support the claims of patients. Your carpet may be bad for your health and you may be better off with bare hardwood floors.

Rosalind Anderson, Ph.D., of Anderson Laboratories in Dedham, Massachusetts, analyzed the effect of gas emissions on laboratory mice, based on over 300 carpet samples obtained through retail stores, carpet mills, or from patients' homes. All carpets had been in use from one week to 12 years and none were older than 40 years. To get her disturbing results, Dr. Anderson performed over 500 different experiments.

She found that carpet emissions decreased the breathing rate of mice immediately on contact, from a norm of 280 times per minute to a low, after 8 minutes of exposure, of 235. When the mice were removed from exposure to the carpet emissions, their respiration rates became normal again. Dr. Anderson next learned that one or more exposures by the mice to the carpet samples produced a range of alarming symptoms, including swollen face, hemorrhaging beneath the skin surface, altered posture, loss of balance, hyperactivity, tremors, limb paralysis, convulsions, even death.

Then she analyzed 125 carpet samples for signs of neurotoxicity, that is, emissions that harm brain cells or the nervous system. Dr. Anderson found that 90% produced at least one toxic effect and 60% produced 3 or more "severe neurotoxic effects" in at least 25% of the mice. Over 200 different chemicals have been identified in the typical modern carpet, says Dr. Anderson, and these can produce "diverse toxic effects" in humans including headaches (lasting up to 16 weeks), flu-like symptoms, muscle pain, fatigue, tremors, memory loss, and concentration difficulties. When it comes to negative health effects from carpets, "This is not a psychological phenomenon," says Dr. Anderson.

SOURCE— "Toxic Emissions from Carpets," Rosalind C. Anderson, Ph.D., *Journal of Nutritional & Environmental Medicine* 5:4 (1995), 375-386. Available from: Carfax Publishing Co., P.O. Box 25, Abingdon, Oxfordshire OX14 3UE, Great Britain.

migraine especially after emotional outburst); *Belladonna* (right-sided migraine); *Iris* (right-sided migraine with vomiting); *Lycopodium* (right-sided migraine when pain is worst from 4 to 8 p.m. and accompanied by excessive gas); *Pulsatilla* (right-sided migraine, worse from heat); *Sanguinaria* (right-sided headaches that occur around menstruation or when relief occurs after vomiting); *Cheladonium* (right-sided headaches with right-sided pains); *Lachesis* (left-sided migraines that are worse in the morning or just prior to menstruation); *Spigelia* (left-sided migraine, particularly when the head is sensitive to the touch and triggered by cold or wet weather).

For Headaches without Symptoms Characteristic of a Particular Remedy—*Aconitum nappellus* (taken at onset of any acute headache); *Apis mellifica* (migraines accompanied by swelling); *Secale cornutum* (migraines); *Serotoninum* (congestive headaches, particularly with unstable blood pressure).

ICE AND HEAT

One tried-and-true method that has been around for centuries is applying hot or cold packs. A steamy towel or a bag of ice may be enough to end your head pain. Heat works at the onset of a tension headache, while ice applied to the forehead at first sign of a migraine has been known to stop it from occurring, particularly if you imagine your hands getting warmer as the ice is applied. Ice packs or cold towels are also effective ways to get through the pain while you are waiting for herbs or other remedies to work.

Ice helps because it constricts blood vessels and reduces the sensitivity of painful nerve endings, but it is generally effective only when used at the first sign of a headache. Apply a flexible ice pack or cold gel pack directly onto the back of the neck, forehead, or temples so that it molds to your shape; leave on for about 20 to 30 minutes.

Heat is more effective as a soother than a reliever, but it feels good applied on tight neck muscles for 20 to 30 minutes. A hot shower massager also may bring some relief. Other relief techniques include taking a hot shower or bath with a warm washcloth draped over the back of your neck or with a cold washcloth on top of your head.

JOURNAL WRITING

Journal writing is an excellent way to release the frustrations that can accompany headaches. A journal is an ear that never gets tired of listening, and, no matter what you write, you will not be rejected or told to stop complaining. A journal gives you a chance to express how your headaches feel and to learn to be with whatever comes up, without judgment. Over time, journal writing provides perspective, helping you to see the emotions, patterns, images, and dramas that are linked to your headache; you can compare it to your headache diary to reveal patterns and events that you may not otherwise have considered. Furthermore, journal writing is a great excuse to take time for yourself.

All you need is a pen, some paper, and your thoughts. Write without worrying about whether you are saying anything important. You don't need good grammar or perfect spelling because all that matters in this exercise is that you are open and honest about your feelings and thoughts. As you reach to the healer within, you'll be surprised at how much you have to say—and how good it feels to write it.

LIFESTYLE CHANGES

No matter what kinds of alternative practitioners you consult, chances are they will tell you that the only way to find lasting relief from your headaches is to look closely at your life and let go of or change the things that are not serving your mind and body. Depending as much on your personality as on your condition, this could be as simple as throwing away your cigarettes, eating better, starting an exercise program, finding a creative outlet, learning how to express your emotions, or getting a dog to walk every night.

Your life is a series of choices, some of them healthy, others unhealthy—only you know what makes you feel good. It may not be necessary to give up all of your vices and bad habits, but it is important to strive for moderation. Once you make the commitment to finding your personal balance, you will be amazed at the peace of mind you experience the more you achieve that balance. Soon, you will find that changes have helped not only to take your mind off your headaches but to take the ache out of your head altogether.

MASSAGE

Sometimes a headache strikes when there is no one around to give you a massage. So, rather than sitting around in pain until your bodyworker or your massage buddy has a free hour, you can learn a few simple techniques for giving yourself a massage. Remember, you do not have to wait for your next headache to try these techniques, as many of them are designed simply to help relax your head, shoulders, and neck, the areas where you hold the most tension.

Why not try waking up to a light shoulder massage or ending your day with a few neck rubs to release your worries before you go to sleep? The following are a few examples of effective techniques for administering your own relief.

To give yourself the feeling of being pampered by a massage, dim the lights and play soft, meditative, or relaxing music before you perform the techniques described below.

Carotid Artery Massage

This helps to relieve brain congestion and stimulate the stomach meridian, relieving headaches associated with digestion problems, congestion, high blood pressure, and stress. Located on both sides of the neck, the carotid arteries can be found by finding your carotid pulse, which is located at the spot between the Adam's apple and the neck muscles just below the jaw. Using 4 fingers, massage the arteries one at a time, gently stroking from the jawbone down.

Neck and Shoulder Massage

Start by sitting in a chair with your head tipped back slightly (to relax the muscles), cradle the back of your neck with your hand, and squeeze it gently, moving from the base of your skull downward. After 5 squeezes (approximately 30 seconds), increase the pressure and repeat. To massage the shoulder, grab the shoulder with the right hand and knead toward the neck, first lightly, then deeply. Reverse hands and grasp the other shoulder, and repeat. With both of these techniques, find the most sensitive, tender parts of the muscles (often the place where the neck and shoulders meet) and press steadily for up to a minute until the pain begins to modify or ease.

Sinus Massage

If your headache is accompanied by sinus-type symptoms, try this simple massage. With your thumb and index finger, use a circular motion to gently massage the bridge of your nose for about 30 seconds. Next, take your

Heavy Metal Food

Researchers at McGill University in Montreal have confirmed that you can help your body neutralize radiation and lead, mercury, and cadmium poisoning by eating algin, a derivative of kelp, which can be found in many health food stores and in products containing magnesium alginate, sodium alginate, and other alginates.

If you specifically suspect that you are being exposed to lead or want to protect yourself in any case, John Miller, Ph.D. suggests eating $1/4$ to $1/2$ cup of vegetarian baked beans daily. The sulfhydryl substance in baked beans helps chelate the lead for more efficient removal from the body. Dr. Miller recommends the following sugar-free applesauce as an excellent remedy for mercury exposure.

Mercury-busting Applesauce

- 5 apples (with peels if organic, otherwise peeled)
- $1/2$ cup water or apple juice
- cinnamon to taste

Hollow out the apples and cut them into small pieces. Place all ingredients in a medium saucepan and cook over medium heat until soft. Mash with fork.

Constipation

Since many chronic diseases often begin with constipation (along with its close cousin, headaches), a change in eating habits is one of the best defenses against further damage and the onset of more debilitating illnesses. Here are some steps you can take to prevent constipation.

- Eat a 60/40 diet in which 60% of your total food consumption is fruits and vegetables, and the remaining 40% is composed of 20% carbohydrates, 15% proteins, and 5% fats.

- Eat more alkaline foods, such as fruits and vegetables, rather than acidic foods, such as meats, dairy products, and sugars; alkaline foods have a natural laxative effect.

- Include more raw foods and water-retaining foods (leafy greens, apples, carrots, and melons) and fiber (grains, psyllium, fruit pectin, and vegetable fibers) in your diet to keep your stool soft and bulky.

- Drink 6 to 8 glasses of purified water each day to aid bowel function and flush out toxins.

- Don't hold in your bowel movement; go when nature calls.

- Drink prune juice or herbal teas with a laxative effect.

- Get some form of exercise every day, preferably in the morning, either before or after breakfast.

- Take an acidophilus supplement to add bulk and ease elimination.

- Try taking an Epsom salt bath; the salts increase circulation and relax tension, allowing for a natural bowel movement.

thumb and press into the area along the brow line where your nose meets your forehead and hold with a steady pressure for about 15 seconds. Finally, move up a little bit, halfway to the center of your forehead, and, again using a circular motion, massage for about 30 seconds.

MEDITATION

This self-help tool has been around for thousands of years, and it is one of the most effective ways to experience unity of mind, body, and spirit. To put it simply, meditation is an activity or exercise that anchors your mind in the present moment, which is particularly helpful for those with headaches. When suffering from head pain, you have a tendency to live in a contracted sense of time, minutes seeming to take hours to pass. Meditation is designed to lift you from the chattering of the mind. When you are not dwelling on the past or anticipating the future, your sense of timelessness expands, allowing you to enter a state in which it instead takes minutes for hours to pass.

Meditation has been credited with a broad range of benefits, both physiological and psychological. It can reduce stress, tension, and pain, regulate blood pressure and pulse, enhance immune functioning, and alleviate the accompanying effects of terminal illnesses. Over the last few decades, scientific studies on meditation have been so overwhelmingly positive and conclusive that M.D.s are joining the ranks of alternative therapists in suggesting it to their patients.

Since there are many styles of meditation, it should be easy for you to find one that matches your needs—the one you find the most relaxing and enjoyable. The 2 main branches of meditation are concentrative meditation and mindfulness mediation. Concentrative medication is like sharpening your mind into the fine point of a pencil. This can be done by focusing on the breath, a sound (mantra), an image, or anything else that allows you to selectively attune your mind into a state of quiet clarity.

The second style, mindfulness meditation, is more like stretching your mind to encompass everything in the universe. This is accomplished by staying objectively detached as you watch the ever-rolling movie of thoughts, worries, sensations, images, feelings, sounds, smells, amusements, and distractions that pass through your mind. The idea is not to get caught up in any of them, but to see them all appear and dissolve in the constant ebb and flow of awareness.

Doing stretching or breathing exercises before meditating helps prepare the mind for quiet sitting. It is best if you sit up straight, either cross-legged on a cushion or in a chair with both feet flat against the floor. Your eyes can be either open or closed (open helps to keep you alert; closed helps to block out distractions). You may also lie down, but realize that it is easier to fall asleep this way. It is generally best to meditate on an empty stomach, since the digestive process can make you sleepy.

NUTRITIONAL THERAPY

In a society in which a candy bar is as easy to find as an apple, it is no wonder people are suffering from chronic illnesses. Good health is not fully possible without good nutrition. In today's world of fast food and packaged convenience, it is becoming harder and harder to eat quality, nutrient-dense food. One USDA study reveals that a significant portion of the population consumes less than 70% of the recommended daily allowance of C and B-complex vitamins and the essential minerals calcium and magnesium—all nutrients involved in the prevention of headaches.

Good nutrition can be approached as 3 D's: detection, detoxification, and diet. Detection, through such methods as an elimination diet or kinesiology allergy testing, is the first step in ridding yourself of diet-related headaches, since it enables you to discover what in your diet is triggering your headaches. Second, you must cleanse your body of the offending substance, through such methods as juice therapy (discussed below) or

Detoxification Therapy (see Chapter 17, An A-Z of Alternative Medicine). Finally, you need to provide your body with the best possible fuel through dietary changes, juice therapy, and nutritional supplements.

Dietary Changes

The single, easiest headache factor you can control is your diet. The following is a reminder of some of the dietary changes that will help you to realize relief from your headaches.

- Limit or eliminate alcohol and caffeine consumption.
- Avoid all trigger foods.
- Check all foods for food additives, and avoid those which contain them.
- Don't overeat; it interferes with digestion and creates an enlarged, overworked liver.
- Vary your food choices: too much of one thing can be toxic to the liver and gallbladder, especially if this substance is alcohol, chemicals, drugs, fats, fried oils, or meat.
- Drink lots of water: Not only does this prevent constipation and dehydration-related headaches, but it also flushes out toxins.
- Eat more fiber to stimulate digestion and improve the efficiency of the bowels.
- Avoid junk food, sugar, and refined carbohydrates, which cause blood sugar levels to soar, then crash, making headaches worse.
- Limit fat intake, especially greasy, fried foods, since fat is difficult to digest and can cause stomachaches and headaches.
- Eat plenty of raw fruits and vegetables.
- Supplement your diet with herbs and vitamins.

Sample Elimination Diet

The following diet can help you discover whether your headaches are related to your diet. This type of elimination diet is generally used for 3 to 6 weeks as a trial. However, we have listed it here only as a suggestion, since dietary requirements can vary considerably depending upon your specific needs and sensitivities. To get maximum benefit from an elimination diet, it is wise to consult with your practitioner before beginning.

BREAKFAST

- Lemon juice and water
- One piece of fruit (pear, apple, kiwi)
- Warm oatmeal, granola (sugar free, wheat-free, corn-free) or rice cereal with rice or soy milk, and/or wheat-free muffin or one slice of pure rye, rice, or spelt (*Triticum spelta*, a type of wheat) bread

SNACK

- Unsalted nuts or sunflower seeds

LUNCH

- Choice of raw mixed vegetable salad with lemon and oil dressing (no corn oil) or broiled chicken, tuna, salmon, trout, or halibut on a bed of fresh lettuce
- ½ to 1 cup whole grain (rice, millet, quinoa, spelt, amaranth, or buckwheat) or 2 slices of pure rye, rice, or spelt bread (you can use vegetables and broiled meat to make a sandwich if you wish)

SNACK

- One glass of fresh vegetable juice (carrot, beet, celery, or green mix) or goat milk yogurt

DINNER

- A light meal of vegetable salad or stir-fried vegetables with

Supplements for Headache Relief and Prevention

Before starting any B vitamin therapy, begin taking between 50 and 100 mg a day of B complex, since taking extra doses of the isolated B vitamin can upset the overall balance of B vitamins.

Vitamin B2 (thiamin)—up to 400 mg daily (migraine, cluster, allergy/sensitivity)

Vitamin B3 (niacin or niacinamide)—50 to 250 mg (time-released) once a day with meal (migraine, cluster, allergy/sensitivity, tension)

To abort a vascular headache attack, take a 50 to 300 mg niacin tablet (not time-released niacin or niacinamide) at the first sign of headache and lie down immediately afterward. Try one more dose if you do not feel the flush within 20 minutes. This works best on an empty stomach.

Vitamin B5 (pantothenic acid)—50 to 200 mg daily

Vitamin B6 (pyridoxine)—100 to 200 mg daily

Vitamin C—1,000 to 3,000 mg daily (general, migraine, cluster, allergy/sensitivity)

Vitamin E—200 to 800 IU daily (general, migraine, tension)

Calcium—1,000 to 2,000 mg daily

Chromium—50 to 100 mg twice a day (digestion, food allergy)

Magnesium—300 to 400 mg daily (vascular, tension, migraine, hormonal)

Potassium—100 mg daily (hypoglycemic)

Zinc—30 to 50 mg daily (hypoglycemic)

Acidophilus—200 to 300 mg up to 3 times per day (digestion, food allergy)

Essential Fatty Acids (EFA)—2 grams each of EPA, GLA, and flaxseed oils or 3 to 4 mg of fish oil, evening primrose oil, or black currant oil daily (vascular, migraine, hormonal, allergy/sensitivity)

The Braly Supplement Plan for Headache Sufferers

In addition to a basic multivitamin, James Braly, M.D., of Fort Lauderdale, Florida, recommends taking the following supplements daily:

Vitamin C—2 to 8 g divided into 3 doses

Vitamin E—400 to 800 IU

Niacinamide (a form of vitamin B3)—500 mg

Calcium/Magnesium—600 mg of each

Evening Primrose Oil—3 to 4 capsules at breakfast and again at dinner

DL-phenylalanine (an amino acid)—275 mg 2 to 3 times daily between meals

chicken or fish or whole grains (rice, millet, quinoa, spelt, amaranth, or buckwheat) with steamed vegetables

SNACK

- Raw pumpkin or sunflower seeds and/or rye or rice crackers

Over the past 10 to 15 years, the American public has become increasingly aware of the important connection between food and health. Books advocating one diet plan or another fill bookstore shelves, but rarely do they address the importance of dietary individualization. A diet that is healthy for one person may not be so for someone else. A nutritionist, naturopath, Ayurvedic doctor, or other practitioner can help you determine the diet that is best suited to your particular constitution and nutritional needs. However, a few dietary guidelines are healthful for everyone:

- **Feed your body good, high-quality food.** This means reading labels carefully and avoiding foods that have been processed, chemicalized, or refined. Buying organic and only choosing fruits and vegetables in season is the best way to ensure that you are getting the healthiest food available.

- **Eat 5 or more servings of fruits and vegetables daily.** Both conventional and alternative doctors agree that fruits and vegetables are an excellent source of vitamins, minerals, and fiber. (Fiber is essential because it not only prevents and relieves constipation, but escorts excess estrogen out of the body via the stool.) To get a wide range of nutrients, choose different varieties and colors of produce.

- **Increase your intake of raw foods.** The nutritional value of raw foods is higher than that of cooked foods and raw foods require less work to digest, freeing extra energy for other processes. However, some people cannot handle the intensity of raw foods. If that is the case, be sure not to overcook your food and avoid microwaving, which lowers the nutitional value even more.

- **Get your protein from vegetable sources whenever possible.**
  While it is unnecessary to quit, as it were, cold turkey, a plant-based, vegetarian diet is preferable to eating meat. One of the primary reasons for this is that animal products are laden with antibiotics, growth hormones, and other drugs, as well as pesticides from the heavily-sprayed foods they are fed; plant products, on the other hand, especially if organically grown, are far less contaminated. Furthermore, animal products tend to be high in fat, which can increase the toxicity of the chemicals that are lodged in them, rendering them even more hazardous. A 1995 study published by the Physicians Committee for Responsible Medicine shows that medical costs directly attributable to meat consumption are between $28 and $61 billion.[7] Legumes, soy products, and grain and vegetable combinations are excellent sources of plant-based proteins.

- **Eat more complex carbohydrates.** Foods such as grains, vegetables, seeded breads, and pasta are dense, nutrient-rich sources of calories. Because they provide bulk and fiber, they are also more filling, leaving you more satisfied and less inclined to overeat. Complex carbohydrates also tend to decrease sugar cravings.

- **Make sure your oils are of the polyunsaturated variety.**
  Sunflower, safflower, corn, grape seed, olive, sesame, and flaxseed oils contain essential fatty acids, which are "good" fats that help keep the blood healthy.

Juice Therapy

Like an intravenous injection of living nutrients, drinking raw juice floods the system with easily digestible nutrients. When a fruit or vegetable is juiced, the fibrous cell wall is cut open, releasing all the material from the cell, including vitamins, proteins, enzymes, minerals, carbohydrates, sugars, and other nutrients. Juice allows you to consume all these nutrients without all the mass, meaning you can drink a quart of carrot juice and get the benefits of 5 pounds of carrots.

Moreover, drinking fruit and vegetable juice does much more than supplement your diet, for juices are also powerful antioxidants and detoxifiers, particularly when incorporated in a fasting program. Juices strengthen your immune system, help carry away toxins, and reduce blood pressure.

Since many juices have a high sugar content and ferment rapidly once they reach the stomach, persons with hypoglycemia should drink juices only with food. In any event, juices are best diluted with an equal part of water. Vegetable juices are used more frequently in fasting because they have less sugar and a higher vitamin and mineral content; however, fruit juices are easier for the body to absorb.

When making juice at home, use fresh, organic fruits and vegetables and drink the juice immediately after making it. If you purchase juices, it is best to buy them at a health food store on the same day they were made. The following juices are particularly beneficial to those with headaches relating to allergies or digestive disorders:

- **Carrot/beet/celery**—This delicious combination provides a rich source of important nutrients, including beta carotene, vitamin C, vitamin E, folic acid, antioxidants, potassium, magnesium, and other minerals.

- **Wheat grass**—The grass grown from wheatberries is rich in chlorophyll, a substance nearly identical to the hemoglobin (the body's oxygen carrier) in human blood, thus it helps to oxygenate the cells and aid in the detoxification process. This sweet green juice is pressed from freshly cut, young wheat plants and contains over 100 vitamins, minerals, and other nutrients. Wheat grass has 60 times more vitamin C than oranges, and 8 times more iron than spinach. It contains all of the 8 essential amino acids, plus 11 others, as well as the vitamin compounds called bioflavonoids that are believed able to neutralize toxic substances. It also stimulates and regulates the bowels.

- **Apple**—An apple a day becomes much more potent when consumed as a juice. It provides a gentle, natural laxative.

- **Apple/ginger/carrot**—This juice is excellent for digestive worries or constipation; because of ginger's strong flavor, it is best to start off with only a little ginger until you are used to its taste.

- **Tomato/celery/onion**—When made in a ratio of 2 parts tomatoes, 1 part celery, and 2 teaspoons onion and taken a cup at a time every 2 hours, this juice can mitigate a headache attack associated with fatigue, nervous tension, hangover, or stomach problems.

- **Aloe vera juice**—Three to 4 ounces diluted in water and taken 15 to 20 minutes before mealtime will aid digestion.
- **Carrot / celery, carrot / beet / cucumber or carrot / celery /spinach/parsley:** These are other good juice combinations.

Nutritional Supplements

Vitamins, minerals, and other nutrients are vital to good health because they help to regulate metabolism, assist in the processes that carry energy throughout the body, and defend against the damages of drugs, alcohol, and chemical and environmental pollutants. Because research suggests that many people with headaches are nutrient-deficient, vitamin and mineral supplements can help to fill the void and accelerate the body's return to health.

An estimated 46% of Americans are taking nutritional supplements. Many health practitioners, however, believe that they are not really effective because most people do not assimilate them properly. Some supplements may even cause potential risks if taken over prolonged periods. Therefore, to get the most benefit from nutritional supplementation, it is wise to have your diet analyzed to determine what is lacking and exactly what will be most beneficial in healing your headaches. Although megadoses can be helpful, they are advisable only under the care of a qualified nutritionist because excessive intake of any nutrient, defined as more than 300% of the Recommended Daily Allowance (RDA), can affect functioning or cause secondary deficiencies.

When choosing among the many products on the market today, it is

In a 1995 study conducted at the New York Headache Center, 40 patients suffering from acute migraines underwent intravenous magnesium sulfate treatment (1 g over a period of 5 minutes). Patients who had low pre-treatment levels of magnesium responded better, with lasting relief occurring in 865 of the cases, while 16% of those with normal pre-treatment levels responded favorably. In all, 35 of the 40 participants said they experienced a complete reduction in head pain within 15 minutes, and complete relief occurring in 9 cases. Almost none had any pain recurrence over the next 24 hours.[8] Another study found that the migraines of 80% of the women tested disappeared after they supplemented their diet with daily magnesium.[9]

CAUTION

Before taking any nutritional supplement in doses beyond recommended amounts, visit a qualified practitioner such as a nutritionist, naturopath, or traditional Chinese medical doctor to receive individualized guidance. This ensures that you gain maximum benefit from the supplements you purchase and avoid any allergic or toxic reactions.

best to purchase natural rather than synthetic supplements. Although laboratory vitamins and minerals mimic the properties of the real thing, many of them also contain artificial colorings, sugars, coal tars, preservatives, and other additives. The last thing you want to ingest is another substance that makes your body work more than it has to. Buy hypoallergenic and yeast-free supplements whenever possible.

Unless specified otherwise, vitamins and minerals should be taken with meals. Water-soluble vitamins, such as B complex and C, are generally taken between or after meals, while fat-soluble vitamins, such as E, as well as the essential fatty acids, should be taken before meals. Mineral supplements should be taken with the meal containing the least fiber, since fiber decreases mineral absorption. Amino acids should be taken on an empty stomach an hour before or after a meal.

If you are taking high doses of any nutritional supplement, divide them into smaller doses you can take throughout the day. Always drink plenty of water to prevent nausea and other side effects; if you still get nauseated, try taking supplements in a liquid form, diluted in juice or water.

Weight, body type, age, activity level, health conditions, hereditary proclivities, and actual nutritional needs are all factors in determining the proper dosage of any supplement. For example, if you are small in stature and weight, you may want to decrease the recommended dosage; on the other hand, older people may want to take more than the suggested amount to compensate for the fact that, with age, the digestive track loses its ability to absorb nutrients. Pregnancy, stress, hospitalization, surgery, competitive sports, and depression can also affect dosage levels.

Essential Vitamins

Basic Multiple Vitamin: A daily multiple vitamin can help to make sure that you will not become imbalanced in other vitamins. However, pay attention to the RDA amounts of each vitamin and factor that into your dosage of supplemental nutrients.

Vitamin A: Although it can be toxic or trigger headaches if taken in excess, if taken in sensible, daily recommended amounts, vitamin A can be particularly healing to mucous membranes in sinuses and to eyes, skin, and general health (sinus, migraine, allergy/sensitivity, cluster, vascular).

B complex: B vitamins are among the most helpful supplements for headache sufferers. They help the body cope with stress and help metabolize food into usable energy. The following B vitamins are especially important for the prevention of headaches, particularly migraines and other headaches related to blood vessel constriction and immune suppression.

B2 (thiamin) helps prevent headaches through a mechanism involved in cell energy production. In one study, 49 recurrent migraine sufferers were given 400 mg a day with breakfast for 3 months, after which the average number of migraine attacks fell by 67% and migraine severity improved by 68%.[10]

B3 (niacin or niacinamide) dilates blood vessels, sometimes causing a side effect of hot and itchy skin known as the "niacin flush," and can help prevent a vascular headache brought on by constricted blood vessels. B3 can also help ease depression and anxiety, especially when they are attributable to blood sugar fluctuations. A 1979 report showed that, in high doses, the effects of B3 actually resemble those of anti-anxiety drugs such as Valium, Xanax, and Librium, suggesting that B3 can be used as a preventative as well. To self-administer, take 50 to 200 mg in a time-release capsule once a day with meals, or as much as 1,000 mg a day when under the guidance of a medical professional.

B5 (pantothenic acid) strengthens the adrenal glands, helps to stabilize the production of hormones, and is involved in food metabolism and cell energy release.

B6 (pyridoxine) enhances the production of neurotransmitters and acts as a natural diuretic. Therefore, it is effective in vascular-type headaches and those that are related to water retention, such as hormonal or allergy/sensitivity headaches. B6 is also believed to ease the withdrawal period of rebound headache sufferers. B6 can cause nerve damage in doses over 500 mg daily, but discontinue taking it if you experience any negative effects at a smaller dosage.

Vitamin C: Aiding in the body's natural detoxification process, this protective antioxidant offers relief for headache sufferers, especially when headaches are related to food allergies or toxic contamination. Vitamin C also acts as an antihistamine, helps the body to absorb other nutrients, and boosts the immune system.

Vitamin E: Vitamin E lubricates circulation, reduces platelet clustering, improves blood flow, stops inflammation, and enhances the immune system, partly because it protects cell membranes from the destructive effects of oxygen and thereby increases the life expectancy of cells. If you have high blood pressure or are allergy-prone (especially if allergic to wheat, since Vitamin E capsules are often prepared with wheat germ oil), see a nutritionist.

Essential Minerals

Calcium: Calcium relaxes blood vessels, and calms muscle tension, and helps to ensure that nerves are effectively sending their messages throughout the body. This makes calcium a good preventative when taken in normal amounts (between 1,000 to 2,000 mg daily), but it can also provide an abortive effect when taken in megadoses (up to 4,000 mg a day, although not recommended unless under the supervision of a knowledgeable practitioner). When taken with vitamin D, calcium also serves to prevent PMS and hormonally related headaches. Chelated forms of calcium are the most usable.

Chromium: Very difficult to derive from foods, this mineral is especially effective for headaches associated with blood sugar fluctuations because it stabilizes insulin production, thereby regulating the body's ability to convert and process glucose for energy. Either chromium picolinate or chromium nicotinate should be taken by those with food sensitivities because these forms are yeast free.

Copper: Copper helps to produce, operate, and break down the brain chemicals that cause blood vessels to dilate and constrict. This explains why foods that contain high levels of copper (chocolate, nuts, wheat germ, and shellfish), foods that increase the intestinal absorption of copper (citrus fruits), and foods that bind and transport copper (MSG) have all been implicated in headaches. Studies have shown that people with abnormal copper metabolism are especially sensitive to these trigger foods and are thus more likely to get headaches and/or suffer from anemia.

Iodine: Iodine deficiencies can cause headaches because iodine regulates the metabolic rate, enzyme system, fat metabolism, and sodium-potassium ratio. Besides headaches, symptoms of an iodine deficiency include feeling cold, particularly in the hands and feet, constipation, exhaustion, tendency to gain weight, PMS, memory lapses, and depression. The standard dose of iodine is 50 to 300 mg a day, but since it can cause indigestion or skin problems in sensitive people, dietary sources of iodine are also recommended, such as cod liver oil, haddock, shrimp, perch, halibut, kelp, chard, turnip greens, cantaloupe, sunflower seeds, and sea salt.

Iron: Iron is essential to red blood cell synthesis, oxygen transport, and energy production through food metabolism. When iron is deficient, the amount of blood and oxygen that flows into the brain decreases, leading to headaches and fatigue. Dosages tend to be between 10 and 30 mg of iron a day, taken along with Vitamin C to increase iron absorption.

Be careful when taking iron because excess iron can blacken stools and cause stomachaches and constipation. A better source of iron comes from eating iron-rich foods, such as kelp, blackstrap molasses, lecithin, pumpkin seeds, sesame seeds, sunflower seeds, pistachio nuts, walnuts, almonds, oats, millet, and parsley.

Magnesium: As American soils become continuously depleted of magnesium, the daily intake of magnesium has decreased, from 450 to 485 mg per day in the early 1900s to between 185 and 235 per day today, even though the RDA is at least 350 mg daily. Because magnesium helps to regulate blood vessel dilation as well as neurotransmitter and enzymatic responses to pain, deficiencies in this important mineral have been linked to headaches, especially those related to vascular irregularities and hormonal imbalances. Magnesium thins the blood and tones and relaxes blood vessels, thus calming overall muscle tension.

Although relief from acute attacks comes primarily with magnesium administered intravenously (often mixed with calcium, vitamin C, and B12 for better absorption and use within the body), oral doses can be a good preventative as long as the supplement is chelated and a highly absorbable form, such as brands with high concentrates of elemental magnesium like magnesium orotate, magnesium apartrate, magnesium citrate, or taurate.

Potassium: Besides soothing nerves, potassium balances sodium assimilation, thus helping to prevent excess water retention, a source of undue pressure on the brain. Headaches and other conditions related to hypoglycemia are remedied by potassium intake, since potassium is depleted by low blood sugar. Take 100 mg daily or make a potassium tonic: wash and place an assortment of seasonal, organic vegetables, skins and all, in a large pot of cold water. Cover the pot and bring the water to a full boil, then simmer for 8 to 10 minutes. When the mixture cools, strain the liquid into a glass container. Drink one cup a day, refrigerating the rest.

Zinc: This essential mineral is involved in many enzymatic processes and reactions, including those regulating digestion and insulin production, making it especially useful for headaches related to hypoglycemia.

Headache sufferers and hypoglycemics are often low in serum zinc. But since excessive zinc can cause copper deficiencies, a daily dose of zinc should not exceed 30 to 50 mg.

Lipids

Essential fatty acids (EFA): Essential fatty acids are vitamin-like compounds that cannot be made in the body but must be ingested through the foods you eat. Your body needs EFAs because without them, your organs cannot manufacture prostaglandins, substances that are key regulators of immune, digestive, cardiovascular, and reproductive functions. Furthermore, cell membranes consist mainly of lipids (fats), and since lipids are highly susceptible to free-radical damage, EFAs help to protect against this damage. EFAs also help thin the blood and prevent blood clots from forming and aid in reducing the release of serotonin.

Research has shown that EFA supplementation is effective in reducing headaches. Charles Glueck, M.D., and Timothy McCarren, M.D., of the University of Cincinnati College of Medicine conducted a study in which participants taking 15 grams of a fish oil preparation containing EPA each day cut the incidence of severe migraines in half, while lessening the pain and severity of each attack. Interestingly, men were shown to benefit more from fish oil than women.

Supplemental forms of EFAs include omega-3 fatty acid EPA and DHA found in fish oils, linoleic acid, GLA (gamma-linolenic acid), evening primrose oil, borage oil, hemp seed oil, and flaxseed oil. EPA, DHA, GLA, and evening primrose oil are especially good for vascular-type headaches, as well as any headache related to hormones or allergy/sensitivity problems. Two grams each of EPA, GLA, and flaxseed oils is a common recommendation, although 3 to 4 mg of fish oil daily with meals, and/or adding fatty fish, like salmon, tuna, and mackerel to your diet can produce longer term benefits to brain chemistry. (The fishy smell of fish oil tablets is mitigated by refrigerating them.) Cod liver oil is not recommended because of its high Vitamin A content.

Other Useful Nutrients

Acidophilus: A beneficial bacteria naturally found in the intestine, acidophilus acts as an antibiotic, fights yeast infections, and helps to improve overall intestinal health. It is particularly important for those whose headaches are related to digestive-tract disturbances, such as food allergies, candida, constipation, and overeating, and toxic contamination, especially from pharmaceutical drugs. Since the directions for acidophilus vary, with some requiring dosage 30 minutes before a meal and others 30 to 60 minutes after a meal, be sure to read directions carefully. Although acidophilus is available in freeze-dried forms, it is better to buy the form that requires refrigeration. There are several types of acidophilus, so try alternating several types (for example, acidophilus bifidus and laterospore).

Blue-Green Algae: Two capsules daily of this potent supplement provides a super protein that gives you sustainable energy and without the crash of rebound that stimulants such as caffeine involve. Blue-green algae is loaded with folic acid, pantothenic acid, biotin, essential fatty acids, vitamins, and minerals. Studies have shown that it helps liver detoxification by facilitating the elimination of pharmaceutical drugs and mercury. It also fosters the growth of healthy intestinal bacteria.

Bioflavonoids: Generally derived from citrus fruits, these are highly soluble natural antioxidants which help to increase the absorption of vitamin C. Take between 500 and 1,500 mg a day.

Choline: Research has shown that some people who suffer from chronic headaches have low blood levels of the nonessential nutrient choline, particularly those with cluster headaches. Choline is also a good platelet inhibitor, particularly when taken with omega-3 fatty acids and fish oils. Take 500-1,000 mg daily.

Coenzyme Q10: A close relative of B complex, this nonessential nutrient improves oxygenation, supports metabolism, and helps to convert food into cellular energy. Take 30 mg twice a day.

Pycnogenol: This special class of bioflavonoid is derived either from grape seeds or from the maritime pine. Studies have shown that as an antioxidant it is 20 times more powerful than vitamin C and 50 times more powerful than vitamin E. It is especially beneficial for liver protection and blood vessel tone. Take between 25 and 50 mg twice a day.

REFLEXOLOGY

Headache Relief in Your Hands and Feet

When giving yourself a foot reflexology treatment, your feet should be bare and elevated just slightly above the body; the best way to do this is to sit in a comfortable position and cross one knee over the other. When working with areas on the hands, rest the receiving hand comfortably in your lap and stimulate with the other hand. As you massage, use your index fingers and the flat parts of your thumb, pressing firmly, rubbing into each reflex area for at least 10 seconds.

Especially tender areas denote sensitivities or weakness in their cor-

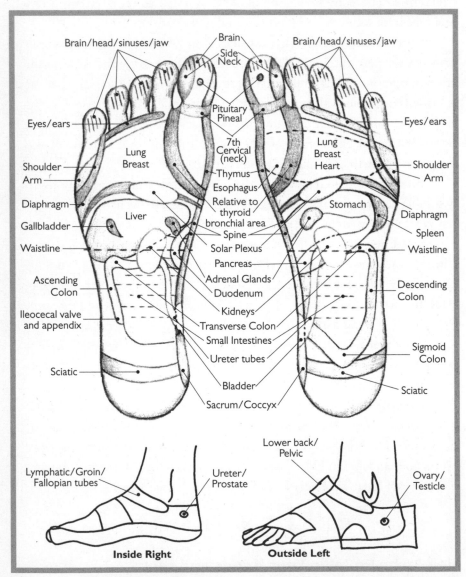

Figure 16.2—Reflexology areas of the feet.

responding organs; don't worry, this is a normal discovery in reflexology. As you move from area to area, maintain contact with your skin by sliding your fingers rather than lifting them. Make sure that you balance your treatment by repeating whatever you did on the other foot and/or hand.

The following areas are the most effective for headaches and their underlying causes. While they are generally used for emergency relief, regular reflexology in these areas can also selectively strengthen and build up weak areas of the body.

Brain: all headaches, circulation, and overall body function

Head: all headaches, stress, shoulder and neck tension

Pituitary: hormones, allergy/sensitivity, digestive, migraine, cluster: regulates all the hormones in the body

Sinuses: sinus, allergy

Eyes: vision, stress

Heart: vascular, circulation, hypertension

Jaw: stress, TMJ

Neck: tension, physical and emotional stress

Arms and shoulders: physical and emotional stress and muscle tension

See Chapter 17, An A-Z of Alternative Medicine, Reflexology, for general information on how reflexology works.

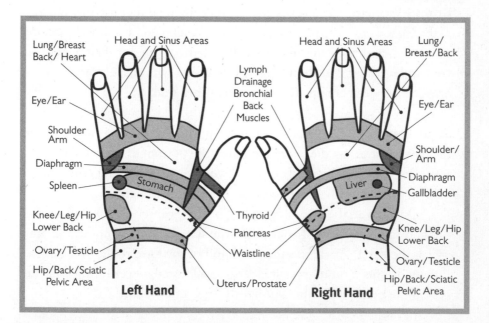

Figure 16.3—Reflexology areas on the hands.

Spine: all headaches, trauma, stress, tension, digestion

Solar Plexus: all headaches, stress, anxiety, digestion

Adrenal Gland: hypertension, hormones, digestion, toxicity

Stomach: digestion, sensitivity/allergy, migraine

Pancreas: hypoglycemia, digestion

Intestines: digestion, sensitivity/allergy, migraine

Kidney: vascular, allergy/sensitivity, toxicity, migraine

Liver: digestion, circulation, toxicity

Reproductive: menstrual disorders, hormones

The brain, the solar plexus, and the spine are intricately involved in the mechanism of head pain, no matter what the underlying cause. The brain controls all of the neurological functions of your body; the solar plexus, the nerve network that connects the trunk and limbs, functions as the brain's middle manager, overseeing and directing many of the body's functions; and the spine is the body's lifeline, relaying information to and from the brain like a highly sophisticated switchboard. Because of the intimate connection among these 3 areas of the body, you should begin every reflexology session by working on these 3 areas.

Brain—Work the brain reflex area by stimulating either the tips and pads of the big toe or the tip pads of the thumb, working one at a time, by pulling, squeezing, and rhythmically massaging them gently but firmly between your index finger and thumb. Do this 7 times without letting up on the pressure between counts. Repeat on the other side.

Solar Plexus—On the hands, the solar plexus corresponds to a point on the palm, just below the fleshy mound at the bottom of the middle finger; stimulate this point by pressing it with your thumb; as you do this the fingers on the hand will start to curl but keep them straight.

On the feet, the solar plexus point is in the center of each foot, around the bottom of the ball of your foot; stimulate the foot point in the same way as the hand. Working either the hand or the foot, rotate your pressed thumb; do this 7 times, pressing harder each time, never lifting your finger off the point but letting up slightly after each count.

Spine—On the hands, the spine reflexes are located along the inside edge, extending from the top of the thumb all the way down to the wrist; when working the hands, start at the thumbnail and work your way down in one steady motion.

On the feet, the spine corresponds to the inside ridge of the foot, all the way from the tip of the big toe to the end of the foot; work the feet in the same fashion as the hands, starting at the toenail and working your way to the edge of the heel. Work either your hands or feet and do this exercise 7 times, increasing the pressure of your touch each time; repeat on the other foot or hand.

RELAXATION EXERCISES

Taking time out every day to do something you love is a great way to relax. Whether it is lying down in a dark room, making a big pot of soup, soaking in a hot bath with candles, or listening to your favorite CD, relaxation helps you to handle your stress and eases the emotional tension that contributes to and worsens headaches. If you want extra help relaxing, or if you just feel too exhausted to come up with a technique of your own, go to a bookstore and look for a good relaxation video or cassette. Generally, relaxation videos combine peaceful images of nature with soothing music, encouraging you to breathe and let go; cassettes do the same without images.

Relaxation techniques help your body relax its blood flow, decrease muscle pain and tension, ease emotional stress, and alter brain chemicals. A study revealed that 96% of the patients who learned relaxation techniques during a 2-month period, were able to lower the frequency, intensity, and duration of their headaches.

Like meditation, biofeedback, and creative visualization (which are relaxation methods in and of themselves), relaxation techniques help to relax blood flow, decrease muscle pain and tension, ease emotional stress, improve sleep, and alter brain chemicals. In a joint study conducted by psychologists at Ohio University and the State University of New York, 96% of the patients who learned relaxation techniques during a 2-month trial were able to lower the frequency, intensity, and duration of their headaches.

The following 2 exercises, progressive relaxation and cue-controlled relaxation, are wonderful tools not only because they are effective but because they are easy and can be done nearly anywhere. (One patient says she has been known to lie on the bathroom floor at her in-laws' house.) If you have difficulty with intruding thoughts, imagine yourself placing them in a special closet for safekeeping until you are finished with the exercise. Unless you want to fall asleep, don't do this exercise immediately after a meal, in the morning, or just before bedtime.

Progressive relaxation

1) Lie down on the floor, couch, or bed with your shoes off; play soft music or light candles if you like, anything that will help set the stage for relaxation.
2) Spend a few moments watching your breath, paying attention to each inhalation and exhalation, taking at least 5 full-belly breaths.
3) Relax the muscles in your body, group by group, starting with your feet and working your way up to your neck, face, and head.

Cue-controlled Relaxation

1) Either sit with your back straight or lie down on your back with your arms next to your sides.
2) Get in touch with your breath and begin to breathe in through your nose and out through your mouth, emptying all your air as you exhale and allowing your stomach to rise as you inhale. Place one hand on your stomach and the other hand on your chest, making sure that only your stomach is moving.
3) Breathe at a slow and regular rate, inhaling to a count of 4, holding your breath for a count of 1, and exhaling to a count 4, then holding your breath for 1 before starting again; get in touch with the movement of your stomach going down as you breathe out.
4) Now, as you breathe, repeat the statement "I am relaxed," saying "I am" as you inhale, "relaxed" as you exhale; do this for 5 minutes or longer.

For assistance in finding a support group or forming one, see Appendix A: Resources, Support Groups.

SUPPORT GROUPS

Joining a headache support group gives you the opportunity to discuss your pain with others who know what you are going through and who would never dream of calling you a hypochondriac. Support group members are people who sympathize with and share your agony. Sometimes just voicing your feelings can make your headache better. In addition, support groups provide another way to expand your knowledge and learn what others are doing to deal with their headaches.

RECOMMENDED READING

Alternative Medicine: The Definitive Guide. Compiled by the Burton Goldberg Group. Tiburon, CA: Future Medicine Publishing, 1994.

Braly, James, M.D. and Torbet, Laura. *Dr. Braly's Food Allergy and Nutrition Revolution.* New Canaan, CT: Keats Publishing, Inc., 1992.

Carper, Jean. *Food: Your Miracle Medicine* New York: HarperCollins, 1993.

Clark, Linda, M.A. *A Handbook of Natural Remedies for Common Ailments.* Greenwich, CT: The Devin-Adair Company, 1976.

Donovan, P. "Bowel Toxemia, Permeability and Disease—New Information to Support an Old Concept." *A Textbook of Natural Medicine.* Edited by J.E. Pizzorno and M.T. Murray. Seattle, WA: John Bastyr College Publications, 1989.

Faber, William J., D.O. *Pain, Pain Go Away.* San Jose, CA: ISHI Press International, 1990.

Howell, E., M.D. *Food Enzymes for Health and Longevity.* Woodstock Valley, CT: Omangod Press, 1980.

Jevning, R., Wallace, R.K., and Beidebach, M. "The Physiology of Meditation: A Wakeful Hypometabolic Integrated Response." *Neuroscience & BioBehavioral Reviews* 16:3 (Fall 1992), 415-424.

Kayser, H.W. and Istanbulluoglu, S. "Treatment of PMS without Hormones." *Hippokrates* 25:25, 717.

Kunz, Kevin and Kunz, Barbara. *Hand Reflexology Workbook.* Albuquerque, NM: RRP Press, 1994.

Lee, R.H., ed. *Scientific Investigations into Chinese Qi-Gong.* San Clemente, CA: China Healthways Institute, 1992.

Lilienthal, Samuel, M.D. *Homeopathic Therapeutics.* New Delhi: Jain Publishing Co., 1996.

Manahan, William, D., M.D. *Eat for Health.* Tiburon, CA: H. J. Kramer, Inc., 1988.

Natural Health Secrets from around the World. Boca Raton, FL: Shot Tower Books, 1996.

Nespor, K. "Pain Management and Yoga." *International Journal of Psychosomatics,* 38:1-4 (1991), 76-81.

Randolph, T.G. *Human Ecology and Susceptibility to the Chemical Environment.* Springfield, IL: C.C. Thomas, 1981.

Reed, Daniel. *A Handbook of Chinese Healing Herbs.* Boston, MA: Shambhala Publications, 1995.

Rick, Stephanie. *The Reflexology Workout.* New York: Harmony Books, 1986.

Rothschild, Peter R., M.D., Ph.D. and Fahey, William. *Free Radicals, Stress, and Antioxidant Enzymes: A Guide to Cellular Health.* Honolulu, HI: University Labs Press, 1991.

Schmitt, Walter, Jr., D.C. "Molybdenum for Candida albicans: Patients and Other Problems." *Digest of Chiropractic Economics* 31:4 (1991), 56-63.

Simpson, Kristine, et al., eds. *The Experts Speak 1996: The Role of Nutrition in Medicine.* Sacramento: Kirk Hamilton PA-C, 1996, 121-122.

Steel, J. "Brain Research and Essential Oils." *Aromatherapy Quarterly* 3 (Spring 1994).

Stromfeld, Jan and Weil, Anita. *Free Yourself from Headaches: The Natural Drug-Free Program for Prevention and Relief.* Palm Beach Gardens, FL: The Upledger Institute, Frog, Ltd., 1995.

Wilson, Roberta. *Aromatherapy for Vibrant Health & Beauty.* Garden City Park, NY: Avery Publishing Group, 1994.

Chapter 17

An A-Z of Alternative Medicine

"*The natural force within each one of us is the greatest healer of disease.*"

—Hippocrates

"*The art of healing comes from nature and not from the physician. Therefore, the physician must start from nature with an open mind.*"

—Paracelsus

This chapter provides detailed explanations of the many therapies we have referred to throughout the book. At this point, you may already have an idea which of the numerous alternatives available you want to include in *your* treatment package. Remember, many of these approaches enhance one another, so a combination may be your best solution to becoming headache free.

As you read about these therapies and consider which treatments would be right for you, take into account your total health, not just your headache. As we have emphasized repeatedly, different modalities work for different people, even if they suffer from the same type of headache. If one therapy does not produce the results you are looking for, try another; the only side effect you will get from this approach is better overall health.

However, it is important to be patient with alternative therapies because, while some people may experience healing immediately, others do not. The lack of immediate results does not necessarily mean the therapy is not working. Unlike drugs, alternative therapies are subtle and often take longer to produce a significant change. That is because the healing is not just eliminating symptoms, but addressing the underlying causes as well. Qualified practitioners can provide supplemental techniques to keep you comfortable in the meantime.

Keep in mind that all of the treatments listed below are tools. In the long run, your commitment and attitude are your best health care modality: the key to becoming headache free is your willingness to commit yourself to making the changes that will bring wellness back into your life.

For easy access, we list the therapies alphabetically, rather than in the categories of metabolic/biochemical/bioenergetic-based, structurally oriented, and psycho/emotional therapies as they appear in previous chapters. However, each is labeled for cross-referencing purposes as follows:

MBB—metabolic/biochemical/bioenergetic-based therapies

SO—structurally oriented therapies

PE—psycho/emotional therapies.

For more information on how to locate a qualified alternative doctor, see Chapter 4, Finding the Right Practitioner, *Alternative Medicine: The Definitive Guide.*

For a listing of alternative practitioners by therapy type and geographical location, see *Alternative Medicine Yellow Pages.*

Consult with a qualified health practitioner before beginning any therapy.

ACUPUNCTURE AND TRADITIONAL CHINESE MEDICINE (MBB)

Originating in China over 3,000 years ago, Traditional Chinese Medicine (TCM) is a comprehensive system of medical practice that treats the body according to the principles of nature. According to the World Health Organization (WHO), $1/4$ of the world's population makes use of one or more of TCM's therapies, and TCM has been selected by WHO as one of the favored medical systems for meeting the health-care needs of the 21st century. TCM has proven to be an effective treatment for a full range of human illnesses, including the prevention and relief of chronic headaches of all types.

TCM and acupuncture, which is one of its branches, treat illness as imbalances in the *qi* (pronounced chee, also spelled *ki* or *chi*) or energy that circulates through the body along 12 major pathways, or meridians. Each meridian is linked to specific internal organs and/or organ systems, creating a network for the movement of energy. Whenever this energy flow is blocked, overactive, or stagnant—through internal problems, external factors, or thoughts and attitudes—the body develops symptoms and becomes susceptible to disease.

Another important concept of Chinese medicine is the interrelationship of the organs, each of which is also designated as "*yin*" or "*yang*" to describe the kind of energy that characterizes them. *Yang* is akin to action and its organs, such as the stomach, intestines, and bladder, are classified as hollow, where energy passes through; *yin* is more passive energy and its organs, such as the heart, spleen, lungs, kidney, and liver, are solid and substantial.

If TCM treatment could be summed up in a few simple phrases, they might be: if the energy flow is deficient, tonify and unblock; if it is excessive, detoxify and disperse. These corrections are accomplished through a variety of tried and proven techniques which, along with acupuncture, include diet and lifestyle changes, herbs, massage techniques, and moxabustion (the burning of special "moxa" or herbs above the skin in correspondence to a specific acupuncture point).

In TCM, the head is believed to be the meeting place of the *yang* channels, where both the *qi* and the blood of 11 organs come together. Thus a headache is often classified as a disharmony of the internal organs, one that results from either external pathogens or internal injury.

TCM doctors also consider the location of pain as an indication of the origins of the headache. For example, pain over the eyes or forehead is linked to the meridians of the large intestines and stomach and often indicates overconsumption of yin-type foods, such as fruit juices, sugar, caffeine, and alcohol (unless this pain is felt in conjunction with a funny taste in the mouth, which means a blockage in the spleen meridian). A dull, constant headache in the back or side of the head is generally related to an overconsumption of yang-type foods, especially meat, eggs, and salt, and corresponds to a blockage in the gallbladder or bladder meridians. Pain on top of the head, particularly if it feels like the head is exploding, comes from liver blockage. Pain on the back of the neck indicates a bladder or kidney blockage, and temple pain corresponds to the gallbladder meridian.

Pulse-reading is the main method of diagnosis used in acupuncture and Chinese medicine in general. This involves checking the patient's 12 radial pulses (6 on each wrist). By placing fingers on the patient's wrists, the acupuncturist can "read" the pulses and determine the location of energy blockage and the organs affected.

Acupuncture restores and enhances energy flow through hair-thin, stainless steel needles inserted slightly into the skin at acupoints along the meridians. There are more than a thousand acupoints (called *Qi* "holes" or "wells," as *Qi* can accumulate here) within the meridian system, each corresponding to a specific function, allowing the acupuncturist to rebalance the entire body. The treatment is essentially painless, although a slight pricking sensation is felt as the needles first enter the skin. (If there is pain, the acupuncturist should be told immediately because a slight adjustment of the needle will make it go away.)

The needles (anywhere from 12 to 50 presterilized disposable needles per treatment) are then left in place while the patient rests comfortably or even falls asleep for 20 to 60 minutes. The number and frequency of treatments depends upon the condition of the patient and can vary from once a month to twice a week. Most headache sufferers feel some relief within 1 to 3 sessions.

Acupuncture is gaining considerable respect in the West, particularly because it is helping those who had been labeled by conventional medicine as "untreatable." WHO has listed 104 different health conditions, including headaches, that can benefit from acupuncture. WHO has also listed acupuncture as a valuable treatment for environmentally induced illnesses, such as those due to radiation, pesticide poisoning, environmentally toxic compounds, and air pollution.

One reason acupuncture works well for headaches is that it treats your body on both energy and biochemical levels, correcting both the symptoms and the imbalances that lie beneath them. Properly placed needles activate natural headache relief by bioenergetically stimulating "painkillers" in the brain, such as endorphins and enkephalins. They can also work on disturbances such as digestive, hormonal, and circulatory problems; structurally, on painful conditions such as arthritis, trauma, and back pain; and emotionally, on imbalances resulting from anxiety, stress, depression, or addiction.

Chinese medicine products can be purchased at Mayway Corporation, 1338 Mandela Parkway, Oakland, CA 94607; tel: 800-2-MAYWAY or 510-208-3113; fax: 510-208-3069.

ALPHABIOTICS (SO)

Developed 65 years ago, by Virgil Chrane, Sr., M.D.C., and refined by his son Virgil Chrane, Jr., D.C., the Alphabiotic Alignment Process is a painless structural aligning method specially designed to reset the central nervous system and synchronize the hemispheres of the brain. Although it evolved from chiropractic, the process is different: instead of working with individual vertebra, alphabiotics focuses only on the brain stem, which is the direct link to the entire nervous system. Because it does not target specific symptoms but works with the body as a whole, it has proven useful for many conditions—physical, mental, and emotional—including headaches.

Considered more a tool than a treatment method, alphabiotics—which means "first life"—normalizes and relaxes brain waves, balancing energy and paving the way for the body to heal itself. Your brain and nervous system work on a priority basis, meaning the energy is sent where it is needed most. If energy channels are blocked, your body has little energy left to heal itself because it is expending much of its energy trying to unblock these channels. The Alphabiotic alignment process frees up this energy and allows it to go where it is most needed.

Taking less than 5 minutes, the alignment, which is similar to a light neck adjustment, instantaneously puts you into an alpha state, the brain wave associated with a calm, meditative, and creative state, which is the state researchers believe to be optimal for healing. After an alignment, the effects of the body working to correct itself are felt immediately in a relaxed, tingling sensation. Over a series of alignments, the body is guided back to its more natural state.

AYURVEDIC MEDICINE (MBB)

Literally translated as "science of life," Ayurvedic medicine is a 5,000-year-old Indian system of medicine which uses a blend of mind, body, and spirit therapies to restore the body to a healthy state of balance. Today, Ayurvedic medicine is practiced all over the world and is recognized and supported by the World Health Organization. In the U.S., Ayurvedic medicine has begun to be integrated, though on a modest level, with other healing practices such as naturopathy, chiropractic, and even conventional medicine.

The cornerstone of Ayurvedic medicine is the concept of *doshas*, or the 3 body types—*vata*, *pitta*, and *kapha*—each of which is used to describe specific physical attributes and their corresponding metabolic and emotional tendencies. For example, a *vata* person is generally slim with cool, dry skin, tends to be moody and vivacious, and is prone to constipation, arthritis, and nervous disorders. The *doshas* allow the Ayurvedic doctor to personalize treatments to suit the overall constitution of the patient. In Ayurvedic medicine, good health means the doshas are balanced and the mind, body, and spirit are in harmony; when this is not the case, the body becomes susceptible to illness.

According to Ayurvedic theory, 7 factors can disrupt health: genetic, congenital, internal, seasonal, and magnetic/electrical influences; external trauma; and natural tendencies/habits. For diagnosis, Ayurvedic practitioners rely on patient interviews and physical observation, which includes palpating the body, listening to the heart, lungs, and intestines, and an examination of the tongue, eyes, nails, urine, and 12 radial pulses (6 on each wrist). Once a diagnosis has been made, the practitioner restores health using the 4 curative pillars of Ayurvedic medicine: cleansing and detoxification, palliation, rejuvenation, and mental hygiene.

The methods employed in cleansing and detoxification include herbal-oil massage, steam bath, bowel purging, vomiting, nasal douching, enemas, blood cleansing, and herbal and food supplements. Both curative and preventative, palliation deals with cleansing, using herbs, fasting, stretching and breathing exercises, and meditation; it is often prescribed when a patient is too ill or emotionally weak to endure the more rigorous methods of cleansing and detoxification.

Once the cleansing process has been completed, the rejuvenation process is employed to restore vitality to the body. This is a physiological tune-up consisting of herbs, minerals, and stretching and breathing exercises. Mental hygiene is introduced with specific meditations aimed at releasing long-held psychological stress, emotional worry, prejudices, and negative thought patterns and beliefs.

For **Ayurvedic products**, contact MAPI, P.O. Box 49667, Colorado Springs, CO 80949-9667; tel: 800-255-8332 or 719-260-5500; fax: 719-260-7400.

BEHAVIORAL OPTOMETRY (SO)

A rapidly growing field of medicine, behavioral optometry is founded upon the idea that imbalances in the visual perception system do not cause just vision problems but a wide range of disorders, from headaches and travel sickness to depression and learning disabilities. The visual perception system, which includes the muscles and nerves serving your brain and eyes, is a key link between your eyes and brain, as it determines how your brain interprets visual messages. If this system is not working properly, your brain is unable to understand what your eyes are telling it, forcing both brain and eyes to work harder to communicate their signals, until both are so exhausted that headaches and other symptoms emerge.

Fully schooled and capable of practicing all the techniques available to conventional optometrists, behavioral optometrists take their practices a few steps further to encompass the principles of alternative healing. They are trained to do much more than prescribe a pair of glasses or contact lenses. They seek to uncover and treat the underlying visual problem, one which often creates symptoms other than problematic vision.

A treatment starts with an eye exam followed by a series of tests to determine the function of your visual perception system. These tests measure your ability to focus, control the accuracy and speed of your eye movements, and to team your eyes so vision is comfortably shared with both. These tests take at least 45 minutes longer than a conventional eye exam.

Based on the test results, the behavioral optometrist creates an individualized program to teach you how to use your eyes more efficiently. This may include a number of tools, such as corrective lenses and prisms (which bend light, forcing you to realign your eyes before you can focus through them), and simple exercises which are designed to enable the eye-focusing and teaming systems to work more efficiently. These techniques enhance awareness and alignment more than build up the eye muscles. According to Anne Barber, O.D., of Santa Ana, California, your eye muscles are already 50 to 100 times stronger than necessary. Eventually, with dedication and effort on your part, you will retrain your eyes, so that they become more relaxed, allowing your brain to receive clear visual signals.

BIOFEEDBACK (PE)

Founded on the idea that you can learn to consciously regulate the bodily functions that are generally regarded as automatic, biofeedback is like a mirror that helps you to see the relationship between your mind and body. Although primarily used for relaxation and pain relief, biofeedback is also used in conjunction with other alternative therapies to treat and prevent stress-related disorders, such as temporomandibular joint syndrome (TMJS), headaches, insomnia, hypertension, gastrointestinal problems, and most other conditions made worse by psychological factors.

Biofeedback is a learning technique in which electrodes are attached to your head; they are hooked up to equipment that emits visual or auditory signals to identify physiological changes that would otherwise go unnoticed. You are asked questions and guided in various relaxation and creative visualization exercises to elicit stressed and non-stressed states of mind. The biofeedback machine detects and monitors bodily responses such as blood flow beneath the skin (skin temperature, ST), the electrical conductivity of the skin (galvanic skin response, GSR), muscle tension (electromyogram, EMG), brain waves (electroencephalogram, EEG), and heart rate (electrocardiogram, EKG).

Once you have been trained, through repeated sessions, to recognize and voluntarily control some of the internal processes of your body, you are taken off the instrument and encouraged to practice biofeedback techniques on your own whenever you are under stress or feel a headache coming on.

The goal of this practice is to make you more aware of your own physical processes so that you can stop symptoms before they become serious problems. Two types of biofeedback are currently used to treat headaches: thermal biofeedback, which helps vascular-type headaches, and EMG (electromyogram, monitoring muscle tension) biofeedback, which controls headaches involving muscle contraction.

Thermal Biofeedback—Here you learn to mentally direct blood flow from the swollen vessels in your head to less problematic parts of the body, such as your hands and feet. This technique is particularly helpful for women with migraines, as they often have cold hands; research demonstrates that when women use thermal biofeedback to warm their fingertips to 96 ° F at the first sign of migraine, a headache is aborted up to 80% of the time.[1]

EMG (electromyogram) Biofeedback—The most common type of biofeedback in use today, EMG biofeedback can relieve headaches and all types of muscle spasm, tension, and pain. In this technique, the patient wears headphones and electrical leads from a machine are attached to the patient's forehead. The patient is then asked to relax the forehead because, as it relaxes, the muscles of the scalp, neck, and upper body also relax. As long as the forehead stays tense, the machine sends an uncomfortable, high-pitched sound through the headphones, but as the patient relaxes, the sound becomes lower and more soothing, enabling the patient to learn to listen to the muscles.

Like other alternative therapies, biofeedback is neither a passive technique nor a cure-all. It takes hours of practice to learn the technique and must be practiced regularly to remain effective, which is why biofeedback is most successful when used by those who are motivated to get in touch with the inner workings of their bodies.

BIOLOGICAL DENTISTRY (SO)

Focusing on the role that dental health plays in the body, biological dentistry combines the skills and tools of conventional dentistry with the knowledge and insight offered by alternative diagnostic tools and treatment therapies. Research has shown that dental problems, such as cavities, infections, root canals, allergy-producing or toxic filling materials (mercury), and misalignments of the teeth and jaw, have effects that extend far beyond their localized environments, causing chronic and degenerative disorders. These include headaches, allergies, toxic poisoning, chronic fatigue syndrome, arthritis, and autoimmune disorders.

Biological dentistry recognizes this connection and treats the teeth, jaw, and related structures not as isolated problems that need fixing, but as a means of gaining more insight into overall body imbalance. Biological dentists use diagnostic methods such as applied kinesiology and electrodermal screening to identify problems, such as hidden infections from root canals, that are often overlooked by conventional dentistry.

Once problems are uncovered, the biological dentist may employ or recommend acupuncture, bodywork, light therapy, detoxification therapy, homeopathy, jaw realignment (using orthopedic appliances), neural therapy (with offending teeth as trigger points), or nutritional therapy, in addition to conventional dentistry.

CAUTION

The safe removal of mercury fillings requires a dentist who specializes in the procedure and is trained in safety precautions to prevent mercury leakage.

Some biological dentists deal primarily with patients suffering from the chronic problems associated with mercury amalgam fillings. After testing for mercury poisoning, these dentists safely extract the offending mercury and refill the tooth with less hazardous materials. They then may put the patient on a detoxification program and use oral acupuncture, bodywork, or homeopathy to help speed up the repair process.

BODYWORK (SO)

Bodywork is an all-encompassing term used to describe healing modalities that work with the structure of the body. While there are hundreds of different bodywork techniques, the majority of them fall into 1 of 3 general categories: therapeutic massage, movement therapies, and energy balancing. Although touch is one of the oldest healing methods, bodywork has gained considerable attention in the past 10 years as scientific evidence has shown it to be a beneficial treatment for a number of conditions, including musculoskeletal problems brought about by injury or trauma, muscle spasm and pain, headaches, temporomandibular joint syndrome, and PMS. Furthermore, bodywork is an excellent preventative, as it helps keep muscles relaxed and improves circulation and the elimination of waste.

Chronic patterns of stress, whether due to skeletal misalignments, prolonged muscle tension, or emotional worries, compress the nerve fibers of the muscles and block the normal flow of energy. If these patterns are not interrupted, natural acids called metabolic wastes build up and accumulate in the muscles and, because tense muscles do not allow enough blood to circulate to wash out waste, the pain-sensitive nerves become irritated, leading to muscle fatigue, spasm, and pain.

Most bodywork techniques use some combination of hands-on pressure, deep tissue massage, movement education, body awareness exercises, breathing, and emotional expression to alter the muscular and/or soft tissue structures of the body and restore energy flow. When dealing with headaches, bodyworkers often give extra attention to the shoulders, neck, abdomen, and spine. In addition to Swedish or other standard type of massage, the following are the some of the most popular forms of bodywork.

Acupressure—Referred to as *Amma* in Japan and *Tui Na* in China, this ancient Chinese massage technique is similar to acupuncture except it does not involve the use of needles. In acupressure, fingers press directly on the meridian points to stimulate the internal organs and open up energy pathways. Many acupressure techniques are designed to be self-administered.

For information about self-administering acupressure, see Chapter 16, An A-Z of Self-care Options.

The Alexander Technique—Pioneered by Frederick Matthias Alexander, this simple bodywork technique rebalances the body through breath, awareness, movement, and touch. It is designed to bring unconscious movement patterns and faulty breathing habits to light and to facilitate proper motion, balance, and posture. In addition to headaches, the Alexander Technique can be effective for back injury, chronic back, shoulder, or neck tension, TMJS, and recovery from back surgery or slipped disk.

Aston-Patterning—Developed by Judith Aston in 1977, this technique is designed to balance body movement and structure, thereby improving coordination and helping the patient to manage pain. Using a combination of movement reeducation, massage, soft tissue bodywork, fitness training, stretching, and ergonomic design (such as a computer keyboard and desk chair designed for the user's health), patients are given tools to connect with their bodies and regain fluidity and ease of movement.

The Feldenkrais Method—After experiencing a sports injury that left him in incredible pain, Moshe Feldenkrais, D.Sc., was able to combine his knowledge of martial arts, physiology, anatomy, psychology, and neurology into a movement technique that completely restored his body's function. He developed this technique into a highly individualized reeducational tool called the Feldenkrais Method. The method is composed of 2 stages, a group process called Awareness through Movement, and a one-on-one technique that uses hands-on touch and movement exercises called Functional Integration. This method is different from other forms of bodywork because there is no attempt to structurally alter the body; instead, the practitioner uses nonmanipulative touch to introduce patients to their own bodies. Feldenkrais can be effective for headaches, TMJS, and neck, shoulder, and back pain. It also has been known to produce greater mental clarity, improve breathing and sleep, and enhance vitality.

Hanna Somatics—Developed by Thomas Hanna, Hanna Somatics is an educational movement technique designed to facilitate the release of chronic muscle tension and pain. It is designed to reverse a process that Hanna calls sensory motor amnesia (SMA). SMA occurs when conscious control of contracted muscles is lost, meaning the brain continues to tell the muscles to contract even when you want to relax. The brain is forcing the body to compensate for the habitual tightness by rearranging posture and body movements. Unfortunately, this effort only worsens the problem, bringing further pain, tension, and dysfunction.

Hanna Somatics breaks this painful impasse through a series of simple movement exercises that retrain the brain by moving the muscle toward the contraction, shifting the level of control back to the voluntary brain.

Hellerwork—Joseph Heller believed that the physical changes achieved by manual manipulation alone are not enough to bring about permanent realignment in the body, that the mind and emotions must also be balanced. To this end, he created a bodywork technique called Hellerwork. It consists of 11 sessions, each of which addresses a specific component in achieving balance in the physical, psychological, and emotional realms. For example, the first session is designed to unlock tension and unconscious holding patterns in the chest to allow for fuller and more natural breathing. The practitioner engages the client in a dialogue regarding emotions and attitudes that are affecting the client's breathing.

Hellerwork employs this verbal dialogue, along with deep touch and movement education, to achieve emotional release, increase flexibility, improve body alignment, minimize the mechanical stress of movement, maximize the use of the body's energy, and foster a healthy mind/body relationship.

Myotherapy—Frequently used to treat people with trauma-related and TMJ headaches, myotherapy (from "myo," meaning muscle) was developed in the mid 1970s by Bonnie Prudden. Myotherapy is a technique that uses deep, sustained pressure on a trigger point—a highly irritable spot in a muscle—to release a contracted or painful muscle. Although they are not sure why, researchers suggest that myotherapy works because pressure applied by fingers, knuckles, or elbows deprives the trigger point of oxygen, thereby easing the pain. This procedure is supplemented by gentle stretches and movements, as well as by self-myotherapy techniques that can be done at home.

Polarity Therapy—A hands-on technique developed by Randolph Stone, D.C., D.O., N.D., polarity therapy is a comprehensive approach that seeks to restore overall health and well-being on the physical, mental, and emotional levels. It uses joint and muscle manipulation, massage, pressure point stimulation, breathing, exercise, reflexology, dietary and lifestyle changes, and emotional release to unblock energy and restore natural flow.

Rolfing—Developed by biochemist Ida P. Rolf, Ph.D., in 1970, Rolfing, formally known as Structural Integration, is based on the principle that human functioning is improved when all the segments of the body are properly aligned. This technique uses massage to manually manipulate and stretch the fascial tissues of the body, tissues that surround every muscle, bone, blood vessel, nerve, and organ. Although it is highly effective, Rolfing can be painful because its practitioners exert considerable pressure with fingers, knuckles, and elbows to reorganize the rigid fascial tissue into the proper structure.

Reflexology—Reflexology is based on the belief that the feet and hands provide maps of the body, with each area linked to a specific organ, gland, and/or energy pathway. It uses gentle pressure on the feet and hands to stimulate the corresponding areas in the body. The fact that the foot contains 7,200 nerve endings may account for how reflexology works. Foot reflexology has proven an effective method for improving blood circulation, easing digestive disorders, calming the system, and providing better overall functioning.

See Chapter 16, An A-Z of Self-Care Options, for information on self-administering reflexology.

When treating a headache, most reflexologists work with the areas corresponding to the head, solar plexus, and diaphragm (reflex areas that are involved in stress control and relaxation), the brain, shoulders, and arms (areas that accumulate tension), and the spine and spinal cord (areas that help determine nervous system responses).

Therapeutic Touch—A synthesis of many practices, therapeutic touch is an energy-healing system now used in many hospitals and clinics in the U.S. Based on the concept that the therapist possesses a healing force that is capable of affecting the patient's recovery and cure, this technique uses energy from the therapist's hands to "read" the patient's energy field, release blockages, and stimulate the flow of energy. Therapists rarely touch the patient directly and instead place their hands 2 to 6 inches away from the patient's body as the patient relaxes. More than 37,000 doctors, nurses, and health practitioners in the U.S. are currently using this technique to help relieve pain and stress.

The Trager Approach—In 1927, Milton Trager, M.D., discovered that rhythmical touch combined with movement exercises can effectively help a person to recognize and release habitually held patterns of tension. This relaxing technique applies gentle rocking, pulling, and rotational movements to manipulate the patient's head, torso, and limbs. This helps to loosen tense muscles and joints and trigger a sensory-motor feedback response in the central nervous system which stimulates positive changes in the mind and muscles. In addition, Trager practitioners teach patients a set of free-flowing dance-like exercises called Mentastics—or mental gym-

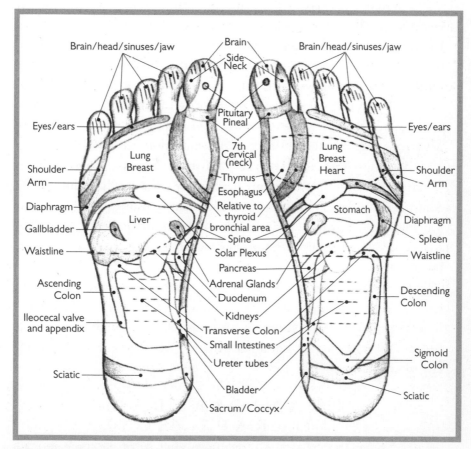

Figure 17.1—Reflexology areas of the feet.

nastics—to increase body awareness and improve flexibility and range of motion. Trager can be beneficial for headaches, especially migraines, low-back problems, asthma, chronic pain syndromes, and degenerative muscular disorders.

CHIROPRACTIC (SO)

Chiropractic was developed in 1895 by Daniel David Palmer. In the U.S., there are over 50,000 chiropractors treating an estimated 15 to 20 million patients each year; one in 15 Americans sees a chiropractor at least once during a 12-month period. Furthermore, a recent Gallup poll reveals that 90% of these patients view their chiropractic care as effective, 80% consider treatment costs reasonable, and 70% say they would make another appointment.

Chiropractic is concerned with the relationship between the spinal column and the musculoskeletal structure of the body, and how these relationships affect the nervous system and organs. Chiropractors regard correct alignment as essential to health and view the spinal column as a "switchboard" for the nervous system. If bones move out of place (called subluxation) as a result of soft tissue injuries, allergies/sensitivities, tension, or toxic buildup, nerve interference can cause chronic illness and pain, including headaches, digestive disturbances, PMS, and emotional problems.

The chiropractor's job is to keep the spine aligned, freeing the nerves to carry out their proper functions. Chiropractors generally perform spinal adjustments and manipulations with their hands, using a combination of touch (called palpation), active motion (getting the patient to bend and stretch in different ways), and passive movement (helping the patient to bend and stretch).

Some chiropractors use special tools, such as the Activator, a hand-held device that is used to gently and painlessly move the vertebrae, while others combine spinal adjustment with other healing modalities, such as massage, energy therapy, nutritional therapy, acupuncture, exercise, and environmental medicine.

CRANIOSACRAL THERAPY (SO)

"Cranio" refers to the head and "sacral" to the base of the spine and tailbone. The craniosacral system consists of the brain, the spinal cord, the

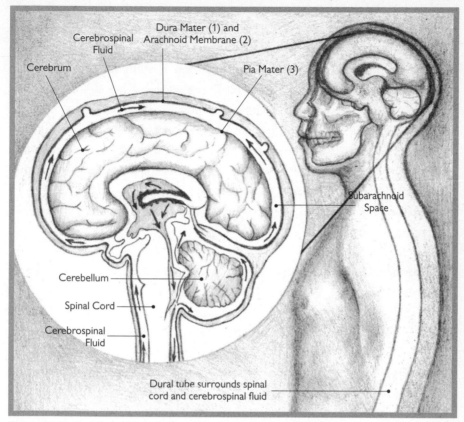

Figure 17.2—Craniosacral system and the 3 layers of the meninges.

cerebrospinal fluid, the membranes (meninges) that surround the brain, and the bones of the spine and skull that house all of the above. There is a rhythmic motion in the craniosacral system created by the rise and fall of cerebrospinal fluid pressure. Contrary to common belief, the bones of the skull and spine are not rigid and static, but move to accommodate the pressure exerted by an increase in fluid and return to their original position when the fluid is reabsorbed into the bloodstream. This cycle occurs from 6 to 10 times per minute.

For information about craniosacral therapy applied to infants, see *Digest* #12, "Healing Hands On a Baby's Head," p. 34.

Injuries, stress, or dysfunction in other parts of the body can interfere with the free motion of the bones in this natural rhythm. Then the craniosacral system does not receive a healthy flow of oxygenated blood, which throws the nervous system and the entire body out of balance. Headaches are only one of the physiological or psychological problems that can result.

Cranial therapists use their hands on a patient's head to feel the motion of the craniosacral system and diagnose the areas of restriction. The therapist then exerts gentle pressure to clear the restrictions and restore the normal rhythm of the craniosacral system, thereby restoring health to all the systems of the body. This therapy works especially well for headaches arising in conjunction with trauma, temporomandibular joint syndrome, tension, allergies, hypertension, and chronic musculoskeletal conditions. Since craniosacral imbalances can begin at birth, craniosacral therapeutic techniques are often an effective way to treat headaches in children, especially newborns and infants.

Craniosacral therapy is divided into three approaches: sutural, meningeal, and reflex.

Sutural approach—Sutures are the lines on the skull where the separate cranial bones meet. Sutural craniosacral therapy focuses on manipulating the sutures to ease pressure and gain more mobility in the cranial bones. Cranial osteopathy is the most widely recognized sutural approach.

Meningeal approach—This technique involves releasing the restrictions of the cranial sutures and the underlying membranes, the meninges. Here, the therapist manipulates the meningeal membranes to restore the normal position of the cranial bones.

Craniosacral Therapy, developed in the 1970s by osteopath John Upledger, D.O., O.M.M., is the most widely practiced meningeal approach. Its efficacy in treating head pain was proven by a study conducted by Dr. Upledger in which relief was experienced by 80 to 85% of patients suffering from chronic disabling headaches who had previously been resistant to therapy.

Reflex approach—The reflex approach uses touch to stimulate the nerve endings in the scalp and between the sutures, thereby inducing the nervous system to turn off its stress signals. This technique often is combined with other craniosacral approaches for a more comprehensive treatment. For example, the Sacro-Occipital Technique (S.O.T) or craniopathy, combines sutural, meningeal, and reflex techniques to remove restrictions, reestablish structural integrity, and enhance neurological functioning.

DETOXIFICATION
THERAPY (MBB)

Detoxification therapy, the treatment method designed to pave the road for good health by helping to rid the body of chemicals and pollutants, is a cornerstone of alternative therapy. If performed *before* serious health problems arise, detoxification can keep the immune system and vital organs thriving and prevent the chronic symptoms and sicknesses that are characteristic of today's society.

As the Earth becomes more polluted, your body is forced to handle more unwanted substances entering it via food, water, and air. Taxed by pesticides, food additives, excess animal proteins, industrial chemicals, drug residues, anesthetics, and heavy metals, your body's normal methods of cleansing (sweating, breathing, sleeping, urination, bowel emptying, and in emergency situations, vomiting, diarrhea, and fever) are often no longer sufficient to maintain your health. Your blood, tissues, cells, and organs, especially your liver and intestines, become toxic dumping grounds. Eventually, your entire system becomes toxic. At this point, before disease sets in, your body needs some extra help to cleanse and detoxify.

Known to reduce stress on the immune system, increase vitality, reduce blood pressure, and improve the assimilation of nutrients, detoxification therapy is particularly important for those who suffer from chronic headaches, because headaches—along with mental dullness, fatigue, anxiety, depression, and constipation—are among the most obvious signs of toxic buildup. There are many ways to detoxify the body, including colonic therapy, chelation therapy, fasting, herbal bowel cleansers, hyperthermia, heavy metal detoxification, and specific diets.

Keep in mind that toxins will circulate through the body before they are expelled, which means that you may experience some adverse sensations as you cleanse your system. Some people get rashes, others experience tingling, excess mucus formation, and/or nausea and cramping. These are generally just temporary symptoms which can be alleviated with plenty of pure water.

Colon Therapy—A healthy colon (large intestines) is necessary for the proper absorption of nutrients and the elimination of toxins. Colon therapy consists mainly of colonic irrigation, a technique in which a trained professional uses a colonic machine to introduce purified water, sometimes containing vitamins, herbs, friendly bacteria, and/or oxygen, directly into the rectum. Unlike an enema, which cleanses only the lower 8 to 12 inches of bowel, this technique cleanses the entire large intestine.

For more information, about chelation and DMPS, see *Digest* #13, "Health Hazard In Your Teeth," pp. 40-44.

A single session lasts from 30 to 45 minutes, and sometimes a series of treatments are necessary. Colonic irrigation is generally supplemented with colon strengthening exercises, massage, acupuncture, homeopathy, and special diets consisting of fibers, herbs, and nutritional supplements.

Chelation Therapy—Derived literally from the word *chele*, "to claw," chelation (pronounced key-LAY-shun) therapy operates like a claw that grabs onto an unwanted substance and drags it out of the bloodstream. Chelation is based on the knowledge that many chronic health problems and degenerative diseases are caused by toxic buildup, platelet clustering, and poor blood circulation that can be reversed by removing toxins and restoring blood consistency and circulatory efficiency.

In this safe and proven medical procedure, chelating substances are introduced into the bloodstream to bind up and remove toxins, heavy metals, and waste products from the internal organs. The most common intravenous chelators are DMPS (di-mercaptopropane sulfonate; trade name, Dimaval) and EDTA (ethylenediaminetetraacetic acid). DMPS is the best chelator for the removal of mercury from the body. EDTA works well for eliminating lead and is also used in treating heart conditions because it removes the calcium plaque that is a feature of atherosclerosis.

Chelators can also be taken orally in the form of more natural substances such as chlorella, spirulina, garlic, vitamin C, or L-acetylcysteine. However, because chelation can also remove wanted substances, such as important minerals, it is necessary to be treated by a trained practitioner who knows how to safeguard against risks.

Enemas—Often combined with other cleansing/detoxification programs, such as fasting, colon therapy, herbal bowel cleansing, and special diets, enemas are a quick flush of the lower, or sigmoid, colon. Coffee is often used in the enema because it has been proven to speed up the detoxification process by quickening the bowel, which in turn speeds up the emptying of the liver ducts holding the waste from the blood and tissues. Most of the coffee never goes directly into the system, so even people with sensitivity to coffee rarely have a side effect. Nonetheless, organically-grown coffee is recommended.

The number of enemas a person requires is individual, but those who use enemas frequently should have medical supervision. Coffee enemas can often abort an oncoming headache when administered at first sign of attack.

Fasting—Fasting is a basic component of many cleansing/detoxification programs as it gives the body a break from the process of digestion. Scientific research shows that fasts work in the treatment of headaches. In a 1985 study, 80% of participants significantly reduced the incidence and severity of their migraines by undergoing a nutritionally supported fast coupled with food sensitivity management.[2]

CAUTION

Fasts longer than 2 days should not be attempted without the ongoing participation of a health-care practitioner.

For **herbal bowel cleansers**, contact Nature's Secret, 4 Health, Inc., 5485 Conestoga Court, Boulder, CO 90301; tel: 303-546-6306; fax: 303-546-6416. For products that encourage the growth of "friendly" bacteria in the intestines, contact GTC Nutrition Co., 1400 W. 122nd Avenue, Suite 110, Westminster, CO 80234; tel: 303-254-8012; fax: 303-254-8201.

Among the different types of fasting programs, juice fasting and water fasting are the most popular. Before a fast, it is generally necessary to go on a super-healthy, whole foods, pre-cleanse diet free of meat, dairy, junk food, and stimulants such as caffeine, tobacco, and sugar. Following this regimen for a week, then reducing your food consumption for 2-3 more days is a good way to prepare your system for going without food.

Some therapists have patients supplement their diets with special herbs and root teas, acidophilus, and multivitamins. The length of the actual fast depends upon the condition of the individual, usually ranging from 1 to 7 days.

Fasts work because when you reach a certain level of caloric deprivation, generally under 500 calories per day, your body starts to burn up waste. Your blood sugar drops and the enzymes that normally are used to break down foods go to work on toxins. Enemas are sometimes used in conjunction with fasts since they can help to speed up the detoxification process and lessen the unpleasant side effects, such as bloating, fatigue, and dizziness. When fasting, avoid strenuous exercise, stress, and anything else that would take energy away from the detox process. At the end of the fast, resume eating slowly, starting first with clear soups, fruit, and vegetable juices, then working your way up to more solid foods.

Special Detoxification Baths

Naturopathic physician Hazel Parcells, N.D., D.C., Ph.D., (106 years old when she died in 1995) recommended special baths to detoxify the system. The combination of heat and detoxifying substances pulls the toxins out through the skin. Dissolve the substance(s) in a tub of hot water and soak until the water cools.

For general toxic contamination: 1 pound sea salt and 1 pound baking soda.

For poisoning caused by irradiated food: 2 pounds of baking soda.

For heavy metals, pesticides, and carbon monoxide: 1 cup of Clorox.

CAUTION

Some people, particularly those who are underweight or physically weak, may not be well enough to undertake a rapid, active detoxification process. There are many different ways to detoxify, some gentle, some extreme, so it is wise to consult a qualified practitioner to make sure you choose the one that is right for your needs.

Hyperthermia—Hyperthermia, also known as heat stress detoxification, was used as long ago as 500 B. C. and is still in use all over the world for relaxation and to stimulate healing. Native Americans have sweat lodges; the Finnish take saunas; Russians opt for steam baths; Hawaiians sit in volcanic steam vents.

When performed by an alternative practitioner, hyperthermia incorporates full-immersion baths, saunas, steam, and blanket packs to increase body temperature and produce a fever-like state. When the body is heated in this fashion, the immune system is stimulated, antibody production is increased, and toxins are released from the fat cells. This treatment must be used with extreme care and overseen by a qualified professional because the body sometimes goes into a healing crisis while throwing off toxins.

Herbal Bowel Cleansers—Herbal bowel cleansers are cleansing and purifying supplements that you take orally 2 or 3 times a day for a period of time ranging from a week to a month, depending on the product. Although more expensive than other methods, herbal cleansers are preferred by busy people because they allow you to detoxify without interrupting your normal routine. While they work better with an organic, whole foods diet, it is not a requirement for a good cleanse. Health food stores carry various herbal cleansers, most containing herbs, roots, and barks that have been dried, blended, and pressed into tablets.

Special Detoxification Diets—Detoxification can be accomplished by special diets. Practitioners of various therapy modalities offer particular dietary programs that alternate 24- to 36-hour fasts with 2 to 3 days of a modified diet consisting, for instance, of only whole foods, only raw foods, only organic fruits and vegetables, or only brown rice, buckwheat, or millet. Some practitioners advocate eating with the seasons, since Nature provides the right balance of nutrients with each cycle and can keep the body healthy and cleansed without throwing it into a "must-do" situation.

Another diet, the Alkaline-Detoxification Diet, is a 3- to 4-week plan designed to detoxify body tissues by removing the acidic residue which is often left as a by-product of toxic buildup. Developed by Elson Haas, M.D., Director of the Preventive Medicine of Marin, Inc. in San Rafael, California, this diet requires that you eliminate acid-forming foods such as tomatoes and citrus, eat a diet primarily of vegetables, with some fruit, fresh sprouts, and whole grains (eaten only in the morning), and drink pure water. All food must be thoroughly chewed (30 to 50 times per mouthful) and eaten before 6:30 p.m.

ENERGY MEDICINE (MBB)

Energy medicine is a field of therapy that uses sophisticated energy devices to diagnose—often before they can be detected by conventional procedures—and treat imbalances in the body. Practitioners of energy medicine use a broad range of devices which employ waves of electrical, magnetic, sonic, acoustic, microwave, or infrared energy to ferret out energy imbalances and to rebalance them by sending specific electromagnetic signals to counteract the affected frequencies.

Energy medicine is based on the principles of the acupuncture meridian system and the modern understanding of electromagnetic energy signals emitted from the body. Whenever there is a problem in the body, energy flows get disturbed and the body begins sending out abnormal electromagnetic readings. Since acupuncture points emit measurable electrical conductivity—a measurement that changes only when health deteriorates—it is possible to read them to determine a person's health. High readings mean there is an irritation or inflammation in the corresponding organ or system; low readings indicate the organ or organ system is suffering from fatigue or degeneration.

The following are energy medicine treatment devices:

MORA—Created by Franz Morrel, M.D., this device was designed in keeping with the concept that all biological processes are made up of electro-

For the **Electro-Acuscope**, contact Electro Medical, Inc., 18433 Amistad, Fountain Valley, CA 92708; tel: 800-422-8726 or 714-964-6776. For the LBG, contact Marika von Viczay, N.D., Ph.D., 16 Arlington St., Asheville, NC 28801; tel: 704-253-8371; fax: 704-258-1350. Also for the LBG, along with the Sound Probe and Teslar Watch, contact ELF Teslar, State Route 1, Box 21, St. Francisville, IL 62460; tel: 618-948-2393; fax: 618-948-2650.

magnetic signals that can be read as a complex wave form, smooth waves being healthy, erratic waves diseased. The MORA interprets the body's electromagnetic signals, modifies the aberrant waves by either raising or lowering them to create normal ones, and then sends them back into the body through the acupuncture point. MORA uses only those signals that are coming directly from the patient. It is generally used for headaches, muscular aches and pains, and circulation problems.

TENS (transcutaneous electrical nerve stimulation) Unit— Geared primarily for pain relief, this device is used mainly by physical therapists, although it can be purchased for home use. It works by sending an electrical current to the irritated nerves through electrodes placed on the skin above the pain sites, blocking the nerves' ability to transmit pain and, in some cases, stimulating the production of natural pain-relieving endorphins. This device is useful for TMJ headaches, tension headaches, muscle aches and pains, and other problems with a direct correlation between nerve input and pain.

Electro-Acuscope—Using a very low electrical current, the Electro-Acuscope (or Electroacupuncture Biofeedback Device) reduces pain by stimulating tissue repair. This device requires considerable skill to use because the current must be continually adjusted to match the resistance of the damaged tissue. It is useful in chronic problems such as headaches, especially those of a structural nature, strains and sprains, arthritis, and carpal tunnel syndrome.

LBG (Light Beam Generator)—By radiating units of light directly into cells, the LBG helps to restore cells to their normal state and thereby to help build up the body's ability to heal. It can be used for many problems, since it is capable of penetrating organs and structures deep within the body. The LBG stimulates the lymphatic system, improves blood circulation, reduces swollen tissues, and frees stored toxins for elimination and is therefore especially helpful for headaches caused by metabolic imbalances.

Infratonic QGM—Developed in Beijing in the early 1980s by Lu Yan Fang, Ph.D., this massage-like device directs low frequency electro-acoustical waves, known as secondary or infratonic sound, into the body to alleviate pain. It is used primarily to relieve headaches, increase circulation, and relax muscles.

Sound Probe—Emitting a pulsed tone of 3 alternating frequencies, this device works by destroying any frequency (such as that of a virus, bacteria, or toxin) that is not in resonance with a healthy body. This treatment is often used in conjunction with the LBG, since one is capable of destroying the problem, while the other is used to clear the system.

Teslar Watch—While devised primarily to minimize the harmful effects of low-frequency electromagnetic pollution, the Teslar Watch has enhanced the immune response of those who have worn it. It is especially helpful to those whose headaches are caused by allergies, because allergies make one prone to the adverse effects of electromagnetic overload.

For information about the elimination diet, see Chapter 10, Allergy/Sensitivity Headaches.

ENVIRONMENTAL MEDICINE (MBB)

In the past 20 or 30 years, an alarming number of people have begun to develop diseases and symptoms that can be traced to exposure to environmental pollutants, foods, chemicals, mold, pollens, and other reaction-causing substances. Nearly every chronic physical and emotional illness—asthma, depression, PMS, learning disabilities, ulcerative colitis, canker sores, and headaches—has been linked to the after-effects of an allergy or sensitivity.

Environmental medicine, previously known as clinical ecology, attempts to determine the role dietary and environmental allergies/sensitivities play in health and illness. The basic steps of the environmental medicine approach to allergies are: testing, identification, and elimination or neutralization. Today's allergy-induced illnesses are much more complicated to unravel and treat than they were when doctors first began practicing environmental medicine. Due to the increasing numbers of environmental and food-based chemicals, plus the growing ranks of people on medications, the solution to

QUICK DEFINITION

Electrodermal screening is a form of computerized information gathering, based on physics, not chemistry. A noninvasive electric probe Is placed at specific points on the patient's hands, face, or feet, corresponding to points at the beginning or end of acupuncture energy meridians. Minute electrical discharges from these points are seen as information signals about the condition of the body's organs and systems, useful for a physician in evaluation and treatment design.

See Chapter 16, An A-Z of Self-Care Options, for information on self-administering flower essences.

For more information on **flower essences**, contact: Flower Essence Services, P.O. Box 1769, Nevada City, CA 95959; tel: 800-548-0075 or 916-265-0258; fax: 916-265-6467; or Ellon USA, Inc. (formerly Ellon Bach USA), 644 Merrick Road, Lynbrook, NY 11563; tel: 516- 593-2206.

allergy-induced headaches is seldom as simple as finding a single cause and eliminating it.

Environmental medicine practitioners use a variety of techniques such as elimination diet and electrodermal screening to identify allergies/sensitivities. Treatment requires the full cooperation and commitment of the patient in implementing a combination of dietary, lifestyle, and environmental changes in order to heal.

FLOWER ESSENCE THERAPY (PE)

Developed in the 1930s by Edward Bach, D.Hom., flower essence therapy is a form of healing that uses carefully refined herbal infusions to influence emotional states in order to help bring about physical and psychological well-being. Although not intended to treat physical conditions directly, flower essences have a wide range of applications, working to balance the negative feelings and stress that often impede health and recovery. As emotions stabilize, a more positive outlook is achieved, triggering an immune system response that stimulates physical healing.

Flower essences are used to treat the patient and not the disease, so are often used in conjunction with other therapies, such as psychotherapy, bodywork, chiropractic, acupuncture, naturopathy, and nutritional therapy. Many alternative practitioners consider them a valuable complement to their practices because they heal through a subtle energy that enhances the effectiveness of other techniques. Some use them to replace pharmacological drugs such as antidepressants, sedatives, and tranquilizers.

One to 12 weeks of flower essence therapy is generally required to unblock emotional states, but deeply rooted problems can take longer. Although nontoxic and nonaddictive, their potency diminishes as the patient achieves a state of emotional balance. Flower essences are administered according to individual needs, the strength and method varying from person to person. A combination of remedies is sometimes needed to deal with the issue at hand, although no more than 5 essences should be taken at one time; fewer remedies make it easier to assimilate the emotional processes they stimulate.

HERBAL MEDICINE (MBB)

Herbs have always been an essential part of medicine. Early humans used plants to treat physical complaints long before written history. Most drugs on the market today were discovered because of the use of herbs, but now, instead of trees, shrubs, or herbs, the active substances are chemicals specifically designed to mimic the properties of nature.

One of the reasons conventional medicine may have strayed from the use of pure herbs is that they are harder to control, cannot be patented, and are therefore less profitable. Substances grown in the fresh outdoors are generally far superior to, less expensive, and much easier on the system than medications concocted in laboratories. With herbs you can treat a headache with no side effects for about 10¢ to 25¢ a day, compared to the $2 to $8 a day it costs to treat a headache with prescription drugs.[3]

See Chapter 16, An A-Z of Self-Care Options, for information on self-administering herbal supplements.

Herbal medicine (also called botanical medicine or, in Europe, phytotherapy or phytomedicine) is the medicinal use of any plant substance—stem, root, blossom, leaf, fruit, seed, or bark. According to the World Health Organization, it is the third most widely used form of medicine in the world. Herbs are one of the primary treatment methods used in Ayurvedic medicine, naturopathy, and traditional Chinese medicine, and many other alternative practitioners use them in supplemental treatments.

The effect of herbs ranges from mild to powerful, with some having a prolonged effect and others an immediate one. Like conventional drugs, herbs contain biochemical properties which interact with the chemical structure of the human body; however, herbs enter the bloodstream indirectly and therefore do not act as quickly.

Many practitioners prefer liquid extracts or tinctures over capsules and tablets because the body can assimilate liquid more quickly. However, if you are sensitive to alcohol, you can buy powdered herbs and turn them into a liquid tonic by mixing a teaspoon of the herb with a little warm water and swallowing it immediately. Whenever you take an herb for an extended period of time, it is necessary to periodically review your progress and adjust herb selections and dosages as needed.

HOMEOPATHY (MBB)

Homeopathy is based on the principle of treating a health problem with a highly diluted form of a plant, mineral, or animal substance that would cause the same problem if taken in stronger, grosser doses. Derived from the Greek word *homios* meaning like or similar, homeopathy acts as a catalyst, stimulating the body to initiate its own healing process. In other words, the same substance that in stronger doses produces the symptoms of an illness, in minute doses cures it; or even more simply put, like cancels like.

Homeopathic remedies are prepared through a series of dilutions; the more a substance is diluted, the higher the potency. The end product of these dilutions, in most cases, contains no molecular trace of the substance. Researchers studying the effectiveness of homeopathic remedies have concluded that the high dilutions result in the "energy" quality or essence of the original substance being imprinted in the remedy. Homeopathy affects the body first on an energy, then on a biochemical, level.

Most homeopaths who prescribe high potencies of a given remedy insist that, in order for the treatment to work, all other medications must be avoided because they cloud the symptom picture. Therefore, homeopathy does not work well if combined with drug therapy. Other homeopaths disagree and use low-potency medications as an intermediary along with drug therapy until the patient improves and medication can be discontinued.

According to the World Health Organization, homeopathy is the second most widely used form of medicine in the world. In England, homeopathic hospitals and outpatient clinics are part of the national health system. In the United States, about 20% of pharmacists are directing their patients to over-the-counter homeopathic remedies, on an average of 6 times per month.

See Chapter 16, An A-Z of Self-Care Options, for information on self-administering homeopathic remedies.

One of the reasons homeopathy works so well is that treatment is based on the total symptom picture and individuality of the patient. Homeopathic evaluation is comprehensive, taking into consideration the physical, emotional, and mental aspects of the person. A homeopath looks at all the symptoms to build a complete picture and match the remedy to the picture. Rather than just getting rid of your headache, the remedy safely addresses and can eliminate the underlying causes. For this reason, homeopathy is particularly welcome in an age of toxic drugs and dangerous side effects.

Although homeopathic remedies are available in most health food stores, it is not wise to use them the way you would over-the-counter drugs.

We recommend that you consult a homeopathic practitioner or naturopath, chiropractor, or holistic physician trained in homeopathy and the modes of action of each remedy.

≋CAUTION≋

Although safe for most people, it is important to undergo hypnosis only under the direction of a qualified practitioner.

HYPNOTHERAPY (PE)

Hypnotherapy uses the power of suggestion to induce trance-like states that enable the patient to access deep levels in the mind and body, bringing about positive changes in emotional, physical, and psychological problems. Hypnotherapy is so powerful that doctors and dentists have used it occasionally in lieu of anesthetic (one 15-year-old girl underwent a successful, 4-hour open heart operation under hypnosis).

Research has shown that it can successfully treat a wide range of conditions, including headaches, respiratory problems, sleep disorders, stress, and chronic pain. One study determined that 94% of those who undergo hypnotherapy derive benefit, even if it is only relaxation.

Since you must have the desire to be hypnotized in order for it to work, all hypnosis is, in a sense, self-hypnosis. It offers a chance to communicate with the subconscious mind. Whether or not you realize it, it is often the subconscious mind that determines how you are dealing with life. Furthermore, because the subconscious mind is highly suggestible and non-critical, hypnotherapy is able to help you see deeply buried emotional issues and accept ideas and feelings that may seem impossible during the normal waking state. The hypnotherapist then reinforces these positive attitudes, clearing the way for a new life. For example, an early event can create a response pattern that results in a headache; through hypnosis, this pattern can be uncovered and replaced by a headache-free response.

People who have been suffering from chronic headaches for years often forget what it feels like to live without pain. They perceive headaches as part of their identity, and they no longer believe it is possible to live without them. With hypnosis, it is possible to locate that pain-free time and experience what it felt like to live without head pain.

A typical hypnotherapy session lasts 45 to 90 minutes; the number of sessions required to produce results varies from 6 to 12 weekly visits.

LIGHT THERAPY (MBB)

Light, be it sunlight, full-spectrum, ultraviolet, color, or laser light, can help reestablish the body's natural rhythm and balance energy flows, helping to heal chronic disorders. When light rays enter the retina of the eye, they are translated into nerve currents known as photocurrents. These electrical impulses travel along the optic nerve to the brain, where they spark a range of bodily functions that regulate activity and maintain both physiological and psychological health.

Obviously, sunlight is the most recognized form of light therapy. In this high-tech age, however, numerous forms are now available to supplement nature. The following are particularly effective in reducing or eliminating head pain.

Full-Spectrum Light Therapy—This treatment employs either the direct skin application of sunlight or a full-spectrum lighting device to achieve relief from headaches and other chronic symptoms such as depression, insomnia, PMS, and hypertension.

Ultraviolet Light Therapy—This therapy isolates part of the UV-A wavelength (ultraviolet rays from the sun being divided into 3 parts: UV-A, UV-B, and UV-C) and sends it into the skin, where it helps to relieve, among other things, headaches, fatigue, and autoimmune dysfunction.

Syntonic Optometry—Scientific evidence suggests that different colors have different effects on the body, which has led researchers to postulate that some colors stimulate hormone production or balance the nervous system, while others work directly on diseases and chronic ailments such as headaches. By stimulating the eyes with the appropriate colored light, syntonic optometry is able to improve the functioning of the higher brain centers and increase the body's ability to heal itself. This is generally done with a device called the Lumatron Light Stimulator.

Cold Laser Therapy—Also known as soft or low-level laser therapy, cold laser therapy uses laser light to initiate enzymatic reactions and bioelectric events to stimulate healing at a cellular level. It can also be used to stimulate acupoints, rendering it a good alternative for headache sufferers who are leery of the needles used in traditional acupuncture. Besides being beneficial for problems associated with chronic pain, this therapy is used by some dentists to treat infections hiding underneath teeth.

MAGNETIC FIELD THERAPY (MBB)

The planet pulsates with magnetic fields, some generated by solar storms and weather changes, others by the Earth itself. These natural fields are compounded by the ever-increasing creations of modern technology—televisions, computers, lights, hair dryers, and the power lines that supply them. In the last few decades, scientists have discovered that, because the cells of the body also hold a magnetic charge, these external fields can and do affect the health and balance of the body. Magnetic field therapy developed out of this discovery.

Magnets for use in magnetic field therapy can be purchased through Philpott Medical Services, 17171 S.E. 29th St., Choctaw, OK 73020; 405-390-3009.

Magnetic field therapy is a treatment method that uses the energy of magnets to relieve symptoms and retard the further weakening of bodily functions. This is achieved through the use of magnets and/or electrical devices that generate controlled magnetic fields. Negative magnetic fields enhance health and positive fields tear it down. Therefore magnetic field therapy uses negative magnetic energy to penetrate the body, affecting the functioning of organs and the overall body system—all without harmful side effects. It increases the amount of oxygen available to cells, balances fluid levels, normalizes

CAUTION

Since the body's electromagnetic fields are sensitive to even minor alterations, magnetic field therapy should be applied only under the supervision of a qualified practitioner.

pH, cancels out free radicals, eliminates toxins, and stimulates metabolism; it is especially useful for chronic problems such as headaches, allergies, constipation, fatigue, bone fractures, muscular aches and pains, circulatory disorders, and environmental stress.

Magnetic therapy can be applied in different ways, ranging from small, simple magnets to massive machines capable of producing huge fields (used mainly to treat fractures and joint problems). Beds, blankets, pillows, and headbands have also been constructed with strategically placed magnets. Treatments, many of which can be self-administered, can last from a few minutes to overnight, and, depending on the problem, may need to be applied several times a day for weeks or months at a time.

NATUROPATHIC MEDICINE (MBB)

Naturopathic medicine (also called naturopathy) was originally formulated in Europe in the 18th and 19th centuries and is the foundation of mod-

The 6 Pillars of Naturopathic Medicine

Nature has the **power to heal.** With a little help from the naturopath, the body is capable of healing itself.

The cause, not the effect, must be treated. To a naturopath, a headache is the body's way of trying to heal itself, so to suppress it is to ignore the body's innate wisdom.

Under no circumstances may the naturopath cause the patient harm. Instead, naturopaths are dedicated to safe and proven natural therapies.

Only the whole person can be treated. Rather than viewing the body as divisions, naturopaths look for the physical, mental, emotional, and spiritual causes of illness.

The naturopath is a teacher and patients are responsible for their own healing. Naturopaths are dedicated to empowering patients by providing the tools, education, and motivation to heal.

The most effective cure is prevention. Naturopaths advocate diet, exercise, and lifestyle changes, encouraging patients to adopt healthy habits.

ern alternative medicine. It is now recognized as a legitimate, licensed medical specialty in 12 states in the U.S. and the World Health Organization is recommending that naturopathy be incorporated into conventional health care systems.

Naturopathy treats health conditions by utilizing the body's inherent ability to heal. Naturopathic physicians aid the healing process by incorporating a variety of alternative methods based on the patient's individual needs. Treatment may include nutritional therapy, homeopathy, acupuncture, hydrotherapy, herbal medicine, lifestyle counseling, massage, and bodywork, among others.

Naturopathic medicine is most effective for treating chronic conditions such as headaches, digestive disorders, chronic fatigue, and other immune system imbalances because naturopaths are trained to look for the underlying cause and to treat it by natural means, honoring the body's innate healing ability.

NEURAL THERAPY (SO)

Also known as trigger point injection, neural therapy uses anesthetic injection to unblock neural pathways and deliver energy to cells that have been short-circuited by disease or injury. This method of treatment normalizes cellular function, helps the body to restore itself to a state of health, and has been used successfully to treat many conditions, including allergies, asthma, chronic pain, circulatory disorders, depression, headache, hormonal imbalances, injuries, muscle spasm, PMS, and sinusitis. It is often the method that works when all others fail.

Neural therapy is based on the biological energy and ground theories. Biological energy theory maintains that cells are charged with electricity, each with its own specific frequency range. When the body is healthy, energy is conducted via frequencies in the normal range, but if interference causes the frequency to become too high or too low, the cells become stressed, and the body will eventually become sick.

According to ground theory, the interference itself is the main cause of illness and the connective tissues between the cells (called the ground system) are the true regulators of health; when they cannot communicate properly, the body cannot function the way it should.

Interference can occur any time the body experiences trauma. Scars, swollen glands, fractures, sunburns, toxic buildup, tense or strained muscles, excess fat tissues, and infections can all produce a field of interference, which, depending upon its location, can cause more serious problems elsewhere, including the symptoms of a headache.

These interference sites—called trigger points—can lie undetected for years, until a trauma or some other condition stresses the system and activates them, making them painful and sensitive to the touch. Trigger points are frequently described as little knots within the muscle.

CAUTION

Neural therapy cannot reverse structural damage and should not be used as a replacement for orthopedic medicine. Also, it should not be used by persons with cancer, diabetes, coagulation disorders, or allergies to local anesthetics.

A neural therapist generally relies on patient interviews and applied kinesiology to uncover interference fields and their corresponding trigger points. Once they are found, a saline solution mixed with the anesthetic procaine or lidocaine (because both are easily broken down and eliminated by the body) is injected directly into these irritated points, or, in cases in which the exact location of the interference field is still unclear or the field itself is too sensitive, into related interference fields, until the original interference is found.

See Chapter 16, An A-Z of Self-Care Options, Nutritional Therapy, for information on diet, juice therapy, and nutritional supplements.

A headache is sometimes healed in a single treatment, but it usually takes between 1 and 6 treatments given twice a week to restore cells to a state in which they can generate health.

NUTRITIONAL THERAPY (MBB)

There are numerous kinds of nutritional therapy and often a combination can be useful in addressing individual nutritional needs. In addition to the enzyme and amino acid therapies discussed below, nutritionists also employ dietary recommendations, juice therapy, and nutritional supplements, among other techniques.

Enzyme Therapy

Enzymes are catalysts that trigger chemical reactions. You would not be alive today if it were not for enzymes. Not only would you be unable to derive nutritive benefit from your food, but without enzymes you would not have been born—since 2 of the most essential synthesizing enzymes are DNA and RNA.

Each enzyme depends upon other enzymes, especially those you derive from the foods you consume. Unfortunately, plant enzymes are now being altered by mass manufacturing to retard ripening and lengthen the shelf-life of produce. This deprives food of vital nutrients, likewise depriving the body. Physical and emotional stress, prescription drugs, and environmental pollutants can also contribute to enzyme deficiency. Enzyme deficiencies can result in water retention, inflammation and pain, food allergies, chronic digestion problems, and degenerative diseases.

CAUTION

Amino acids often need other nutrients to function, and taking one amino acid can render the others ineffective. Amino acids should be taken only in the proper amounts and combinations, under the recommendation and supervision of a qualified nutritionist.

Enzyme therapy involves the use of enzyme supplements to vitalize normal functioning and thereby eliminate problems caused or triggered by enzyme deficiencies. The 3 primary types of enzymes are plant enzymes, pancreatic enzymes, and antioxidant enzymes. Plant enzyme supplements bring about the assimilation of food nutrients and are usually taken with meals in conjunction with a whole or raw foods diet to aid digestion. When taken on an empty stomach, plant enzymes enter the bloodstream and break down toxins. Pancreatic enzymes are produced in your body to aid in digestion. Antioxidant enzymes strengthen the immune system and help to eliminate the waste products of metabolism.

Individual conditions vary considerably, so it is impossible to recommend specific doses; instead, your dose should be administered by a qualified practitioner as part of a total nutritional program.

Amino Acid Therapy

As the building blocks of protein, amino acids help to produce what the body needs to build, repair, and maintain body tissues, make cells and antibodies, carry oxygen, create hormones and enzymes, and fight infection. Amino acids also initiate the synthesis of other body chemicals, including neurotransmitters (such as serotonin) and natural painkillers (enkephalins and endorphins), meaning that when amino acids are not present in the right ratios, these important brain chemicals become imbalanced and neurological function is impaired. Delivered as supplements, amino acids can correct deficiencies and restore ratios to their proper balance.

OSTEOPATHY (SO)

Osteopathy is a treatment method that blends conventional medical practices with manipulative therapies. Like other alternative musculoskeletal therapies, osteopathy is based on the principles that the structure of the body is inextricably tied to the function of its systems and organs and that disruptions in one can cause problems in the other, making both subject to a wide range of disorders.

Osteopathy is effective in treating pain and chronic illnesses. Osteopathic doctors identify reflex patterns and use a combination of therapies to normalize the body's mechanical structure and allow it to operate more freely. Research suggests that few conditions do not benefit from osteopathy; some studies demonstrate that it improves conditions that conventional doctors are unable to remedy through medication and surgery.

In a typical osteopathic examination, the doctor will begin by evaluating the patient for obvious mechanical problems. This is done in a number of ways, including the following:

- Observing the way the patient stands, sits, and walks
- Testing various parts of the body for restrictions in range of motion
- Looking for asymmetry in the body, such as one leg longer than the other or an abnormally curved spine
- Inspecting the soft tissues of the body for tenderness, knotted muscles, reflex activity, fluid retention, temperature and skin changes, or other signs of restriction

After evaluation, the osteopath corrects identified problems through one or more of the osteopathic therapies, such as joint manipulation, bodywork (see above), craniosacral therapy (see above), articulation (similar to chiropractic adjustments), physical therapy, and/or postural reeducation (such as Feldenkrais; see Bodywork above).

Another technique, called SomatoEmotional Release, encourages patients to stay in touch with their emotions during treatments so that powerful feelings, such as past trauma or repressed emotions locked into the body, can be activated and released during the session. Like other alternative therapists, osteopaths typically involve patients in the healing process by asking them to change their diets and incorporate breathing and relaxation exercises into their daily routines.

OXYGEN THERAPY (MBB)

Although doctors have been treating patients with oxygen for over a hundred years, few people are aware of the range of therapies that use oxygen to promote healing. Falling under the general label of oxygen therapy, these therapies—which include hyperbaric oxygen therapy, hydrogen peroxide therapy, and ozone therapy—have been proven clinically effective in treating conditions such as circulatory problems, chronic fatigue syndrome, candida, cancer, allergies, and headaches.

IMPORTANT

Although European medical practitioners have been treating people with oxygen therapy for many years, it has yet to be approved by the FDA and is still controversial in the U.S., in which only certain states approve its use. Currently it is administered in hospitals and select clinics throughout the country. Oxygen therapies must always be administered by a trained professional.

All of your cells, tissues and organs need oxygen to function, so adding oxygen under strictly controlled therapeutic conditions boosts cellular function and helps the body to detoxify and repair itself. The 2 basic methods of oxygen therapy are oxidation (creating a reaction that splits off electrically charged particles that selectively destroy pathogens) and oxygenation (adding oxygen directly to the blood).

Hyperbaric oxygen therapy (HBOT)—This is an oxygenation process that delivers pure oxygen through specially designed chambers; HBOT therapies can be especially beneficial for those with headaches associated with traumatic injuries, toxic poisoning (especially carbon monoxide), and circulation problems.

Hydrogen peroxide therapy—This oxidation process is one of the least expensive therapies; it is generally administered intravenously and is used to combat vascular headaches, such as migraines and clusters, as well as those arising from allergies, candida, and chronic fatigue syndrome. Diluted hydrogen peroxide is sometimes injected into trigger points to reduce nerve and muscle pain. Oral hydrogen peroxide, which is very diluted, may also be taken, with possible benefits.

Ozone therapy—This treatment uses medical-grade ozone, a substance common in nature that is much purer than the air-polluting by-product of manmade combustion. Ozone therapy is a combination of oxygenation and oxidation, and provides the benefits of both methods. Because it enhances the body's overall metabolic processes, it is a very effective treatment for chronic headaches of most types, including those associated with digestive disorders, circulation problems, allergies, infections, and swollen tissues, muscles, and nerves.

PSYCHOTHERAPY (PE)

Psychotherapy can be an effective tool for relieving stress and getting to the core of emotional issues. Many different forms of therapy are available today. You do not necessarily have to spend hours on a couch discussing the trials and tribulations of childhood; instead, you can look for one of the growing number of psychotherapists who are using alternative therapies to complement their practices. The world of contemporary mental health care abounds in useful options, including creative visualization (see Chapter 16), hypnotherapy (see above), cognitive therapy, Gestalt, inner child therapy, and neurolinguistic programming (NLP).

Therapists will not blame you for your headache, they will look for its emotional components. The therapist may ask questions about your job, relationships, leisure time, or creative releases. You will also be asked questions to dis-

5 Healing Steps You Can Take Right Now

Christiane Northrup, M.D., honors the dictum "do unto yourself as you (usually) do unto others" in offering these 5 easy steps as a way to prevent emotional turmoil:

1. Say no: Draw boundaries and get rid of the "shoulds," guilt trips, and people-pleasing habits.

2. Listen to your body: Rest when you are tired, eat when you are hungry, and realize that your body has an innate, internal wisdom and always knows exactly what you need.

3. Let go of whatever is not working: To heal, you must be willing to let go of things that no longer serve you (bad relationships, old ideas and beliefs, a stressful job) and make room for healthy things (physical well-being, positive people, new opportunities).

4. Accept yourself "as is": Pat yourself on the back for coming as far as you have, and realize that healing only begins when you love yourself for who you are today, right this moment.

5. Say "yes" to feeling good: Believe you can feel better and take steps to make it so.[4]

cover whether your headache is serving you in some subconscious way. For example, headaches can be a way to get time away from work, attention from family and friends, or a reprieve from challenges and responsibilities that seem overwhelming. Sometimes just the process of airing your feelings provides relief.

As in other areas of alternative healing, many psychotherapists employ a number of techniques to provide clients with the benefits of a multimodal therapy. The following are just a few of the many psychotherapeutic options available.

Cognitive Therapy—Cognitive therapy is based on the theory, simply put, that if you change your thoughts and perceptions from negative ideas to positive ones, you will create health and harmony in your body and in the world around you.

Gestalt Therapy—Emphasizing individual growth and awareness, Gestalt, which means "the whole picture," is a system of therapy that focuses on bringing your attention into the present moment. This process is achieved by teaching you how to integrate and accept the 3 levels of awareness, which include the inner zone of body sensations and emotions, the middle zone of fantasies, ideas, and thoughts, and the outer zone of the 5 senses and the surrounding world.

Inner Child Therapy—This relatively new approach to therapy suggests that many of your negative feelings and emotions are rooted in ignored or repressed childhood beliefs and experiences. These feelings manifest themselves in veiled forms in an attempt to get your attention and find some relief. Inner child therapy takes you back to your childhood through drama, role play, art therapy, and discussion, so that you can reexperience the feelings in their original form and release them.

Neurolinguistic Programming (NLP)—Often described as the study of how you think, NLP is a technique that teaches you to harness your mind, use your imagination, and gain access to its wider potential.

RECOMMENDED READING

Akerele, O. "Summary of WHO Guidelines for the Assessment of Herbal Medicines." *HerbalGram* 28 (1992), 13-16. Available as Classic Botanical Reprint 234.

Alternative Medicine: The Definitive Guide, Compiled by the Burton Goldberg Group. Tiburon, CA: Future Medicine Publishing, 1994.

"Arthritis unyielding to drugs." *Medical Advertising News* (May 1991), 26-27.

Bannerman, R.H. and Wen-Chieh, C., eds. *Traditional Medicine and Health Care Coverage.* Geneva: World Health Organization, 1983.

Benson, Paul, D.O. "Biofeedback and Stress Management." *Osteopathic Annals* 12 (August 1984), 20-26.

Braly, James, M.D. and Torbet, Laura. *Dr. Braly's Food Allergy and Nutrition Revolution.* New Canaan, CT: Keats Publishing, Inc., 1992.

Carper, Jean. *Food, Your Miracle Medicine.* New York: HarperCollins, 1993.

Chatfield, K.B. "The Treatment of Pesticide Poisoning with Traditional Acupuncture," *American Journal of Acupuncture* 13 (1985), 339-345.

Clark, Linda, M.A. *A Handbook of Natural Remedies for Common Ailments.* Greenwich, CT: The Devin-Adair Company, 1976.

Di Concetto, D., M.D. and Sotte, L. "Treatment of Headaches by Acupuncture and Chinese Herbal Therapy: Conclusive Data Concerning 1000 patients." *Journal of Traditional Chinese Medicine* 2:3 (September 1991), 174-176.

Donovan, P. "Bowel Toxemia, Permeability and Disease—New Information to Support an Old Concept." *A Textbook of Natural Medicine.* Edited by J.E. Pizzorno and M.T. Murray. Seattle, WA: John Bastyr College Publications, 1989.

Faber, William J., D.O. *Pain, Pain Go Away.* San Jose, CA: ISHI Press International, 1990.

Farnsworth, N.R. et al. "Medicinal Plants in Therapy." *Bulletin of the World Health Organization* 63:6 (1985), 965-981.

Farr, C.H., M.D., White, R., and Schachter, M., M.D. "Chronological History of EDTA Chelation Therapy." Presented to the American College of Advancement in Medicine, Houston, TX, May 1993.

Farr, C.H., M.D. "The Use of Dilute Hydrogen Peroxide to Inject Trigger Points, Soft Tissue Injuries and Inflamed Joints." International Bio-Oxidative Medicine Foundation (P.O. Box 13205, Oklahoma City, OK 73113), 1992.

Fryman, V.M. "A Study of the Rhythmic Motions of the Living Cranium." *Journal of the American Osteopathic Association* 70 (May 1971), 928-945.

Gard, Z., M.D. and Brown, E. "Literature Review and Comparison Studies of Sauna/Hyperthermia in Detoxification." *Townsend Letter for Doctors* 107 (June 1992), 470-478.

Howell, E., M.D. *Food Enzymes for Health and Longevity.* Woodstock Valley, CT: Omangod Press, 1980.

Jayasuraiya, A. *Open International University's Text Book on Acupuncture.* Columbo, Sri Lanka: Open University, 1987.

Jensen, Bernard, D.C., Ph.D. *Tissue Cleansing through Bowel Management,* 10th ed. Escondido, CA: Bernard Jensen Publishing, 1981.

Jouanny, Jacques, M.D. et al. *Homeopathic Therapeutics: Possibilities in Chronic Pathology.* France: Editions Boiron, 1994.

Kaminski, Patricia and Katz, Richard. *Flower Essence Repertory.* Nevada City, CA: Earth-Spirit, Inc., 1994.

Kaslof, Leslie J. *The Bach Remedies: A Self-Help Guide.* New Canaan, CT: Keats Publishing, Inc., 1988.

Keller, Erich. *The Complete Home Guide to Aromatherapy.* Tiburon, CA: H.J. Kramer, Inc., 1991.

Klinghardt, D.K., M.D. and Wolfe, B., M.D. *Advanced Neural Therapy Workshop.* Santa Fe, NM, December 5-6, 1992.

Leach, Robert A., A.A., D.C., F.I.C.C. *The Chiropractic Theories: Principles and Clinical Applications.* Baltimore, MD: Williams & Wilkins, 1994.

Lilienthal, Samuel, M.D. *Homeopathic Therapeutics.* New Delhi: Jain Publishing Co., 1996.

Lucero, K.M. "The Electro-Acuscope/Myopulse System." *Rehab Management: The Journal of Therapy and Rehabilitation* 4:3 (April/May 1991).

Miller, J.B., M.D. "Intradermal Provocative/Neutralizing Food Testing and Subcutaneous Food Extract Injection Therapy." *Food Allergy and Intolerance.* Edited by J. Brostoff and S. Challacombe. London: Baillier Tindal Publishers, 1987, 932-947.

NADA Newsletter Committee. *National Acupuncture Detoxification Association Newsletter* (Dec. 1992), 1-6.

Natural Health Secrets from around the World. Boca Raton, FL: Shot Tower Books, 1996.

Philpott, W. and Taplin, A. *Biomagnetic Handbook.* Choctaw, OK: Enviro-Tech Products, 1990.

Privitera, James R., M.D. "Clots: Life's Biggest Killer." *Health Freedom News* (September 1993), 22-23.

Randolph, T.G. *Human Ecology and Susceptibility to the Chemical Environment.*, Springfield, IL: C.C. Thomas, 1981.

Reed, Daniel. *A Handbook of Chinese Healing Herbs.* Boston, MA: Shambhala Publications, 1995.

Roos, P.A. "Light and Electromagnetic Waves: The Health Implications." *Journal of the Bio-Electro-Magnetics Institute* 3:2 (Summer 1991), 7-12.

Rothschild, Peter R., M.D., Ph.D. and Fahey, William. *Free Radicals, Stress, and Antioxidant Enzymes: A Guide to Cellular Health*. Honolulu, HI: University Labs Press, 1991.

Rudolph, C.J., D.O., Ph.D. et al. "An Observation of the Effect of EDTA Chelation and Supportive Multivitamin Trace Mineral Supplementation of Blood Platelet Volume: A Brief Communication." *Journal of Advancement in Medicine* 3:3 (Fall 1990).

Schmitt, Walter, Jr., D.C. "Molybdenum for *Candida albicans*: Patients and Other Problems." *Digest of Chiropractic Economics* 31:4 (1991), 56-63.

Sharma, H.M., Triguna, B.D., and Chopra, D. "Maharishi Ayur-veda: Modern Insights into Ancient Medicine." *Journal of the American Medical Association* 266:13 (1991), 2633-2637.

Simpson, Kristine, et al., eds. *The Experts Speak 1996: The Role of Nutrition in Medicine*. Sacramento: Kirk Hamilton PA-C, 1996, 121-122.

Sohdi, V. "Ayurveda: The Science of Life and Mother of the Healing Arts." *A Textbook of Natural Medicine*. Edited by J.E. Pizzorno and M.T. Murray. Seattle, WA: John Bastyr College Publications, 1989.

Stromfeld, Jan and Weil, Anita. *Free Yourself from Headaches: The Natural Drug-Free Program for Prevention and Relief*. Palm Beach Gardens, FL: The Upledger Institute, Frog, Ltd., 1995.

Tinterow, M.M., M.D. "Hypnotherapy for Chronic Pain." *Kansas Medicine* 88:6 (June 1987), 190-192, 204.

Vogel, H.C. The Nature Doctor: *A Manual of Traditional and Complementary Medicine*. New Canaan, CT: Keats Publishing, Inc., 1991.

Resources

**Information on where to
find everything cited in this book—
products, clinics, substances,
herbs, equipment, books, and
practitioners.**

General Headache Information

HELPFUL ORGANIZATIONS
The National Headache Foundation (NHF)
5252 North Western Avenue, Dept. PF
Chicago, IL 60625—312-878-7715 or 800-843-2256

The American Council for
Headache Education (ACHE)
875 Kings Highway
West Deptford, NJ 08096
800-255-ACHE

World Health Organization
15300 Ventura Blvd., Suite 405
Sherman Oaks, CA 91403
818-907-5483

General Mind/ Body Information

HELPFUL ORGANIZATIONS
The Fetzer Institute
9292 West KL Avenue
Kalamazoo, MI 49009
616-375-2000

Center for Mind-Body Medicine
5225 Connecticut Avenue, N.W., Suite 414
Washington, DC 20015
202-966-7338

Books, Tapes, and Videos

Audio Vision
800-367-1604
This company sells relaxation videos and tapes.

Somatics Educational Resources
1516 Grant Avenue, Suite 212
Novato, CA 94945
415-892-0617
They sell books, videos, and audiotapes on
HannaSomatics, yoga, relaxation, and other mind/body
techniques.

Stress Reduction Tapes
P.O. Box 547
Lexington, MA 02173

Tools & Products

AcuPoint, Inc.
7040 W. Palmetto Park Road, 2-554-D
Boca Raton, FL 33433
407-391-2073
This company makes and distributes a doctor-
approved, needle-free acupoint stimulator.

The Cutting Edge Catalog
P.O. Box 5034

Southampton, NY 11969
516-287-3813
This company sells state-of-the-art products in
electromagnetic field protection, full-spectrum lighting,
biomagnetics, water filters, air filters, and more.

Self Care Catalog
P.O. Box 182290
Chattanooga, TN 37422-3371
800-345-3371
This catalog offers a wide variety of useful products,
including a biofeedback device, self-massage tools, heat
and cold therapy devices, pain management devices,
audiotapes, vitamins and herbs.

Tools for Exploration
47 Paul Drive
San Rafael, CA 94903
800-456-9887
This mail order company offers a varied selection of
mind/body tools, devices, videos, books, and tapes.
The blinking red light devices referred to in Chapter 7
and 16 are available from this company.

HEADACHE PRODUCTS
The Headache Band™
Living Arts
P.O. Box 2939
Venice, CA 90291
800-2-LIVING
This company sells a velcro-secured headband, and a
tape of headache relief music derived from the
principles of Oriental medicine.

A-Z Therapies and Self-Care

ACUPRESSURE

HELPFUL ORGANIZATIONS
American Oriental Bodywork Association
6801 Jericho Turnpike
Syosset, NY 11791
516-364-5533
This professional organization offers information, a
practitioner directory and referrals.

RECOMMENDED READING
Acupressure's Potent Points, Michael Gach
(New York: Bantam Books, 1991)

Acu-Yoga: The Acupressure Stress Management Book,
Michael Gach (Tokyo & New York: Japan Publications,
1981)

ACUPUNCTURE

HELPFUL ORGANIZATIONS
American Academy of Medical Acupuncture
58200 Wilshire Blvd., Suite 500
Los Angeles, CA 90036
213-937-5514
This is a professional organization that provides
educational materials, postgraduate courses, and
referrals to M.D.s and D.O.s who are well-trained.

American Association of Acupuncture and
Oriental Medicine (AAAOM)
4101 Lake Boone Trail, Suite 201
Raleigh, NC 27607
919-787-5181
This is a professional trade organization that will
provide referrals.

National Commission for the Certification of
Acupuncturists (NCCA)
1424 16th Street NW, Suite 601
Washington, DC 20036
202-232-1404
The NCCA offers a test that some states use
to verify competency.

National Acupuncture
Detoxification Association (NADA)
3115 Broadway, Suite 51
New York, NY 10027
212-993-3100
NADA offers literature in 8 languages, plus videotapes.

RECOMMENDED READING
Acupuncture Energetics, Joseph M. Helms, M.D.
(Berkeley, CA: Medical Acupuncture Publishers, 1995)

Plain Talk about Acupuncture, Ellinor R. Mitchell
(New York: Whalehall, Inc., 1987)

AFFIRMATIONS/ AUTOSUGGESTIONS

RECOMMENDED READING
You Can Heal Your Life, Louise L. Hay
(Santa Monica, CA: Hay House)

ALPHABIOTICS

HELPFUL ORGANIZATIONS
Alphabiotics International
634 Preston Royal S/C, Suite 206
Dallas, TX 75230
214-369-5100
This organization trains practitioners, performs
alphabiotics, and provides referrals.

AROMATHERAPY

HELPFUL ORGANIZATIONS
National Association for Holistic Aromatherapy
(NAHA)
P.O. Box 17622
Boulder, CO 80308
303-258-3791
This organization offers courses, aromatherapy
products, and referrals.

Aromatherapy Seminars
3379 S. Robertson Boulevard
Los Angeles, CA 90034
800-677-2368/310-838-6122
They train and certify aromatherapy practitioners, both
locally and through a correspondence course.

Lotus Light
P.O. Box 1008
Wilmot, WI 53170
414-889-8501
They offer mail order distribution of aromatherapy
books, videotapes and materials.

RECOMMENDED READING

The Aromatherapy Book: Applications and Inhalations,
Jeannie Rose (Berkeley, CA: North Atlantic Books,
1992)

Aromatherapy for Common Ailments, Shirley Price
(New York: Simon & Schuster, 1991)

Aromatherapy for Vibrant Health & Beauty, Roberta
Wilson (Garden City Park, NY: Avery Publishing
Group, 1994)

The Complete Home Guide to Aromatherapy, Erich Keller
(Tiburon, CA: H.J. Kramer, Inc., 1991)

AYURVEDIC MEDICINE

HELPFUL ORGANIZATIONS
American School of Ayurvedic Sciences
10025 NE 4th Street
Bellevue, WA 98004
206-454-8022
A college that offers training to both medical
professionals and laypeople.

The College of Maharishi
Ayur-Veda Health Center
P.O. Box 282
Fairfield, IO 52556
515-472-5866
A college and treatment center that offers training,
information, and referrals.

Sharp Institute for Human Potential and Mind-Body
Medicine
8010 Frost Street, Suite 300
San Diego, CA 92123
800-82-SHARP
The Institute conducts research to validate the
effectiveness of Ayurvedic medicine, provides
patient care, and offers courses for medical
professionals and laypeople.

RECOMMENDED READING
Ageless Body, Timeless Mind, Deepak Chopra, M.D.
(New York: Harmony Books, 1993)

Ayurvedic Healing, David Frawley, O.M.D.
(Salt Lake City: Morson Publishing, 1990)

Perfect Health, Deepak Chopra, M.D.
(New York, Harmony Books, 1991)

Quantum Healing, Deepak Chopra, M.D.
(New York: Bantam Books, 1993)

BEHAVIORAL OPTOMETRY

HELPFUL ORGANIZATIONS
Optometric Vision Extension Program
1921 East Carnegie Avenue, Suite 3L
Santa Ana, CA 92705
714-250-8070
This is a foundation that provides international referral
lists of doctors who practice behavioral optometry.

BIOFEEDBACK

HELPFUL ORGANIZATIONS
Association for Applied Psychophysiology and

Feedback (AAPF)
and the Biofeedback Certification Institute of America
(BCIA)
10200 West 44th Avenue, Suite 304
Wheatridge, CO 80033
303-422-8436 (AAPF)
303-420-2902 (BCIA)
They provide training, certification, and referral.

Center for Applied Psychophysiology
Menninger Clinic
P.O. Box 829
Topeka, KS 66601
913-273-7500, ext. 5375
This organization provides research, training, and
treatment in biofeedback.

RECOMMENDED READING
Biofeedback: An Introduction and Guide,
David G. Danskin and Mark Crow
(Palo Alto, CA: Mayfield Publishing Co., 1981)

BIOLOGICAL DENTISTRY

HELPFUL ORGANIZATIONS
Foundation for Toxic-Free Dentistry
P.O. Box 608010
Orlando, FL 32860
This nonprofit group educates the public and offers
referrals to biological dentists worldwide. Send a self-
addressed stamped envelope (affix 55 cents postage).

Environmental Dental Association
9974 Scripps Ranch Boulevard, Suite 36
San Diego, CA 92131
800-388-8124/619-586-1208
This membership organization offers information,
books, products, and public referrals.

DAMS (Dental Amalgam Syndrome)
725-9 Tramway Lane Northeast
Alburquerque, NM 87122
505-291-8239
This is a public education, support, and information
organization.

RECOMMENDED READING
The Complete Guide to Mercury Toxicity from Dental
Fillings, Joyal Taylor (San Diego, CA: Scripps Publishing
Co.,1988)

Dental Mercury Detox, Sam and Michael Ziff
(Orlando, FL: Bio-Probe Inc., 1993)

It's All in Your Head, Hal Huggins, D.D.S.
(Colorado Springs, CO: Life Science Press, 1986)

Silver Dental Fillings—The Toxic Time Bomb, Sam Zoff
(Santa Fe, NM: Aurora Press, 1986)

BODYWORK/GENERAL MASSAGE

HELPFUL ORGANIZATIONS
American Massage Therapy Association
820 Davis Street, Suite 100
Evanston, IL 60201
312-761-2682

This association publishes Massage Therapy Journal and
provides information to practitioners and the public on
most aspects of massage and bodywork.

RECOMMENDED READING
BodyWork: What Type of Massage to Get and How to
Make the Most of It, Thomas Claire
(William Morrow & Company, 1995)

The Massage Book, George Downing
(New York: Random House, 1972)

Alexander Technique

HELPFUL ORGANIZATIONS
North American Society of Teachers of the
Alexander Technique
800-473-0620
They offer information, referrals and training.

RECOMMENDED READING
The Alexander Technique, John Gray
(New York: St. Martin's Press, 1991)

Aston-Patterning

The Aston Training Center
P.O. Box 3568
Incline Village, NV 89450
702-831-8228
They train professionals and offer information.

The Feldenkrais Method

Feldenkrais Guild
P.O. Box 489
Albany, OR 97321
503-926-0981
They offer practitioner training, certification, and
information.

RECOMMENDED READING
Awareness through Movement: Health Exercises for
Personal Growth, Moshe Feldenkrais
(New York: Harper & Row, 1972)

HannaSomatics

HELPFUL ORGANIZATIONS
Novato Institute for Somatics Research and Training
1560 Grant, Suite 212
Novato, CA 94945
415-892-0617
This organization offers practitioner training,
information, and referral

RECOMMENDED READING
Biofeedback and Somatics: Toward Personal Evolution,
Eleanor Criswell (Novato, CA: Freeperson Press, 1995)

The Body of Life, Thomas Hanna
(Santa Cruz, CA: Healing Arts Press, 1980)

Somatics: Reawakening the Mind's Control of Movement,
Flexibility, and Health, Thomas Hanna
(Redding, MA: Addison-Wesley, 1988)

Hellerwork

HELPFUL ORGANIZATIONS
The Body of Knowledge/Hellerwork
406 Berry Street
Mt. Shasta, CA 96067
916-926-2500
They offer training, information, and practitioner referral.

RECOMMENDED READING
Bodywise, Joseph Heller and William Henkin
(Berkeley: Wingbow Press, 1991)

Myotherapy

HELPFUL ORGANIZATIONS
The Bonnie Pruden Pain Erasure
3661 North Campbell, Suite 102
Tucson, AZ 85719
800-221-4634
A school that offers training and certification in myotherapy; also provides a list of certified practitioners.

RECOMMENDED READING
Pain Erasure: The Bonnie Prudden Way, Bonnie Prudden
(New York: Ballantine Books, 1982)

Polarity Therapy

HELPFUL ORGANIZATIONS
Polarity Wellness Center
10 Leonard Street, Suite A
New York, NY 10013
212-334-8392
They offer information, publications, and a referral directory.

RECOMMENDED READING
A Guide to Polarity Therapy: The Gentle Art of Hands-on Healing, Maruti Seidman
(Boulder, CO: Elan Press, 1991)

Rolfing

HELPFUL ORGANIZATIONS
International Rolf Institute
P.O. Box 1868
Boulder, CO 80306
303-449-5903
They offer training and information.

RECOMMENDED READING
Rolfing: The Integration of Human Structures, Ida P. Rolf
(New York: Harper and Row, 1977)

Therapeutic Touch

HELPFUL ORGANIZATIONS
Orcas Island Foundation
Box 86, Route 1
East Sound, WA 98245
206-376-4526
They offer training in Therapeutic Touch.

RECOMMENDED READING
Accepting Your Power to Heal: Personal Practice of Therapeutic Touch, Dolores Krieger
(Santa Fe: Bear and Company, 1993)

Tragerwork

HELPFUL ORGANIZATIONS
Trager Institute
33 Millwood
Mill Valley, CA 94941
415-388-2288
They offer training, certification, and information, and publish a practitioner directory.

RECOMMENDED READING
Trager Mentastics: Movement as a Way to Agelessness, Milton Trager and Cathy Guadagno
(Barrytown, NY: Station Hill Press, 1987)

CHELATION THERAPY

HELPFUL ORGANIZATIONS
American College for Advancement in Medicine
23121 Verdugo Drive, Suite 204
Laguna Hills, CA 92653
714-583-7666
They provide courses and referrals for physicans practicing chelation therapy.

CHIROPRACTIC

HELPFUL ORGANIZATIONS
American Chiropractic Association
1701 Clarendon Blvd.
Arlington, VA 22209
703-276-8800
This is a major source of chiropractic information.

World Chiropractic Alliance
2950 N. Dobson Road, Suite 1
Chandler, AZ 85224
800-347-1011
This international association provides information and referrals.

Association for Network Chiropractic Spinal Analysis
P.O. Box 7682
Longmont, CO 80501
303-678-8086
They offer training, information, and referrals

National Upper Cervical Chiropractic Association (NUCCA)
217 West Second Street
Monroe, MI 48161
This organization trains chiropractors and provides referrals.

RECOMMENDED READING
The Chiropractor's Adjustor, Daniel David Palmer
(Davenport, IA: Palmer College Press, 1992)

Today's Health Alternative, Raquel Martin
(Tehachapi, CA: America West Publishers, 1992)

COLON THERAPY

HELPFUL ORGANIZATIONS
American Colon Therapy Association
11739 Washington Blvd.
Los Angeles, CA 90066
310-390-5424
Besides offering national referrals, this association publishes pamphlets and holds

seminars and trainings for professionals
and laypersons.

California Colon Hygienists Society
P.O. Box 588
Graton, CA 95444
707-829-0984
They provide education and referrals to a national
network of colon therapists.

International Association for Colon Therapy
2051 Hilltop Drive, Suite A-11
Redding, CA 96002
916-222-1498
They offer seminars, training, and referrals to their
nationwide network of colon therapists.

Wood Hygienic Institute, Inc.
P.O. Box 420580
Kissimmee, FL 34742
407-933-0009
They offer certification and referral.

RECOMMENDED READING
A Doctor's Guide to You and Your Colon, Martin Plaut
(New York: Harper & Row, 1986)

Tissue Cleansing through Bowel Management,
Bernard Jensen, D.C., Ph.D. (Escondido, CA:
Bernard Jenson, 1981)

CRANIOSACRAL THERAPY

HELPFUL ORGANIZATIONS
Cranial Academy
3500 Depaw Blvd.
Indianapolis, IN 46268
317-879-0713
They teach cranial therapy (sutural approach) and
provide referrals.

SORSI (S.O.T)
P.O. Box 8245
Prairie Village, KS 66208
913-649-3475
They teach postgraduate courses in Sacro-Occipital
Technique and provide referrals to chiropractors
certified in craniopathy.

Upledger Institute
11211 Prosperity Farms Road
Palm Beach Gardens, FL 33410
407-622-4706
They train professionals in CranioSacral Therapy and
offer information and referrals to the public.

RECOMMENDED READING
*Your Inner Physican and You: CranioSacral Therapy
SomatoEmotional Release,* John E. Upledger, D.O.,
F.A.A.O.
(Berkeley, CA: North Atlantic Books, 1992)

CREATIVE VISUALIZATION

HELPFUL ORGANIZATIONS
The Academy for Guided Imagery
P.O. Box 2070
Mill Valley, CA 94941

800-726-2070
They train professionals and offer books and tapes for
both professionals and laypeople.

RECOMMENDED READING
*Healing Yourself: A Step-by-Step Program for Better Health
through Imagery,* Martin L. Rossman
(New York: Pocket Books, 1989)

Minding the Body, Mending the Mind, Joan Borysenko
(Reading, MA: Bantam, 1988)

DETOXIFICATION THERAPY

RECOMMENDED READING
Body/Mind Purification Program,
Leon Chaitow, N.D., D. O.
(New York: Simon and Schuster/Gaia, 1990)

Diet for a Poisoned Planet, David Steinman
(New York: Ballantine Books, 1990)

Staying Healthy with Nutrition, Elson Haas, M.D.
(Berkeley, CA: Celestial Arts, 1992)

ENERGY MEDICINE

HELPFUL ORGANIZATIONS
Tools for Exploration
4460 Redwood Highway, Suite 2
San Rafael, CA 94903
800-456-9887
A mail order catalogue of nonmedical energy
machines and other devices.

RECOMMENDED READING
*The Body Electric: Electromagnetism and the Foundation
of Life,* Robert Becker and Gary Selden
(New York: William Morrow and Company, Inc., 1987)

Vibrational Medicine, Richard Berber, M.D.
(Santa Fe, NM: Bear & Company, 1988)

ENVIRONMENTAL MEDICINE

HELPFUL ORGANIZATIONS
American Academy of Environmental Medicine
P.O. Box 16106
Denver, CO 80216
303-622-9755
For information on physicans practicing environmental
medicine, send $3 and a self-addressed stamped
envelope.

Human Ecology Action League (HEAL)
P.O. Box 49126
Atlanta, GA 30359
404-248-1898
They provide information on support groups that assist
those with environmental illnesses.

Immuno Labs
1620 West Oakland Park Blvd., Suite 300
Fort Lauderdale, FL 33311
800-321-9197
This lab offers specialized allergy testing, plus referrals
to environmental physicans all over the world.

Meridian Valley Clinical Laboratory
24030 132nd Avenue SE
Kent, WA 98042
800-234-6825
This lab offers a wide variety of specialized allergy testing and nutritional analyses.

Natural Lifestyles Supplies
16 Lookout Drive
Asheville, NC 28804
704-254-9606
A catalog offering supplies and books especially prepared for the sensitivities of people with environmental illnesses.

RECOMMENDED READING
An Alternative Approach to Allergies, Randolph Theron, M.D. and R. W. Moss, Ph.D.
(New York: Bantam Books, 1987)

Detecting Your Hidden Allergies, William Crook, M.D.
(Jackson, TN: Professional Books/Future Health, 1988)

Dr. Mandell's 5-Day Allergy Relief, Marshall Mandell, M.D. (New York: Harper & Row, 1988)

Say Goodbye to Illness, Devi Nambudripad, D.C., L.Ac., R.N., Ph.D. (Buena Park, CA: Delta Publishing Company, 1993)

FASTING

HELPFUL ORGANIZATIONS
International Association of Professional Natural Hygienists
Regency Health Resort and Spa
2000 South Ocean Drive
Hallandale, FL 33009
305-454-2220
A professional organization of doctors who specialize in therapeutic fasting.

FLOWER ESSENCE THERAPY

HELPFUL ORGANIZATIONS
Ellon USA, Inc. (formerly Ellon Bach USA)
644 Merrick Road
Lynbrook, NY 11563
516-593-2206
This company makes and distributes a complete line of Bach's original 38 flower essences under the trade name "Traditional Flower Remedies from Ellon."

Flower Essence Services
P.O. Box 1769
Nevada City, CA 95959
800-548-0075
916-265-9163
FES makes and distributes FES Quintessentials, North American Flower Essences and imports Healing Herbs (a full line of Bach's 38 remedies) from England.

Perelandra, Ltd.
P.O. Box 3603
Warrenton, VA 22186
703-937-2153
This company makes and sells its own line of flower essences.

RECOMMENDED READING

The Bach Remedies: A Self-Help Guide, Leslie J. Kaslof (New Canaan, CT: Keat Publishing, 1988)

Flower Essence Repertory, Patricia Kaminski and Richard Katz (Nevada City, CA: Earth-Spirit, Inc, 1994)

HERBAL MEDICINE

HELPFUL ORGANIZATIONS
American Botanical Council
P.O. Box 201660
Austin, TX 78720
512-331-8868
This nonprofit research and education council offers information to both professionals and laypeople.

The American Herbalists Guild
P.O. Box 1683
Soquel, CA 95073
This group is dedicated to help bring herbal medicine to the United States.

Empirical Herbs and Foods
1400 North Main, B2
Cedar City, UT 84720
800-565-6650
This company is a good source for herbal products.

RECOMMENDED READING
The Healing Herbs, Michael Castleman
(Emmaus, PA: Rodale Press, 1991)

The Herbs of Life, Lesley Tierra
(Freedom, CA: Crossing Press, 1992)

Weiner's Herbal, Michael Weiner
(Mill Valley, CA: Quantum Books, 1990)

HOMEOPATHY

HELPFUL ORGANIZATIONS
International Foundation for Homeopathy
2366 Eastlake Avenue East, Suite 301
Seattle, WA 98102
206-324-8230
This organization provides courses and offers referrals.

National Center for Homeopathy
801 North Fairfax, Suite 306
Alexandria, VA 22314
703-548-7790
They offer courses for professionals and laypeople, and referrals.

RECOMMENDED READING
Discovering Homeopathy: Your Introduction to the Science and Art of Homeopathic Medicine, Dana Ulman
(Berkeley, CA: North Atlantic Books, 1991)

Everybody's Guide to Homeopathic Medicines, Stephen Cummings (Los Angeles, CA: Jeremy P. Tarcher, Inc., 1991)

HYPERTHERMIA

HELPFUL ORGANIZATIONS
Bastyr College
144 54th Street NE
Seattle, WA 98105
206-523-9585

A college with a natural health clinic that uses hyperthermia treatments for detoxification.

HYPNOTHERAPY

HELPFUL ORGANIZATIONS
American Society for Clinical Hypnosis
2200 East Devon Avenue, Suite 291
Des Plaines, IL 60018
708-297-3317
A membership organization for M.D.s and dentists who use hynotherapy; send a self-addressed, stamped envelope for referrals.

International Medical and Dental Hypnotherapy Association
4110 Edgeland, Suite 800
Royal Oak, MI 48073
313-549-5594/800-257-5467
They train, certify, and profide referral lists of certified practitioners in the U.S. and Canada.

Society for Clinical and Experimental Hypnosis
129A King's Park Drive
Liverpool, NY 13090
315-652-7299

The National Guild of Hypnotists
P.O. Box 308
Merrimack, NH 03054
603-429-9438
They train, certify, and offer books and tapes on hypnotherapy.

RECOMMENDED READING
The Wizard Within: The Krasner Method of Clinical Hypnotherapy, A.M. Krasner, Ph.D.
(Santa Ana, CA: American Board of Hypnotherapy Press, 1990)

LIGHT THERAPY

HELPFUL ORGANIZATIONS
College of Syntonic Optometry
1200 Robeson Street
Fall River, MA 02720
508-673-1251
This organization offers referrals to practitioners of Syntonic Optometry.

Dinshaw Health Society
100 Dinshaw Drive
Malaga, NJ 08238
609-692-4686
This society gives information and self-help tips for those interested in treating themselves with color therapy.

Environmental Health & Light Research Institute
16057 Tampa Palms Boulevard, Suite 227
Tampa, FL 33647
800-544-4878
They provide information on full-spectrum lighting.

RECOMMENDED READING
Color Therapy, Reuben B. Amber
(Santa Fe, NM: Aurora Press, 1983)

Let There Be Light, Darius Denshaw
(Malaga, NJ: Denshaw Health Society, 1985)

Light: Medicine of the Future, Jacob Liberman
(Santa Fe, NM: Bear & Co. Publishing, 1993)

MAGNETIC FIELD THERAPY

HELPFUL ORGANIZATIONS
Bio-Electro-Magnetics Institute
2490 West Moana Lane
Reno, NV 89509
702-827-9099
This nonprofit ogranization provides information, education, and support.

Enviro-Tech Products
17171 Southeast 29th Street
Choctaw, OK 73020
405-390-3499
This service offers research and self-help information to both practitioners and lay people.

RECOMMENDED READING
Cross Currents, Robert O. Becker, M.D. (Los Angeles: Jeremy P. Tarcher, Inc., 1990)

MEDITATION

HELPFUL ORGANIZATIONS
Institute of Noetic Sciences
P.O. Box 909
Sausalito, CA 94966
415-331-5650
This nonprofit organization is a resource for information on meditation, consciousness, and teachers.

Institute of Transpersonal Psychology
P.O. Box 4437
Stanford, CA 94305
415-327-2066
They offer information about meditation research, activities, and teachers.

Maharishi International University
1000 North 4th Street
Fairfield, IA 52556
515-472-5031
They provide information and training in Transcendental Meditation (TM).

Mind/Body Health Sciences, Inc.
393 Dixon Road
Boulder, CO 80303
303-440-8460
They organize meditation workshops and publish a mail order catalog of meditation books and music.

RECOMMENDED READING
The Meditative Mind, Daniel Goleman
(Los Angeles: Jeremy P. Tarcher, Inc., 1988)

Transcendental Meditation, Robert Roth
(New York: Donald I. Fine, Inc., 1988)

NATUROPATHIC MEDICINE

HELPFUL ORGANIZATIONS
American Association of Naturopathic Physicians
2366 Eastlake Avenue East, Suite 322
Seattle, WA 98102
206-323-7610
They provide information and referral and publish a
quarterly newsletter and a directory of naturopathic
physicians.

The Institute for Naturopathic Medicine
66-¹/₂ North State Street
Concord, NH 03301-4330
603-255-8844
This nonprofit organization promotes research and
offers information to medical professionals, the media,
and the general public.

National College of Naturopathic Medicine
11231 SE Market Street
Portland, OR 97216
503-255-4860
This college offers a degree program and provides
information on naturopathic medicine.

RECOMMENDED READING
Encyclopedia of Natural Medicine, Michael Murray, N.D.
and Joseph Pizzorno, N.D.
(Rocklin, CA: Prima Publishing, 1991)

Textbook of Natural Medicine, Michael Murray, N.D. and
Joseph Pizzorno, N.D.
(Seattle: John Bastyr College Publications, 1989)

NEURAL THERAPY

HELPFUL ORGANIZATIONS
The American Academy of Neural Therapy
1468 South Saint Francis Drive
Santa Fe, NM 87501
505-988-3086
They offer doctor training and provide referrals.

RECOMMENDED READING
Facts about Neural Therapy According to Huneke, A Brief
Summary for Patients, Peter Dosch, M.D.
(Heidelberg, Germany: Karl Haug Publishers, 1985; also
available through Medicina Biologica, 2937 NE Flanders,
Portland, OR 97232; 503-287-6775)

NUTRITIONAL THERAPY

HELPFUL ORGANIZATIONS
American College of Advancement in Medicine
(ACAM)
P.O. Box 3427
Laguna Hills, CA 92654
714-583-7666
They provide information on nutritional
supplementation and publish a worldwide directory of
physicians who have been trained in nutritional
medicine.

RECOMMENDED READING
Grains and Greens, Patrick Wright, Ph.D.
(San Rafael, CA: The Wright Publication, 1991)

Prescription for Nutritional Healing: A Practical A-Z
Reference to Drug-Free Remedies Using Vitamins, Minerals,
Herbs, and Food Supplements, James Balch, M.D. and
Phyllis Balch, R.N.
(Garden City Park, NY: Avery Publishing, 1990)

Staying Healthy with Nutrition, Elson Hass, M.D.
(Berkeley, CA: Celestial Arts, 1992)

HELPFUL ORGANIZATIONS
American College of Nutrition
722 Robert E. Lee Drive
Wilmington, NC 28480
919-452-1222
This is a membership organization that provides
information on nutrition.

Center for Science in the Public Interest
Americans for Safe Food Project
1875 Connecticut Avenue NW, Suite 300
Washington, DC 20009-5728
202-332-9110, ext. 384
They provide a list of organic mail order suppliers and
hormone-free beef suppliers.

Eden Acres
Organic Network
12100 Lima Center Road
Clinton, MI 49236-9618
517-456-4288
They publish directories that list international or
statewide suppliers of organic meats, poultry, fruits,
grains, and vegetables.

RECOMMENDED READING
Diet for a New America, John Robbins
(Walpole, NH: Stillpoint Publishing, 1987)

Diet for a Small Planet, 10th ed., Frances Moore Lappé
(New York: Ballantine, 1982)

Transition to Vegetarianism, Rudolph Ballantine
(Honesdale, PA: Himalayan Publishers, 1987)

Vegan Nutrition—Pure and Simple, Michael Klaper, M.D.
(Maui, HI: Gentle World, 1987)

NUTRITIONAL THERAPY: ENZYME THERAPY

HELPFUL ORGANIZATIONS
Lita Lee, Ph.D.
2852 Williamette Street, Suite 397
Eugene, OR 97405
503-746-7621
This former editor and publisher of a quarterly
nutritional newsletter offers information on doctors
using plant enzyme therapy.

NESS
2903 NW Platte Road
Riverside, MO 64150
800-637-7893
They offer a line of enzyme supplements as well as
information on doctors using plant enzyme therapy.

Tyler Encapsulations
2200-4 NW Birdsdale
Gresham, OR 97030
800-869-9705
They sell a line of enzyme supplements.

RECOMMENDED READING
Enzyme Nutrition, Edward Howell
(Wayne, NJ: Avery Publishing Group, 1985)

Food Enzymes, Humbart Santillo, B.S., M.H.
(Prescott, AZ: Holm Press, 1987)

NUTRITIONAL THERAPY: JUICE THERAPY

RECOMMENDED READING
The Complete Book of Juicing, Michael Murray
(Rocklin, CA: Prima Publishing, 1992)

Juicing for Good Health, Maureen B. Keene
(New York: Pocket Books, 1992)

Juicing For Life, Cherie Calbom and Maureen B. Keene
(New York: Avery Publishing Group, 1992)

OSTEOPATHY

HELPFUL ORGANIZATIONS
American Academy of Osteopathy
3500 DePauw Blvd., Suite 1080
Indianapolis, IN 46268
317-879-1881
This is an affiliation of skilled practitioners.

American Osteopathic Association
142 East Ontario Street
Chicago, IL 60611
312-280-5800
This is a professional membership organization for
national D.O.s.

RECOMMENDED READING
Osteopathic Medicine: An American Reformation, George
Northup (Chicago: American Osteopathic Association,
1987)

Osteopathic Self-treatment, Leon Chaitow, D.O.
(San Francisco, CA: Thorsons, 1990)

OXYGEN THERAPY

HELPFUL ORGANIZATIONS
The American College of Hyperbaric Medicine
Ocean Medical Center
4001 Ocean Drive, Suite 105
Lauderdale-by-the-Sea, FL 33308
305-771-4000
A physicians' group promoting research and offering
information on hyperbaric oxygen therapy.

ECH2O2 Newsletter
9845 NE 2nd Avenue
Miami,FL 33138
305-758-8710
This is a newsletter for all who are interested in the oral
use of hydrogen peroxide and ozone.

International Ozone Association
31 Strawberry Hill Avenue
Stamford, CT 06902

203-348-3542
This is a professional scientific organization that
disseminates information to the public.

Medical Society for Ozone Therapy
Klagen Furtestrasse 4
D. 7000 Stuttgart 30, Germany
They provide comprehensive information for both the
public and professionals.

North Carolina Bio-Oxidative Health Center
4505 Fair Meadow Lane, Suite 111
Raleigh, NC 27606
800-473-9812/407-967-6466 (outside North America)
This is an outpatient facility offering a comprehensive
range of oxygen therapies and other detoxification
therapies.

RECOMMENDED READING
Hydrogen Peroxide Medical Miracle, William Campbell
Douglas (Atlanta, GA: Second Opinion Publishing,
1992; to order call 800-728-2288)

Oxygen Therapies, Ed McCabe (Morrisville, NY: Energy
Publications, 1988)

The Use of Ozone in Medicine, First English Edition,
Siegfried Rilling and Renate Viebahn
(New York: Plenum Publications, Volume 1, 1973,
Volume 2, 1975)

PSYCHOTHERAPY

HELPFUL ORGANIZATIONS
American Psychiatric Association
1400 K Street, N.W.
Washington, D.C. 20005
202-682-6000

American Psychological Association
750 First Street, N.E.
Washington, D.C. 20002
202-336-5700

National Association of Social Workers
750 First Street, N.E., Suite 700
Washington, D.C. 20002
202-408-8600

Center for Cognitive Therapy
Science Center, Room 754
3600 Market Street
Philadelphia, PA 19104
215-898-4100

QIGONG

HELPFUL ORGANIZATIONS
The Healing Tao Center
P.O. Box 1194
Huntington, NY 11743
516-367-2701
This center offers classes in various therapeutic arts all
over the world as well as videotape demonstrations of
qigong.

RECOMMENDED READING
Qigong for Health: Chinese Traditonal Exercise, Masaru
Takahashi and Stephen Brown (Tokyo/New York:
Japan Publication, 1986)

Self-Applied Heath Enhancement Methods, Roger Jahnke
(Santa Barbara, CA: Health Action Books, 1989)

REFLEXOLOGY

HELPFUL ORGANIZATIONS
International Institute of Reflexology
P.O. Box 12462
St. Petersburg, FL 33733
813-343-4811
They offer information and referrals.

RECOMMENDED READING
Better Health with Foot Reflexology, Dwight Byers
(St. Petersburg, FL: Ingham Publishing, 1983)

Hand and Foot Reflexology: A Self-Help Guide, Kevin and
Barbara Kunz (New York: Simon and Schuster, 1987)

RELAXATION

HELPFUL ORGANIZATIONS
Mind Body Medical Institute
Beth Israel Deaconess Medical Centerl
West Campus
1 Deaconess Road
Boston, MA 02215
617-632-9530
The outpatient medical clinic offers relaxation
instruction.

Stress Reduction Clinic
University of Massachusetts Medical Center
55 Lake Avenue, North
Worcester, MA 01655
508-856-2656
They offer training in relaxation and meditative-type
awareness.

RECOMMENDED READING
Full Catastrophe Living, Jon Kabat Zinn
(New York: Delacorte Press, 1990)

Mind Body Medicine, edited, Goleman and Gurin
(Consumer Reports Books, 1993)

SUPPORT GROUPS

HELPFUL ORGANIZATIONS
National Self-Help Clearinghouse
25 West 43rd Street
New York, NY 10036
212-354-8525

American Self-Help Clearinghouse
St. Clares-Riverside Medical Center
25 Pocono Road
Denville, NJ 07834
201-625-7101

TEL-MED the Health Line
952 South Mount Vernon Avenue

Colton, CA 92324
714-825-6034

TRADITIONAL CHINESE MEDICINE

HELPFUL ORGANIZATIONS
American Association of Acupuncture and Oriental
Medicine (AAAOM)
4101 Lake Boone Trail, Suite 201
Raleigh, NC 27607
919-787-5181
This is a professional trade organization which, for a
small fee, provides referrals upon written request.

Institute for Traditional Chinese Medicine and
Preventative Healthcare
2017 SE Hawthorne
Portland, OR 97214
800-544-7504
This organization offers Chinese herbal medicines and
education materials for health-care practitioners.

RECOMMENDED READING
Between Heaven and Earth, Harriet Beinfield, L.Ac. and
Efrem Korngold, L.Ac., O.M.D.
(New York: Ballantine Books, 1991)

Chinese Herbal Medicine, Daniel P. Reid
(Boston, MA: Shambhala Publications, Inc., 1987)

*The Essential Book of Traditional Chinese Medicine
Volumes 1 and 2,* Y. Liu
(New York: Columbia University Press, 1988)

Tao of Nutrition, Ni Maoshing, D.O.M., Ph.D., L.Ac. and
Cathy NcNease (Santa Monica, CA: Seven Star
Communications, 1993)

*The Web That Has No Weaver: Understanding Chinese
Medicine,* Ted Kaptchuk
(New York: Congdon and Weed, 1992)

YOGA

HELPFUL ORGANIZATIONS
International Association of Yoga Therapists
109 Hillside Avenue
Mill Valley, CA 94941
415-383-4587
This nonprofit international organization focuses on
yoga education and research.

Iyengar Yoga
2404 27th Avenue
San Francisco, CA 94116
415-753-0909
They offer training, classes, a mail order catalog, and
referrals.

Yoga Journal
2054 University Avenue
Berkeley, CA 94704
510-841-9200
They publish a monthly magazine and a yearly directory
of over 600 national yoga instructors.

Cranial Yoga
Rick Williams, N.M.T.
371 Forrest Avenue
Fairfax, CA 94930
800-652-8388/415-459-7729

RECOMMENDED READING
The Complete illustrated Book of Yoga, Swami
Vishnudevananda (New York: Harmony Books, 1980)

Hatha Yoga: Manual, 2nd Edition, Samskrit and
Veda (Honesdale, PA: The Himalayan International
Institute, 1985)

Light on Yoga, B.K. Iyengar (New York: Schocken
Books, 1987)

Key to Professional Titles

Ac. Phys.	Acupuncture Physician
B.M.	Bachelor of Medicine
B.M.E.D.	Bachelor of Music Education
B.Sc.	Bachelor of Science
B.S.N.	Bachelor of Science in Nursing
C.A.	Certified Acupuncturist
C.A.M.T.	Certified Acupressure Massage Therapist
C.C.N.	Certified Clinical Nutritionist
Ch.B.	Bachelor of Surgery
C.Ht.	Certified Hypnotherapist
C.M.T.	Certified Massage Therapist
C.N.	Certified Nutritionist
D. Ac.	Diplomate of Acupuncture
D.C.	Doctor of Chiropractic
D.D.S.	Doctor of Dental Science
D.H.A.N.P.	Diplomate of Homeopathic Academy of Naturopathic Physicians
D.Hom.(Med)	Diplomate of Homeopathic Medicine
D.I.B.A.K.	Diplomate of the International Board of Applied Kinesiology
D.I.Hom.	Diplomate of the Institute of Homeopathy
Dipl. Ac.	Diplomate of Acupuncture (NCCA)
Dipl. C.H.	Diplomate of Chinese Herbs
D.M.D.	Doctor of Dental Medicine
D.O.	Doctor of Osteopathy
D.O.M.	Doctor of Oriental Medicine
D.Sc.	Doctor of Science
D.V.M.	Doctor of Veterinary Medicine
Ed.D.	Doctor of Education
F.A.A.E.M.	Fellow of the American Academy of Environmental Medicine
F.A.A.F.P.	Fellow of the American Academy of Family Practice
F.A.A.P.	Fellow of the American Academy of Pediatrics
F.A.A.P.M.	Fellow of the American Academy of Physical Medicine
F.A.C.A.	Fellow of the American College of Allergists
F.Ac.A.	Fellow of the Acupuncture Association (British)
F.A.C.A.I.	Fellow of the American College of Allergy and Immunology
F.A.C.N.	Fellow of the College of Nutrition
F.A.C.S.	Fellow of the American College of Surgeons
F.A.C.O.G.	Fellow of the American College of Obstetricians and Gynecologists
F.A.G.D.	Fellow of the Academy of General Dentistry
F.A.O.A.S.	Fellow of the American Osteopathic Academy of Sclerotherapy

F.I.A.C.A.	Fellow of the International Academy of Certified Acupuncturists
F.I.A.O.M.T.	Fellow of the International Academy of Oral Medicine and Toxicology
F.I.C.A.N.	Fellow of the International College of Applied Nutrition
F.I.C.C.	Fellow of the International College of Chiropractors
F.I.C.S.	Fellow of the International College of Surgeons
F.N.A.A.O.M.	Fellow of the National Academy of Acupuncture and Oriental Medicine
F.N.T.O.S.	Fellow of the Natural Therapeutic and Osteopathic Society
F.R.C.Psy.	Fellow of the Royal College of Psychiatry
H.M.D.	Homeopathic Medical Doctor
L.Ac.	Licensed Acupuncturist
L.C.S.W.	Licensed Clinical Social Worker
Lic. Ac.	Licensed Acupuncturist
L.M.T.	Licensed Massage Therapist
M.A.	Master of Arts
M.Ac.O.M.	Master of Acupuncture and Oriental Medicine
M.D.	Medical Doctor
M.D.C.	Master Doctor of Chiropractor
M.F.Hom.	Member of the Faculty Homeopathy (British)
M.N.I.M.H.	Member of the National Institutes of Medical Herbalist (British)
M.P.H.	Master of Public Health
M.R.C.G.P.	Member of the Royal College of General Practitioners (British)
M.R.C.P.	Member of the Royal College of Physicians (British)
M.S.	Master of Science
M.S.W.	Master of Social Work
NCCA	National Commission for the Certification of Acupuncturists
N.D.	Doctor of Naturopathy
N.M.D.	Naturopathic Medical Doctor
O.D.	Doctor of Optometry
O.M.D.	Oriental Medical Doctor
O.M.M.	Osteopath Manipulative Medicine
P.H.N.	Public Health Nurse
R.C.O.G.	Royal College of Obstetricians and Gynecologists
R.D.	Registered Dietician
rer. nat.	Rerum Naturalium
R.M.T.	Registered Music Therapist
R.N.	Registered Nurse
R.P.T.	Registered Physical Therapist

Notes

Introduction

1. "Many Headaches Aren't Inevitable, Researchers Tell Us." Gannett News Service, November 6, 1994.

2. National Headache Foundation Fact Sheet, (National Headache Foundation, October 1994).

3. D.M. Eisenberg et al, "Unconventional medicine in the United States: Prevalence, costs, and patterns of use," *New England Journal of Medicine* 328 (January 1993), 246-252.

Chapter 1:
Head Pain—What's It All About?

1. Goleman and Gurin, eds. Mind Body Medicine. Mt. Vernon, NY: Consumer Reports Books, 126.

Chapter 2:
What Kind of Headache Do You Have?

1. Mark Mayell, "Headache Relief." East West Journal (May 1982), 28.

2. "National Headache Foundation Fact Sheet." National Headache Foundation (October 1994).

3. "Arthritis unyielding to drugs." *Medical Advertising News* (May 1991) 26-27.

4. Barbara Lewis, "Missed migraine diagnosis often due to lack of communication." *Medical Tribune,* (July 27, 1995).

5. Bonnie Prudden, *Pain Erasure: The Bonnie Prudden Way,* (New York: Ballantine Books, 1980) 59.

Chapter 3:
What Causes Your Headache?

1. "National Headache Foundation Fact Sheet." National Headache Foundation (October 1994).

2. A. Joutel, M.G. Bousser, T.S. Olson, et al, "A gene for familial hemiplegic migraine maps to chromosome 19," *Nat Genet:* 5, (1993) 40-45.

3. Christiane Northrup, M.D. *Women's Health: A Special Supplement to Health Wisdom for Women* (Potomac, MD: Phillips Publishing, Inc.), January 1996.

4. "Newsfront," *Modern Medicine* (July 15, 1977) 26.

5. Richard Leviton, *Brain Builders* (New York: Simon & Schuster, 1995) 88.

6. "Recent advances in headache medicine," ACHE Newsletter, Special Headache Issue (May 1994) 6.

7. *Household Hazardous Waste Wheel* (Mothers & Others for a Livable Planet; 40 West 20th Street, New York, NY 10011).

8. *Simillimum IX:* 3 (Fall 1996), 28.

9. Sharon Faelten et al, *The Complete Book of Minerals for Health* (Emmaus, PA: Rodale Press, 1981) 439.

10. John Mansfield, M.D. *Migraine and the Allergy Connection* (Rochester, VT: Healing Arts Press, 1990) 65-66.

11. D. Steinman, *Diet for a Poisoned Planet* (New York: Ballantine Books, 1990), 203.

12. "819 Cities Exceed Lead Level for Drinking Water," *Environmental Protection Agency Environmental News,* Publication #A-107 (May 11, 1993), 110.

13. Stephen E. Langer, M.D. and James F. Scheer, *Solved: The Riddle of Illness,* (New Canaan, CT: Keats Publishing, 1984) 146.

14. Harold H. Taub, *Keeping Healthy In a Polluted World* (New York: Harper & Row Publishers) 225.

15. Christiane Northrup, M.D. *Women's Health: A Special Supplement to Health Wisdom for Women* (Potomac, MD: Phillips Publishing, Inc., January 1996).

16. Lawrence Galton, "A Brighter Day for Migraine Victims," *Parade* (March 20, 1977) 11.

Chapter 4
Why Alternative Medicine Is Your Best Strategy

1. Dr. Cass Igram, *Who Needs Headaches?* (Iowa Literary Visions Publishing, 1991) 15-16.

2. Faber, William, D.O., "Permanent Biological Reconstruction for Migraine and Neck Pain," *Townsend Letter for Doctors* (June 1991), 4.

Chapter 5
Organic Headaches

1. *Johns Hopkins Symptoms and Remedies,* edited by Simeon Margolis, M.D., Ph.D. (New York: Rebus, distributed by Random House, 1995).

Chapter 6
Tension Headaches

1. O.T. Bonnett, M.D. *Confessions of a Healer* (Aspen, CO: MacMurray & Beck, 1994) 6-7.

2. *The Visual Encyclopedia of Natural Healing,* edited by Alice Feinstein and Prevention Magazine Health Books (Emmaus, NY: Rodale Press, 1991) 223.

3. *The American Family Physician,* vol. 47, no. I (1993) 11.

Chapter 7
Migraine Headaches

1. Joan Didion, *The White Album* (New York: Penguin, 1968).
2. Joseph Egger et al, "Is Migraine Food Allergy?" *The Lancet* 2:8355 (October 15, 1983) 865-869.
3. Anne Remmes, M.D. "Headaches and Sleep," *National Headache Foundation Quarterly* 87 (Winter 1993).
4. Kathleen R. Merikangas et al, "Migraine and Pyschopathology," *General Psychiatry* 47:9 (September 1990) 849-53.
5. Deborah Frances, N.D. "Feverfew for Acute Headaches: Does It Work?" *Medical Herbalism,* vol. 7, no. 4 (Winter 1995-96) 1-4.
6. Dr. Christiane Northrup, *Women's Health: A Special Wisdom for Women* (Potomac, MD: Phillips Publishing, January 1996).

Chapter 8
Cluster Headaches

1. Alan M. Rapoport, M.D. and Fred D. Sheftell, M.D. *Headache Relief* (New York: Simon & Schuster, 1990) 78.
2. J. Raloff. "Hot Prospects for Quelling Cluster Headaches." *Science News* (July 13, 1991) 20-21.

Chapter 9
Trauma Headaches

1. Bonnie Prudden, *Pain Erasure: The Bonnie Prudden Way* (New York: Ballantine Books, 1980) 48.
2. Lita Lee, *Earthletter* 2:4 (December 1992).
3. "Maladjustment May Be Result of Birth Events," *Brain Mind Bulletin* 1:7 (February 16, 1976) 1-2.

Chapter 10
Allergy/Sensitivity Headaches
(Food/Chemical/Environmental)

1. James Braly, M.D. and Laura Torbet, *Dr. Braly's Food Allergy and Nutrition Revolution.* (New Canaan, CT: Keats Publishing, Inc., 1992) 264-65.

Chapter 12
TMJ/Dental Headaches

1. Joseph Schames, D.M.D. *Home Exercise for Headache and Facial Pain* (The Dental Trauma Center, 12243 South Hawthorne Blvd., Hawthorne, CA 90250).

Chapter 14
Rebound Headaches

1. "What Works: A Guide to the Headache Medicine Cabinet," *Life Magazine* (February 94), 75; Alan M. Rapoport, M.D. and Fred D. Sheftell, M.D. *Headache Relief* (New York: Simon & Schuster, 1990), 91-118; and "Controlling Headaches: Questions and Answers" (booklet published by DeKalb Medical Center Headache Treatment), 13-17, 35-38.

Chapter 15
Exertion Headaches

1. Seymour Diamond, M.D. and Bill and Cynthia Still, *The Hormone Headache* (New York: Macmillan, 1995) 117.

Chapter 16
An A-Z of Self-Care Options

1. *Medicine and Science in Sports and Exercise,* vol. 13, no. 2 (1981).
2. Leon Chaitow, D.O., M.R.O. *Osteopathic Self-treatment* (London: Thorsons, 1990) 55-56.
3. *The Visual Encyclopedia of Natural Healing,* edited by Alice Feinstein and Prevention Magazine Health Books (Emmaus, PA: Rodale Press, 1991), 223.
4. *The American Family Physician,* vol. 47, no. I (1993), 11.
5. *Cortlandt Forum* 8:9 (1995).
6. Jacob Liberman, O.D., Ph.D. *Light Medicine of the Future* (Santa Fe, NM: Bear & Company Publishing, 1991) 47.
7. Neal D. Barnard, M.D. et al, "The medical costs attributable to meat consumption" (Washington, DC: Physicians Committee for Responsible Medicine, 1995).
8. Alexander Mauskip et al, "Intravenous magnesium sulfate relieves migraine attacks in patients with low serum ionized magnesium levels: A pilot study," *Clinical Science* 89 (1995) 633-636.
9. Dr. James Braly, "Magnesium and migraines," *Optimum Health Update* 4:1 (May 1989) 1.
10. J. Schoenen et al, "High-dose riboflavin as a prophylactic treatment of migraine: results of an open pilot study," *Cephalalgia* 14 (1994) 328-329.

Chapter 17
An A-Z of Alternative
Medicine

1. Paul Benson, D.O. "Biofeedback and Stress Management," *Osteopathic Annals*, vol. 12 (August 1984) 20-26.

2. E.C. Hughes, Ph.D. et al, "Migraine: A diagnostic test for etiology of food sensitivity by a nutritionally supported fast and confirmed by a long-term report," *Annals of Allergy* 55 (1985) 28-32.

3. *Medical Tribune* (January 1995).

4. Dr. Christiane Northrup, M.D. *Women's Health: A Special Supplement to Health Wisdom for Women* (Potomac, MD: Phillips Publishing, Jan. 1996) 15.

Index

BOOKS *your health* depends on

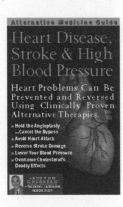
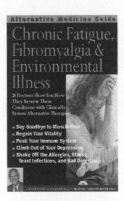
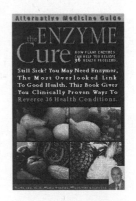
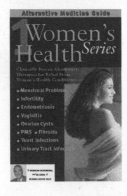
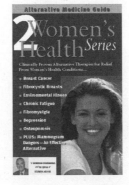
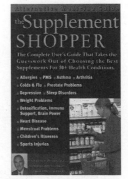

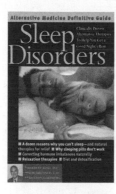
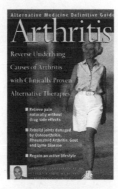
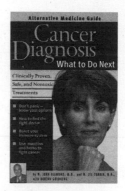
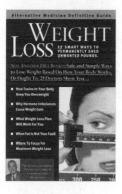
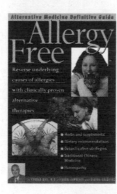
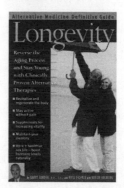

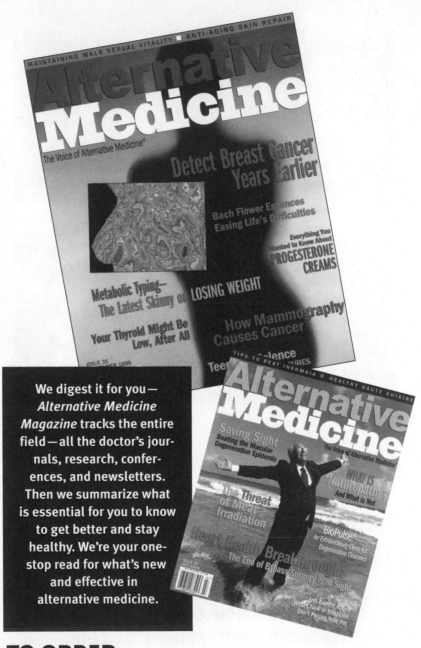